Pharmacokinetics and Metabolism in Drug Design

Pharmacokinetics and Metabolism in Drug Design

Editor: Erica Helmer

AMERICAN
MEDICAL PUBLISHERS
www.americanmedicalpublishers.com

AMERICAN
MEDICAL PUBLISHERS
www.americanmedicalpublishers.com

Cataloging-in-Publication Data

Pharmacokinetics and metabolism in drug design / edited by Erica Helmer.
p. cm.
Includes bibliographical references and index.
ISBN 979-8-88740-375-5
1. Pharmacokinetics. 2. Drugs--Metabolism. 3. Drugs--Design. 4. Pharmacology. I. Helmer, Erica.
RM301.5 .P43 2023
615.7--dc23

American Medical Publishers,
41 Flatbush Avenue,
1st Floor, New York,
NY 11217, USA

ISBN 979-8-88740-375-5 (Hardback)

Contents

Preface ... VII

Chapter 1 **Population Pharmacokinetic Analysis of Tiropramide in Healthy Korean Subjects** ... 1
Seung-Hyun Jeong, Ji-Hun Jang, Hea-Young Cho and Yong-Bok Lee

Chapter 2 **Simultaneous Determination of Chlorogenic Acid Isomers and Metabolites in Rat Plasma Using LC-MS/MS and its Application to a Pharmacokinetic Study Following Oral Administration of *Stauntonia Hexaphylla* Leaf Extract (YRA-1909) to Rats** ... 21
Won-Gu Choi, Ju-Hyun Kim, Dong Kyun Kim, Yongnam Lee, Ji Seok Yoo, Dae Hee Shin and Hye Suk Lee

Chapter 3 **Drying Technologies for the Stability and Bioavailability of Biopharmaceuticals** ... 35
Fakhrossadat Emami, Alireza Vatanara, Eun Ji Park and Dong Hee Na

Chapter 4 **Species Differences in Stereoselective Pharmacokinetics of HSG4112: A New Anti-Obesity Agent** ... 57
In Yong Bae, Min Sun Choi, Young Seok Ji, Sang-Ku Yoo, Kyungil Kim and Hye Hyun Yoo

Chapter 5 **Altered Protein Expression of Cardiac CYP2J and Hepatic CYP2C, CYP4A and CYP4F in a Mouse Model of Type II Diabetes—A Link in the Onset and Development of Cardiovascular Disease?** ... 71
Benoit Drolet, Sylvie Pilote, Carolanne Gélinas, Alida-Douce Kamaliza, Audrey Blais-Boilard, Jessica Virgili, Dany Patoine and Chantale Simard

Chapter 6 **Imbalance of Drug Transporter-CYP450s Interplay by Diabetes and its Clinical Significance** ... 83
Yiting Yang and Xiaodong Liu

Chapter 7 **Augmented Renal Clearance in Critical Illness: An Important Consideration in Drug Dosing** ... 110
Sherif Hanafy Mahmoud and Chen Shen

Chapter 8 **Pharmacokinetics and Intestinal Metabolism of Compound K in Rats and Mice** ... 137
Ji-Hyeon Jeon, Bitna Kang, Sowon Lee, Sojeong Jin, Min-Koo Choi and Im-Sook Song

Chapter 9 **Large Volume Direct Injection Ultra-High Performance Liquid Chromatography-Tandem Mass Spectrometry-Based Comparative Pharmacokinetic Study between Single and Combinatory Uses of *Carthamus tinctorius* Extract and Notoginseng Total Saponins** ... 153
Jinfeng Chen, Xiaoyu Guo, Yingyuan Lu, Mengling Shi, Haidong Mu, Yi Qian, Jinlong Wang, Mengqiu Lu, Mingbo Zhao, Pengfei Tu, Yuelin Song and Yong Jiang

Chapter 10 **Regulation of Hepatic UGT2B15 by Methylation in Adults of Asian Descent** ... 165
Steffen G. Oeser, Jon-Paul Bingham and Abby C. Collier

Chapter 11 **Disposition, Metabolism and Histone Deacetylase and Acetyltransferase Inhibition Activity of Tetrahydrocurcumin and Other Curcuminoids** 179
Júlia T. Novaes, Ryan Lillico, Casey L. Sayre, Kalyanam Nagabhushanam, Muhammed Majeed, Yufei Chen, Emmanuel A. Ho, Ana Luísa de P. Oliveira, Stephanie E. Martinez, Samaa Alrushaid, Neal M. Davies and Ted M. Lakowski

Chapter 12 **A Simple and Sensitive Liquid Chromatography with Tandem Mass Spectrometric Method for the Simultaneous Determination of Anthraquinone Glycosides and their Aglycones in Rat Plasma: Application to a Pharmacokinetic Study of *Rumex acetosa* Extract** 196
Hossain Mohammad Arif Ullah, Junhyeong Kim, Naveed Ur Rehman, Hye-Jin Kim, Mi-Jeong Ahn and Hye Jin Chung

Chapter 13 **A High-Performance Liquid Chromatography Assay Method for the Determination of Lidocaine in Human Serum** 208
Hamdah M. Al Nebaihi, Matthew Primrose, James S. Green and Dion R. Brocks

Chapter 14 **Pharmacokinetic Interaction between Metformin and Verapamil in Rats: Inhibition of the OCT2-Mediated Renal Excretion of Metformin by Verapamil** 216
Seung Yon Han and Young Hee Choi

Permissions

List of Contributors

Index

Preface

This book aims to highlight the current researches and provides a platform to further the scope of innovations in this area. This book is a product of the combined efforts of many researchers and scientists, after going through thorough studies and analysis from different parts of the world. The objective of this book is to provide the readers with the latest information of the field.

Pharmacokinetics (PK) determines the outcome of substances which are administered in the human body and involves drug absorption, distribution, metabolism, and excretion (ADME) processes. Drug absorption is the movement of drug in the bloodstream from its site of administration. It depends on multiple factors, including the formulation and chemical properties of a drug, drug-food interactions and route of administration. Drug distribution is essential for determining drug efficacy and drug toxicity. Drug metabolism is the chemical alteration of the drug by the body. Genetics, age and drug interactions are some factors that affect drug metabolism. In clinical use, an enzyme named cytochrome P450 (CYP450) is responsible for the biotransformation or metabolism of all drugs. It is essential to comprehend the basic mechanisms governing the pharmacokinetics of a drug for designing personalized course of therapy for patients. This book provides comprehensive insights into the role of pharmacokinetics and metabolism in drug design. It is appropriate for students seeking detailed information in this area of study as well as for experts.

I would like to express my sincere thanks to the authors for their dedicated efforts in the completion of this book. I acknowledge the efforts of the publisher for providing constant support. Lastly, I would like to thank my family for their support in all academic endeavors.

Editor

1

Population Pharmacokinetic Analysis of Tiropramide in Healthy Korean Subjects

Seung-Hyun Jeong [1,†], Ji-Hun Jang [1,†], Hea-Young Cho [2] and Yong-Bok Lee [1,*]

[1] College of Pharmacy, Chonnam National University, 77 Yongbong-ro, Buk-Gu, Gwangju 61186, Korea; rhdqn95@naver.com (S.-H.J.); jangji0121@naver.com (J.-H.J.)

[2] College of Pharmacy, CHA University, 335 Pangyo-ro, Bundang-gu, Seongnam-si, Gyeonggi-Do 13488, Korea; hycho@cha.ac.kr

* Correspondence: leeyb@chonnam.ac.kr

† Both authors contributed equally to this work.

Abstract: The purpose of this study was to perform population pharmacokinetic (PPK) analysis of tiropramide in healthy Korean subjects, as well as to investigate the possible effects of various covariates on pharmacokinetic (PK) parameters of tiropramide. Although tiropramide is commonly used in digestive system-related diseases as an antispasmodic, PPK reporting and factors affecting PKs are not clearly reported. Thus, this study for healthy subjects is very significant because it could find new covariates in patients that had not been reported before or predict PPK for patients in the clinic by establishing PPK in healthy adults. By using Phoenix NLME, PK, demographic, and genetic data (collected to explain PK diversity of tiropramide in population) analyses were performed. As a basic model, a one-compartment with first-order absorption and lag-time was established and extended to include covariates that influenced the inter-subject variability. The total protein significantly influenced the distribution volume and systemic clearance of tiropramide, but genetic factors such as *ABCB1* (1236C>T, 2677G>T/A, and 3435C>T), *CYP2D6* (*1 and *10), *OCT2* (808G>T), and *PEPT1* (1287G>C) genes did not show any significant association with PK parameters of tiropramide. The final PPK model of tiropramide was validated, and suggested that some of the PK diversity in the population could be explained. Herein, we first describe the establishment of the PPK model of tiropramide for healthy Korean subjects, which may be useful as a dosing algorithm for the diseased population.

Keywords: tiropramide; healthy Korean subjects; modeling; population pharmacokinetic

---

1. Introduction

Tiropramide is a drug that has been used from the past to the present for symptom relief and treatment of diseases of the digestive system such as acute spastic abdominal pain and irritable bowel syndrome. Tiropramide is a structurally equivalent tyrosine derivative and contains amide functional groups in the structure together with tertiary amines. It has been reported that tiropramide is widely metabolized into various metabolites (hydroxytiropramide, *N*-despropyltiropramide, *N*-desethyltiropramide, and *N*-desethyl-*N*-despropyltiropramide) after oral administration to rats and humans [1–3]. The mechanism of action of tiropramide has been reported to directly affect the smooth muscle cells. That is, tiropramide activates intracellular cyclic adenosine monophosphate (cAMP) synthase (adenylcyclase) to increase the amount of cAMP to regulate calcium ions necessary for muscle contraction, thereby controlling the relaxation and contraction of intestinal smooth muscle cells. This mechanism of action is very important for clinical use. Other antispasmodics include anticholinergics or antimuscarinics that relieve abdominal pain by acting on the intestinal nervous system. However, the mechanism of action on the nervous system may cause systemic side effects such as dry mouth, dry eyes, and drowsiness, which may lower the patients' compliance with medication. As a result, tiropramide has been widely used in the clinic for the treatment of diseases related to the digestive system with the reduction of the systemic side effects.

However, reporting of pharmacokinetic (PK) information of tiropramide for humans is still very limited. Above all, tiropramide's population pharmacokinetics (PPK) have not been reported thus far. Tiropramide has been reported to have hypotension and peripheral vasodilation (as side effects) like other anticholinergic or antimuscarinic drugs only when a high dose is administered. Overall, incidences of tiropramide side effects are very low and a very safe profile in humans has been reported [4]. Although the incidence of adverse effects of tiropramide is reported to be low in humans, optimal dosing algorithm may maximize the therapeutic effect of the drug and reduce its adverse effects by using a PPK model. PPK modeling can enable effective dose setting and individualized pharmacotherapy by quantifying the diversity of the drug concentrations among individuals (in the population) with a variety of related physicochemical factors. In addition, identifying the physicochemical factors affecting PKs of tiropramide will be a significant scientific basis for the clinical application (such as usage and dose settings) and formulation of tiropramide in the future.

Tiropramide is usually administered orally to adults at 100 mg (1 tablet) 2-3 times a day in the clinic. In exceptional cases, it is reported that tiropramide may be additionally administered in cases of less symptomatic relief. However, it is difficult to judge whether these levels of capacity and usage are precise when considering the differences among individuals in the population. More scientific evidence and data on the dose setting and safety of tiropramide are needed. Therefore, we thought that a study of the PPK model of tiropramide was necessary. In addition, it begs the question on how the various physicochemical or genetic factors among individuals in the population affect the PKs of tiropramide. Moreover, even if individual physicochemical or genetic factors affect tiropramide's PKs, it is very doubtful as to how large the effect would be. Finding significant covariates of tiropramide is very difficult due to the lack of detailed PK information on the precise metabolic mechanisms, absorption, distribution, and excretion of tiropramide (especially in humans), and no PPK studies have been reported in the past. Therefore, in this study, we set up a variety of candidate covariates early in the study to establish factors that significantly influence the PK of tiropramide. The process was based on the physicochemical or physiological properties of tiropramide that have been reported to date.

Tiropramide has amine groups in its structure and will be basic at pH (about 7.4) in vivo on the basis of its pKa value (of 3.1) [4]. Therefore, the covariate effect was confirmed by genotyping the *OCT* gene, which is known to be related to the absorption, distribution, and excretion of various organic cations [5]. Tiropramide is a substance derived from the amino acid tyrosine [6]. Therefore, the genotyping of the *PEPT* gene, which is known to be involved in the absorption and distribution of the peptide drugs such as peptides and β-lactam antibiotics, was performed to confirm the covariate effect [7]. P-glycoprotein (P-gp) is a transporter with a broad range of substrate specificities of about 170 kDa and is known to be mainly involved in the efflux of neutral or cationic substances. In addition, *ABCB1* has been reported as a gene that encodes the P-gp. In this study, the covariate effect was confirmed by genotyping *ABCB1* [8]. In the past, the metabolism of tiropramide in the liver was examined [1], and the covariate effect was confirmed by genotyping metabolism-related *CYP2D6*. In particular, we focused on single nucleotide polymorphism (SNP) of the *CYP2D6* gene related to phase I metabolism (oxidation, reduction, hydrolysis, etc.) in the liver, and tried to confirm the correlation with PKs [9]. In addition, we collected information on various physicochemical factors (including general functional indicators of the kidney and liver) and sought to find the major covariates affecting PKs.

We report on PPK modeling of tiropramide in this study, together with factors affecting PK diversity in the population, which have not been reported yet. In the tiropramide final PPK model (of this study), we quantitatively reflected on the total protein, physicochemical, or genetic factors with differences between individuals, suggesting that scientific dose setting can be possible. In these aspects, for clinical applications, the tiropramide's PPK model would be a great advantage. As a result, development of a tiropramide's PPK model for use in healthy Korean subjects was the purpose of this study. The developed tiropramide's PPK model is expected to be useful for determining a valuable dosing algorithm for tiropramide in healthy Korean subjects. In addition, the identification of factors affecting PK of tiropramide is expected to be of great help in related future studies.

2. Methods

2.1. Study Design

Samples obtained from a bioequivalence study of tiropramide in 24 healthy Korean males were included in this analysis. The age of these subjects ranged from 19 to 29 years (mean ± standard deviation (SD), 22.96 ± 2.61 years). Their body weights ranged from 55.2 to 82.8 kg (mean ± SD, 67.60 ± 7.28 kg). Their body surface area (BSA) ranged from 1.58 to 1.97 m^2 (mean ± SD, 1.80 ± 0.11 m^2), and their body mass index (BMI) ranged from 17.89 to 29.06 kg/m^2 (mean ± SD, 22.74 ± 2.72 kg/m^2). Each subject had no hypersensitivity to any drugs or previous history of illness and was physically normal. All subjects provided informed written consent to perform bioequivalence and PK studies. All subjects underwent physical examinations, clinical screening, complete blood count, urinalysis, and analysis of blood chemistry prior to the admission of this study to evaluate their physical health status. If subjects were taking any medications, other drugs, and/or alcohol for at least 1 week prior to this study, they were excluded from this study. The Institutional Review Board of the Institute of Bioequivalence and Bridging Study, Chonnam National University, Gwangju, Republic of Korea, reviewed and approved (Bioequivalence Test no. 875; 01.16.2003) this study protocol. Clinical studies were performed in accordance with rules of good clinical practice and the revised Declaration of Helsinki for biomedical research involving human subjects. Bioequivalence studies were performed as randomized, single-dose, open-label, crossover, and two-way studies. The data from reference formulation were only used for the current analysis. The subjects were hospitalized (Chonnam National University Hospital, Gwangju, Korea) at 7:30 p.m. 1 day before the study. The subjects had a heparin-locked catheter installed in the median cubital vein. A single dose (100 mg) of tiropramide was given orally to all subjects (after an overnight fast) in each study group with 240 mL of water. Before administration (0 h) and at 0.33, 0.67, 1, 1.5, 2, 2.5, 3, 4, 6, 8, and 12 h after oral administration, blood samples (8 mL) were collected into Vacutainer tubes. At the time of blood sampling, about 2 mL of blood was drained each time to completely remove the heparinized saline solution remaining in the IV catheter, and about 8 mL of blood was collected. Following centrifugation (for 20 min, at 5000 × *g*), plasma samples were obtained and transferred to polyethylene tubes. They were then stored at −80 °C until analysis. Another study was repeated in the same manner to complete the crossover design after a washout period of 7 days.

2.2. Determination of Physicochemical Parameters

Plasma samples were used in the determination of physicochemical parameters, including total proteins, aspartate transaminase (AST), albumin, alkaline phosphatase (ALP), alanine transaminase (ALT), and creatinine. The determination of main physicochemical parameters in this study, such as total proteins, albumin, AST, ALT, ALP, and creatinine, was performed in a dry automatic analyzer by microsides VITROS (Ortho Clinical Diagnostics, NJ, USA) operating by reflectance spectrophotometry.

2.3. Determination of Genotypes

The blood samples of 3 mL, obtained from individuals participating in this study, were used for genotyping. The blood samples were centrifuged for 10 min at 1000 × *g*, and deoxyribonucleic acid (DNA) was extracted from the leukocyte layer using a Wizard Genomic DNA purification kit (Promega Co., Madison, WI, USA). The extracted DNA was dissolved in 100 μL of DNA hydration solution and stored at −70 °C until analysis. In order to amplify a portion of gene containing a SNP by polymerase chain reaction (PCR) from the extracted DNA, each primer was prepared according to the variation of allele. Moreover, the genotypes were determined using appropriate methods that have been reported in the past [5,8,10,11]. We conducted experiments three times to acquire exact genotype data.

2.3.1. Identification of ABCB1 1236C>T (in Exon 12), 2677G>T/A (in Exon 21), and 3435C>T (in Exon 26)

Candidate SNPs (1236C>T, 2677G>T/A, and 3435C>T) in the *ABCB1* gene were genotyped by using polymerase chain reaction–restriction fragment length polymorphism (PCR-RFLP). Each primer was prepared according to the variation of allele. Forward primer of 5′-TATCCTGTGTCTGTGAATTGCC-3′ and reverse primer of 5′-CCTGACTCACCACACACCAATG-3′ were used for *ABCB1* 1236C>T genotypes. Forward primer of 5′-TGCAGGCTATAGGTTCCAGG-3′ and reverse primer of 5′-TTTAG TTTGACTCACCT TCCCG-3′ were used for determination of *ABCB1* 2677G>T/A genotypes. Forward primer of 5′-TGTTTTCAGCTGCTTGATGG-3′ and reverse primer of 5′-AAGGCATGTAT GTTGGCCTC-3′ were used for *ABCB1* 3435C>T genotypes. PCR was performed in 20 μL reaction mixture including 1 μL of 10 pmol each primer (forward and reverse), 1 μL extracted DNA, and 17 μL autoclaved distilled water. The PCR program was composed of an initial denaturation at 94 °C for 2 min followed by 35 cycles of denaturation at 94 °C for 30 s, annealing at 59.8 °C for 30 s, and extension at 72 °C for 30 s. The final extension step was performed at 72 °C for 5 min. The DNA fragments amplified by PCR were reacted at 37 °C for 16 h with restriction enzymes *HaeIII* (for *ABCB1* 1236C>T), *Sau3AI* (for *ABCB1* 3435C>T), and *BanI/RsaI* (for *ABCB1* 2677G>T/A), which can recognize and cleave specific sequences. These digested fragments were separated by electrophoresis in 2.5% agarose gel, and were visualized under ultraviolet light after staining the gel with ethidium bromide for 30 min.

2.3.2. Identification of CYP2D6 Alleles

Polymorphisms (*1 and *10) in the *CYP2D6* gene of individuals were determined using DNA sequencing analysis. The primers were designed and prepared using the primer3 software. The PCR was performed in 20 μL reaction mixture including 1 μL extracted DNA, 1 μL of 10 pmol of each primer (forward and reverse), and 17 μL autoclaved distilled water. The PCR program was composed of an initial denaturation at 94 °C for 3 min followed by 35 cycles of denaturation at 94 °C for 20 s, annealing for at 62 °C 30 s, and extension at 72 °C for 20 min. A final extension step was conducted at 72 °C for 5 min. The PCR products were then analyzed by direct sequencing using the ABI PRISIM BigDye Terminator Cycle Sequencing Kit and an ABI Prism 3100 Genetic Analyzer (Applied Biosystems, Foster City, CA, USA).

2.3.3. Identification of OCT2 808G>T

Candidate SNP (808G>T) in the *OCT2* gene was genotyped using pyrosequencing analysis. Each primer was prepared according to the variation of allele. Forward primer of 5′-CGGAGAACAGT GGGGATTTTTTAC-3′, reverse primer of 5′-CACGTAATTCCTTCCGTCTGAAGA-3′, and sequencing primer of 5′-GGTGGTTGCAGTTCACA-3′ were used for *OCT2* 808G>T genotype. Forward primer has a 5′ biotin triethylene glycol label necessary for post PCR processing. PCR was performed in 20 μL reaction mixture including 1 μL extracted DNA, 1 μL of 10 pmol each primer (forward and reverse), and 17 μL autoclaved distilled water. The PCR program comprised an initial denaturation at 94 °C for 5 min followed by 45 cycles of denaturation at 94 °C for 20 s, annealing at 52.1 °C for 30 s, and extension at 72 °C for 20 s. A final extension step was performed at 72 °C for 5 min. The biotinylated PCR products were immobilized on streptavidin-coated Sepharose beads (Amersham Biosciences, Uppsala, Sweden). A total of 37 μL of binding buffer (10 mM Tris HCl, 2 M sodium chloride, 1 mM EDTA, 0.1% Tween 20, pH 7.6; Pyrosequencing AB, Uppsala, Sweden), 3 μL of streptavidin-coated Sepharose beads, and 20 μL of water were added to 20 μL PCR product; then, the solution was vigorously shaken for 10 min at room temperature. A 96 pin magnetic tool (Pyrosequencing AB, Uppsala, Sweden) was used to transfer up to 96 samples at a time to solutions as follows. The beads with bound template were first transferred to 70% ethanol solution and 0.2 N sodium hydroxide solution, then to 1X washing buffer (Pyrosequencing AB, Uppsala, Sweden), and finally into a solution of 1X annealing buffer (20 mM Tris acetate, 2 mM magnesium acetate, pH 7.6), including the appropriate sequencing primer of 10 pmol. Lastly, this mixture was heated for 1 min to 95 °C and then cooled to 50 °C and incubated at room temperature for at least 5 min to bind the sequencing primer to the template. After template preparation, a 96-well plate including the samples was loaded into the instrument (PSQ 96MA; Pyrosequencing AB, Uppsala, Sweden) along with the optimal reagents (Pyro Gold; Biotage AB, Uppsala, Sweden). This instrument sequences the templates by dispensing reagents and deoxynucleotide triphosphates in a user-defined order, achieving real-time sequencing by synthesis in an automated fashion. This is achieved by creating and monitoring an enzyme cascade initiated by nucleotide incorporation that produces light emission. Pyrosequencing data were obtained by using Peak Height Determination Software v2.1 (Pyrosequencing AB, Uppsala, Sweden).

2.3.4. Identification of PEPT1 1287G>C (in Exon 16)

Candidate SNP (1287G>C) in the *PEPT1* gene were genotyped by using PCR-RFLP. Each primer was prepared according to the variation of allele. Forward primer of 5′-CCCTTGTCAGGGTTAAGATGA-3′ and reverse primer of 5′-GCTTCTCTAAATCCTATTATAACAGGG-3′ were used for *PEPT1* 1287G>C genotypes. PCR was performed in 20 μL reaction mixture including 1 μL extracted DNA, 1 μL of 10 pmol each primer (forward and reverse), and 17 μL autoclaved distilled water. The PCR program comprised of an initial denaturation at 95 °C for 5 min followed by 35 cycles of denaturation at 95 °C for 20 s, annealing for at 54.5 °C 30 s, and an extension at 72 °C for 20 s. The final extension step was performed at 72 °C for 5 min. DNA fragments amplified by PCR were reacted at 37 °C for 1 h with restriction enzyme *Sau961*, which can recognize and cleave specific sequences. The digested fragments were separated by electrophoresis in 2.5% agarose gel, and were visualized under ultraviolet light after staining the gel with ethidium bromide for 30 min.

2.4. Determination of Plasma Tiropramide Concentrations

Plasma concentrations of tiropramide were determined using a validated column-switching semi-micro high-performance liquid chromatography (HPLC) method based on a previous study [12].

2.4.1. Chromatographic Conditions

The analytical system consisted of the Nanospace SI-2 series (Shiseido, Tokyo, Japan) with an ultraviolet-visible (UV–VIS) detector 3002, two 3001 pumps, a 3014 column oven, a high pressure six-way switching valve 3012, a 3010 degasser, and a 3023 autosampler. The system operation and signal processing were operated by Syscon (Shiseido, Tokyo, Japan). The columns used in this on-line extraction system include an analytical column (Capcell Pak C_{18} UG120, 150 × 1.5 mm I.D. Shiseido), a pre-column (Capcell Pak MF Ph-1, 10 × 4 mm I.D. 5 μm Shiseido), and an enrichment column (Capcell Pak C_{18} UG120, 35 × 2 mm I.D. Shiseido). The mobile phase for primary separation of tiropramide in the pre-column and concentration in the enrichment column was phosphate buffer (50 mM, pH 7.0)-acetonitrile (88/12, v/v) with a flow rate of 0.5 mL/min. The mobile phase for analytical column was phosphoric acid–phosphate buffer (50 mM, pH 7.0)-acetonitrile (0.04/59.96/40, v/v/v) with a flow rate of 0.1 mL/min. All the columns were maintained at 25–30 °C. The quantification was performed at 230 nm wavelength. The peak with the retention time of tiropramide was verified using a photodiode array detector (2017 Diode Array, Shiseido, Tokyo, Japan).

2.4.2. Analytical Procedures

The performance of column-switching semi-micro HPLC consists of three steps, as follows: sample loading and primary separation, enrichment of analyte fraction, and chromatographic separation. When the column-switching valve was at the precolumn inlet position, an aliquot of filtered (by 0.22 μm,

Millex-GV syringe filter unit, Millipore, Burlington, MA, USA) plasma sample (80 μL) was loaded to the pre-column, and a primary separation of tiropramide from plasma proteins was conducted by using phosphate buffer (50 mM, pH 7.0)-acetonitrile (88/12, v/v). Subsequently, the valve was switched to the enrichment column inlet position, and the tiropramide fraction was eluted from the pre-column and concentrated in the enrichment column by phosphate buffer (50 mM, pH 7.0)-acetonitrile (88/12, v/v). Afterwards, the valve was switched to analytical column inlet position, and tiropramide was finally isolated and quantified by phosphoric acid–phosphate buffer (50 mM, pH 7.0)-acetonitrile (0.04/59.96/40, v/v/v).

2.5. Pharmacokinetic Analysis

Basic PK parameters of tiropramide were obtained from non-compartmental analysis (NCA) through the Phoenix-WinNonlin (8.1 version, Pharsight, Certara Inc., Princeton, NJ, USA) program. Peak plasma concentration (C_{max}) and the time to reach C_{max} (T_{max}) were individually determined using plasma concentration–time curve. The area under the curve ($AUC_{0-\infty}$) was calculated as the sum of AUC_{0-t} and C_{last}/k, where C_{last} is the final measured concentration and k is the elimination rate constant at terminal phase. AUC_{0-t} was calculated using a linear trapezoidal rule from 0 to t (as 24) h after administration. The half-life ($t_{1/2}$) was calculated as 0.693/k, and the volume of the distribution (V_d/F) was calculated as dose/k·$AUC_{0-\infty}$. The clearance (CL/F) was calculated by dividing the dose of tiropramide by $AUC_{0-\infty}$, where F is the bioavailability of oral administration. All PK parameter values were calculated as mean ± SD, and the statistical differences in the group parameters (according to genotype) were confirmed by the analysis of variance (ANOVA) through the Statistical Package for the Social Sciences (SPSS) program (23 version, IBM). A p-value < 0.05 was established as being statistically significant.

2.6. Model Development

PPK analysis was conducted with a non-linear mixed effects model (NLME) approach through the Phoenix NLME (8.1 version, Pharsight, Certara Inc., Princeton, NJ, USA) program. In addition, PPK model development was performed in the first order conditional estimates method with extended least squares (FOCE-ELS) estimation (with η–ε interaction).

As the first step of PPK modeling, data were fitted to two or one compartment disposition models with first order elimination and absorption kinetics without or with absorption lag-time for determining the structural base model (without covariates). In addition, a multiple transit model with a compartment added to the absorption phase was evaluated to establish the structural base model. The final selection of structural base model was performed by the statistical significance between models using goodness-of-fit (GOF) plots, twice the negative log likelihood (-2LL), and Akaike's information criterion (AIC). The initial values for the parameters used in this process were obtained and referenced using NCA and classic compartment models. As a result, the basic PK parameters were as follows: clearance for the central compartment (CL), absorption lag time (T_{lag}), volume of distribution for the central compartment (V), first oral absorption rate constant (K_{a1}), and second oral absorption rate constant (K_{a2}).

The residual variability was determined to additive error model in log transformed (plasma concentration) data, as shown in the following equation: $C_{obs,ij} = C_{pred,ij} \cdot \exp(\varepsilon_{ij})$, where ε_{ij} is the intra-subject variability (including model misspecification and assay error) with mean 0 and variance σ^2, and $C_{pred,ij}$ and $C_{obs,ij}$ are the jth predicted and observed plasma concentrations in the ith subject, respectively.

The inter-individual variability (IIV) in PK parameters of tiropramide was evaluated by using an exponential error model, as shown in the following equation: $P_i = P_{tv} \cdot \exp(\eta_i)$, where η_i is the random variable for the ith individual, which was normally distributed with mean 0 and variance ω^2; P_i is the parameter value of the ith individual, and P_{tv} is the typical value of the population parameter.

As a second step of PPK modeling, candidate covariates (including demographic and genetic information) screened during this study were considered in reflecting the structural base model to account for PK diversity of tiropramide in the population. Height, body weight, age, BMI, BSA, creatinine, albumin, AST, ALT, ALP, creatinine clearance, and total protein were used as demographic candidate covariates. Here, BMI was determined by using the metric unit system [13]. BSA was determined on the basis of the Mosteller equation [14]. Creatinine clearance was determined on the basis of the Cockcroft–Gault equation [15]. There were also *ABCB1* 1236C>T, *ABCB1* 2677G>T/A, *ABCB1* 3435C>T, *CYP2D6* (*1 and *10), *OCT2* 808G>T, and *PEPT1* 1287G>C as genetic candidate covariates. To confirm the correlation between covariates and PK parameters, these potential covariates were plotted against individual post hoc parameters. In addition, the covariates were divided into categorical and continuous types in order to reflect the identified (correlation with PK parameters) candidate covariates in the PK parameters of the model. Continuous covariates (mainly demographic candidate covariates) were normalized by median values (of observed values). On the other hand, categorical covariates (mainly genetic candidate covariates) were reflected as index variables in the model. The effects of each covariate were confirmed using exponential, power, or additive options. By stepwise backward elimination and forward addition procedure, the covariates were included or eliminated. By change in the objective function value (OFV), the inclusion of covariates was determined. Covariates corresponding to a decrease in the OFV value greater than 3.84 ($p < 0.05$) were included in the base model (in the forward addition procedure). In addition, covariates corresponding to the case where the decrease in OFV value was greater than 6.63 ($p < 0.01$) through the backward elimination process were not removed from the model and were included.

2.7. Model Evaluation

The final established models (in this study) were verified and evaluated both visually and numerically. To evaluate the model, visual predictive check (VPC), bootstrapping, and goodness-of-fit (including distribution of residuals) analyses were used. The goodness-of-fit was confirmed by using diagnostic scatter plots as follows: (a) population-predicted concentrations (PRED) versus observed (DV), (b) individual-predicted concentrations (IPRED) versus DV, (c) PRED versus conditional weighted residuals (CWRES), (d) time (IVAR) versus CWRES, and (e) quantile–quantile plot of the components of CWRES.

By using non-parametric bootstrap analysis, the stability of the final model was confirmed, and the bootstrap option of Phoenix NLME was used. A total of 1000 replicates were generated by the repeated random sampling with replacement from the original dataset. The estimated parameter values, such as the standard errors (SE; including confidence intervals) and medians from the bootstrap procedure, were compared with those estimated from the original dataset.

By using the VPC option of Phoenix NLME, VPCs of the final established models were performed. The time–DV concentration data were graphically superimposed on the median values and the 5th and 95th percentiles of the time-simulated concentration profiles. If the DV concentration data were approximately distributed within the 95th and 5th prediction interval, the model was expected to be precise. Normalized prediction distribution error (NPDE) was used to evaluate the predictive performance of the model on the basis of a Monte Carlo simulation with the R package [16]. NPDE results were summarized graphically using (1) quantile–quantile plot of the NPDE, (2) a histogram of the NPDE, (3) scatterplot of NPDE vs. time, and (4) scatterplot of NPDE vs. PRED. If the predictive performance is satisfied, the NPDE will follow a normal distribution (Shapiro–Wilk test) with a mean value of zero (*t*-test) and a variance of one (Fisher's test).

3. Results

3.1. Study Design and Demographic Analysis

The bioequivalence data (from reference formulation) collected from 24 healthy Korean males were used in this PK study for tiropramide. For the PK modelling, a total of 288 tiropramide plasma concentrations were available. There was complete information on height, age, and body weight for the 24 participants. Additionally, we successfully collected information on the total proteins, albumin, creatinine, AST, ALT, ALP, and the creatinine clearance levels of each participant, according to the method described above (Section 2.2). The related demographic information about the participants are shown in Table 1.

Table 1. Demographic information of the studied subjects (n = 24).

Physicochemical	Median (Range)	Mean ± SD
Age (year)	23 (19–29)	22.96 ± 2.61
Weight (kg)	66.8 (52.5–82.8)	67.60 ± 7.28
Height (cm)	171.45 (164.3–185.4)	172.59 ± 5.85
BSA (m^2) *	1.80 (1.58–1.97)	1.80 ± 0.11
BMI (kg/m^2) **	22.63 (17.89–29.06)	22.74 ± 2.72
Albumin (g/dL)	4.6 (4.2–5.4)	4.64 ± 0.27
Total proteins (g/dL)	7.6 (6.7–8.3)	7.59 ± 0.41
ALT (U/L)	20.5 (8–55)	22.29 ± 11.67
AST (U/L)	20 (10–32)	20.88 ± 5.81
ALP (U/L)	76 (49–126)	81.83 ± 20.66
Creatinine clearance (mL/min) ***	118.49 (91.78–159.77)	122.88 ± 22.25
Creatinine (mg/dL)	0.9 (0.6–1.1)	0.91 ± 0.13

* Body surface area (BSA) was determined on the basis of the Monsteller equation as follows: $\sqrt{(\text{height (cm)} \times \text{ weight (kg)}/3600)}$; ** body mass index (BMI) was calculated as follows: body weight (kg)/height^2 (m^2); *** creatinine clearance was determined on the basis of the Cockcroft–Gault equation as follows: [(140-age) × body weight (kg)]/[serum creatinine (mg/dL) × 72].

3.2. Genetic Analysis

Genotyping was performed on all 24 individuals who participated in this study. The analyzed genotypes were *ABCB1* (1236C>T, 2677G>T/A, and 3435C>T), *CYP2D6* (*1 and *10), *OCT2* (808G>T), and *PEPT1* (1287G>C) genes. The results are presented in Table 2. The *ABCB1* 1236C>T genotyping revealed that 6 (25.00%) subjects had the mutant type (TT), 13 (54.17%) subjects had the heterozygous type (CT), and 5 (20.83%) subjects had the homozygous wild type (CC). *ABCB1* 2677G>T/A genotyping revealed that eight (33.33%) subjects had the mutant type (TT or AT or TA or AA), nine (37.50%) subjects had the heterozygous type (GT or GA), and seven (29.17%) subjects had the homozygous wild type (GG). *ABCB1* 3435C>T genotyping revealed that 3 (12.50%) subjects had the mutant type (TT), 12 (50.00%) subjects had the heterozygous type (CT), and 9 (37.50%) subjects had the homozygous wild type (CC). *CYP2D6* genotyping revealed that 6 (25.00%) subjects had the homozygous *10 allele (*10/*10), 14 (58.33%) subjects had the heterozygous *10 allele (*1/*10), and 4 (16.67%) subjects had the homozygous *1 allele (*1/*1). *CYP2D6**2, *4, *5, *14A/B, *36, and *47 alleles were not detected in any of the subjects of this study. We classified the *CYP2D6* genotypes into three groups to investigate the impact of *CYP2D6* genotypes on the PKs of tiropramide as follows: extensive metabolizers (EMs) (*1/*1), heterozygous intermediate metabolizers (IMs) (*1/*10), and homozygous IMs (*10/*10), on the basis of the reports of the difference in *CYP2D6* enzyme activity according to *CYP2D6* genotypes [9,17]. *OCT2* 808G>T genotyping revealed that 8 (33.33%) subjects had the heterozygous type (GT) and 16 (66.67%) subjects had the homozygous type (GG). *PEPT1* 1287G>C genotyping revealed that 3 (12.50%) subjects had the mutant type (CC), 2 (8.33%) subjects had the heterozygous type (GC), and 19 (79.17%) subjects had the homozygous wild type (GG).

Table 2. Genetic information of the studied subjects (n = 24).

Genotypes		No. (Frequency)
ABCB1		
1236C>T (exon 12)	CC	5 (20.83%)
	CT	13 (54.17%)
	TT	6 (25.00%)
2677G>T/A (exon 21)	GG	7 (29.17%)
	GT, GA	9 (37.50%)
	TT, AT, TA, AA	8 (33.33%)
3435C>T (exon 26)	CC	9 (37.50%)
	CT	12 (50.00%)
	TT	3 (12.50%)
CYP2D6	*1/*1	4 (16.67%)
	*1/*10	14 (58.33%)
	*10/*10	6 (25.00%)
OCT2		
808G>T	GG	16 (66.67%)
	GT	8 (33.33%)
PEPT1		
1287G>C (exon 16)	GG	19 (79.17%)
	GC	2 (8.33%)
	CC	3 (12.50%)

3.3. Determination of Plasma Tiropramide Concentrations

After the oral administration of a 100 mg dose, plasma concentrations of tiropramide were determined by a column-switching semi-micro HPLC method (as mentioned in Section 2.4). This method analyzed tiropramide at a run time of 25 min per sample, enabling PK studies on tiropramide. The linearity of calibration curve for tiropramide was excellent (r^2 = 0.99) in human plasma, ranging from 2 to 500 ng/mL. Moreover, the calculation formula of the calibration curve was as follows: $y = 384.51x + 320.45$ ($p < 0.01$), where y is the peak area of tiropramide and x is the concentration (ng/mL) of the tiropramide. In addition, the lower limit of quantitation (LLOQ) for tiropramide was as low as 2 ng/mL, and was sufficient for PK studies after the oral administration of tiropramide tablet to humans. This assay has been validated for specificity, accuracy, precision, and sensitivity in order to be applied to accurate PK studies. There were no significant interferences derived from system or endogenous substances peaks, and we confirmed the identical tiropramide peak spectrum with the diode array detector. Intra-batch (n = 5) accuracies for tiropramide ranged from 100.70% to 113.50% with precision (coefficient of variation, CV) of < 13.57%. Inter-batch (n = 5) accuracies for tiropramide ranged from 98.00% to 111.42% with precision (CV) of < 9.23%.

3.4. Pharmacokinetic (NCA) Analysis

The observed plasma concentration–time profiles of tiropramide in the 24 subjects after oral administration of the 100 mg dose are presented in Figure 1.

In most individuals, the concentration of tiropramide in blood was measured up to 12 h after dosing. The PK parameters of tiropramide according to the genotypes (*ABCB1* 1236C>T, *ABCB1* 2677G>T/A, *ABCB1* 3435C>T, *CYP2D6*, *OCT2* 808G>T, and *PEPT1* 1287G>C) calculated by NCA are presented in Table 3. According to the NCA results for each genotype, the diversity of PK parameters in each group was not significant ($p > 0.05$). Although the higher mean $AUC_{0\text{-}t}$, $AUC_{0\text{-}\infty}$, and C_{max} values but lower mean CL/F values were calculated in the mutant type group (TT) than in the wild homozygous type groups (CC) in the *ABCB1* 1236C>T gene, this was not statistically significant considering the high SD. In the *CYP2D6* gene, higher mean $AUC_{0\text{-}t}$, $AUC_{0\text{-}\infty}$, and C_{max} values were calculated for IMs (*1/*10 and *10/*10) than EMs (*1/*1), but this was also not statistically significant considering the high SD. In addition, although the higher mean C_{max}, $AUC_{0\text{-}t}$, and $AUC_{0\text{-}\infty}$ values and lower mean CL/F value were calculated in wild homozygous type groups (GG) than in mutant type group (CC) in the *PEPT1* 1287G>C gene, this was not statistically significant considering the high SD. The $AUC_{0\text{-}t}$, $AUC_{0\text{-}\infty}$, C_{max}, half-life, and T_{max} values calculated by the NCA analysis of tiropramide were 254.31 ± 197.38 h· ng/mL, 280.34 ± 199.96 h· ng/mL, 69.07 ± 59.74 ng/mL, 3.41 ± 1.99 h, and 1.74 ± 0.63 h, respectively.

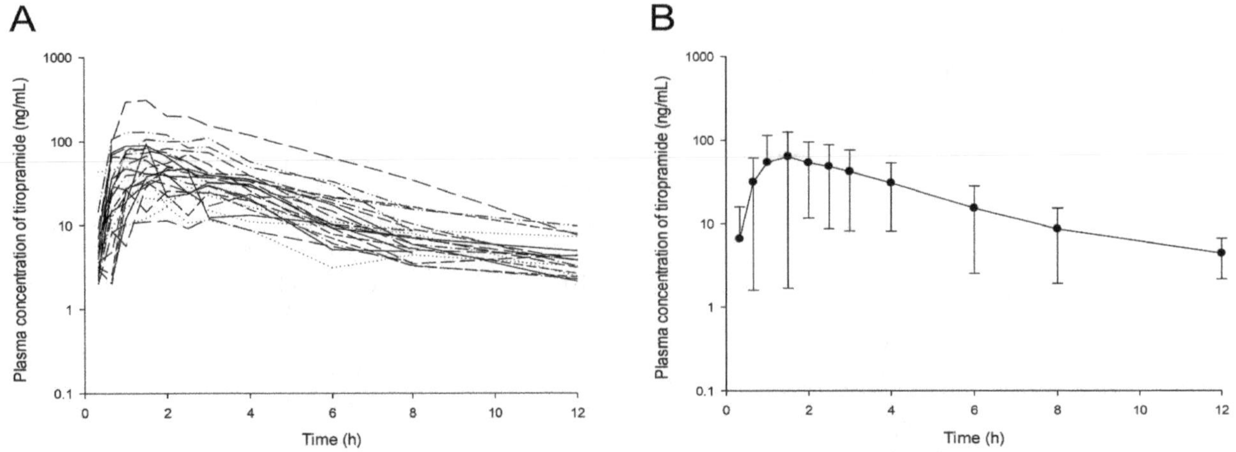

Figure 1. Log-transformed plasma concentration–time profiles of tiropramide in 24 subjects (**A**) and the mean curves (**B**). The vertical bars represent standard deviation of the mean.

Table 3. Pharmacokinetic parameters of tiropramide after a single oral administration of a 100 mg tiropramide tablet according to the genotypes (mean ± SD, *n* = 24).

Genotypes		Half-Life (h−1)	Tmax (h)	Cmax (ng/mL)	AUC0–t (h·ng/mL)	AUC0–∞ (h·ng/mL)	CL/F (L/h)
ABCB1 1236C>T	CC (*n* = 5)	2.91 ± 1.42	1.90 ± 0.42	104.56 ± 117.25	394.51 ± 376.32	419.54 ± 376.69	380.72 ± 246.10
	CT (*n* = 13)	3.80 ± 2.41	1.67 ± 0.70	49.06 ± 23.81	182.00 ± 60.62	209.85 ± 72.09	551.43 ± 263.69
	TT (*n* = 6)	2.99 ± 1.36	1.75 ± 0.69	82.83 ± 39.09	293.01 ± 149.02	317.08 ± 154.99	419.44 ± 292.77
ABCB1 2677G>T/A	GG (*n* = 7)	3.86 ± 3.11	1.38 ± 0.52	52.88 ± 15.94	214.50 ± 69.45	247.94 ± 76.58	439.10 ± 136.89
	GT (*n* = 9)	2.77 ± 0.89	2.06 ± 0.73	88.92 ± 89.16	323.04 ± 294.51	339.44 ± 296.97	481.39 ± 359.30
	TT, AT, TA, AA (*n* = 8)	3.75 ± 1.73	1.69 ± 0.46	60.89 ± 39.69	210.97 ± 122.69	242.22 ± 135.50	522.84 ± 259.46
ABCB1 3435C>T	CC (*n* = 9)	2.82 ± 1.11	1.52 ± 0.46	78.29 ± 88.96	294.77 ± 291.67	317.13 ± 293.75	452.72 ± 201.28
	CT (*n* = 12)	3.44 ± 1.45	1.92 ± 0.70	63.79 ± 38.63	235.35 ± 131.42	259.88 ± 136.73	524.94 ± 338.71
	TT (*n* = 3)	5.10 ± 4.82	1.67 ± 0.76	62.51 ± 23.63	206.48 ± 14.18	251.82 ± 44.95	405.08 ± 67.07
CYP2D6	*1/*1 (*n* = 4)	4.74 ± 4.00	1.25 ± 0.29	63.24 ± 23.66	240.38 ± 75.18	278.97 ± 67.41	379.92 ± 118.76
	*1/*10 (*n* = 14)	3.14 ± 1.17	1.76 ± 0.59	66.73 ± 72.90	258.15 ± 238.14	280.90 ± 240.02	484.79 ± 223.74
	*10/*10 (*n* = 6)	3.17 ± 1.84	2.00 ± 0.77	78.41 ± 45.97	253.49 ± 168.34	279.97 ± 177.22	547.04 ± 420.10
OCT2 808G>T	GG (*n* = 16)	3.62 ± 2.29	1.51 ± 0.53	60.42 ± 29.24	218.24 ± 89.40	247.77 ± 99.03	459.49 ± 166.01
	GT (*n* = 8)	3.00 ± 1.20	2.19 ± 0.59	86.37 ± 96.84	325.60 ± 319.70	345.50 ± 321.06	529.63 ± 414.56
PEPT1 1287G>C	GG (*n* = 19)	3.07 ± 1.38	1.82 ± 0.65	62.40 ± 32.14	226.40 ± 109.97	248.21 ± 115.65	506.33 ± 278.61
	GC (*n* = 2)	6.36 ± 6.07	1.25 ± 0.35	181.48 ± 184.26	621.48 ± 609.37	688.85 ± 546.19	211.72 ± 167.87
	CC (*n* = 3)	3.63 ± 0.41	1.50 ± 0.50	36.36 ± 9.98	183.99 ± 65.49	211.54 ± 80.59	515.08 ± 168.25

3.5. Population Pharmacokinetic Model Development

By a one-compartment disposition model with first order elimination and absorption with an absorption lag time, the plasma concentrations of tiropramide were best expressed. Considering the lag time, the numerical values (such as -2LL and AIC) of the model evaluation and graphical data fitting were more improved than otherwise. Although we tried a two-compartment model, it did not show an improved fit when compared with the one-compartment model. In other words, there was a problem (fail to model fit) in fitting the two-compartment model for some individuals, but in the one-compartment model, all individuals were fitted properly. In addition, the -2LL and AIC values significantly decreased in the multiple (two) transit absorption compartment model in which the additional absorption phase was added to the one-compartment model. However, from two or more transit phases of absorption, there was no significant decrease in the -2LL and AIC values (with increasing number of parameters). As a result, the multiple (two) transit absorption phase-one compartment model with an absorption lag time was selected as the base structure model for tiropramide. The model was parameterized in terms of V/F, T_{lag}, CL/F, K_{a1}, and K_{a2}. When the lag-time or model transit time was given to K_{a2} in the parameterization of the model, no significant model improvement was found with the increasing number of parameters. Therefore, significant model improvement was found when parameterization with lag-time was carried out only at K_{a1}, and the rate constant of substance transit in the absorption compartment. Figure 2 shows a schematic of the disposition compartment model presented for tiropramide.

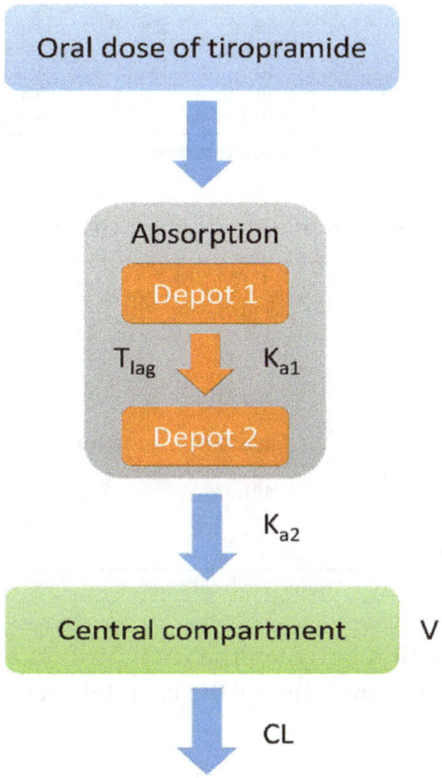

Figure 2. Schematic of tiropramide population pharmacokinetic (PPK) model (two transit absorption phase-one compartment model with an absorption lag time). Depot 1 and 2 represent transit compartments in the absorption phase. K_{a1} refers to the rate constant at which the drug is moved from depot 1 to depot 2. T_{lag} refers to the delay time for the drug to move from depot 1 to depot 2. K_{a2} is the rate constant at which the drug moves from depot 2 to the central compartment. V means the volume of drug distribution in the central compartment, and CL means removal of the drug from the central compartment.

An exponential model was used to describe the IIVs on parameters of T_{lag}, V/F, CL/F, K_{a1}, and K_{a2}. By applying an additive error model on log-transformed data, the residual variability was explained. Table 4 summarizes the steps for developing a basic structural model of tiropramide.

In order to find the covariates affecting the PK parameters of tiropramide, we analyzed the effects of each covariate on the PK parameters. The final potential covariates were selected on the basis of the graphical exploration between candidate covariates and PK parameters. The influence of each selected candidate covariate on the PK parameters of tiropramide was assessed by incorporating the covariates into an established basic structural model. The evaluation was based on OFV, which means model improvement. In this regard, the covariate selection process (according to OFV) to be reflected in the final model of tiropramide is summarized in Table 5.

Table 4. Basic structural model building steps.

Model	Description	n-Parameter	-2LL	AIC	Δ-2LL	ΔAIC	Compared with
	Absorption model						
1	One compartment with first order (no T_{lag})	7	562.27	576.27			
2	One compartment with the first order (add T_{lag})	9	508.80	526.80	−53.48	−49.48	1
3 *	One compartment with the first order (add T_{lag} and additonal absorption transit phase one)	11	420.97	442.97	−87.83	−83.83	2
4	One compartment with the first order (add T_{lag} and additonal absorption transit phase two)	13	419.84	442.11	−1.13	−0.86	3
	Residual error model						
3 *	Log additive	11	420.97	442.97			
5	Additive	11	1964.95	1986.95	1543.98	1543.98	3
6	Proportional	11	1860.33	1882.33	1439.36	1439.36	3
	IIV model						
7	Remove IIV K_{a1}	10	428.64	448.64	7.67	5.67	3
8	Remove IIV K_{a2}	10	428.64	448.64	7.67	5.67	3
9	Remove IIV T_{lag}	10	434.18	454.18	13.21	11.21	3
10	Remove IIV V/F	10	500.86	520.86	79.89	77.89	3
11	Remove IIV CL/F	10	534.10	554.10	113.13	111.13	3

* Selected model.

Table 5. Stepwise search for covariates.

Model	Description	OFV	ΔOFV	n-Parameter	Compared with
1	Base model	420.97		11	
2	Total protein on CL/F	411.72	−9.25	12	1
3 *	Total protein on CL/F and V/F	402.56	−9.16	13	2
4	Total protein on CL/F and V/F, BMI on K_{a1}	400.61	−1.95	14	3
5	Total protein on CL/F and V/F, *PEPT1* (1287G>C) on K_{a1}	402.57	0.01	14	3
6	Total protein on CL/F and V/F, *ABCB1* (1236C>T) on K_{a1}	401.63	−0.93	14	3
7	Total protein on CL/F and V/F, *CYP2D6* (*1 and *10) on K_{a2}	397.15	−5.42	15	3

* Selected final model.

There was a significant correlation between the total protein and tiropramide V/F as well as the total protein and tiropramide CL/F. Figure 3 shows the correlation between the final selected covariates and CL/F of tiropramide.

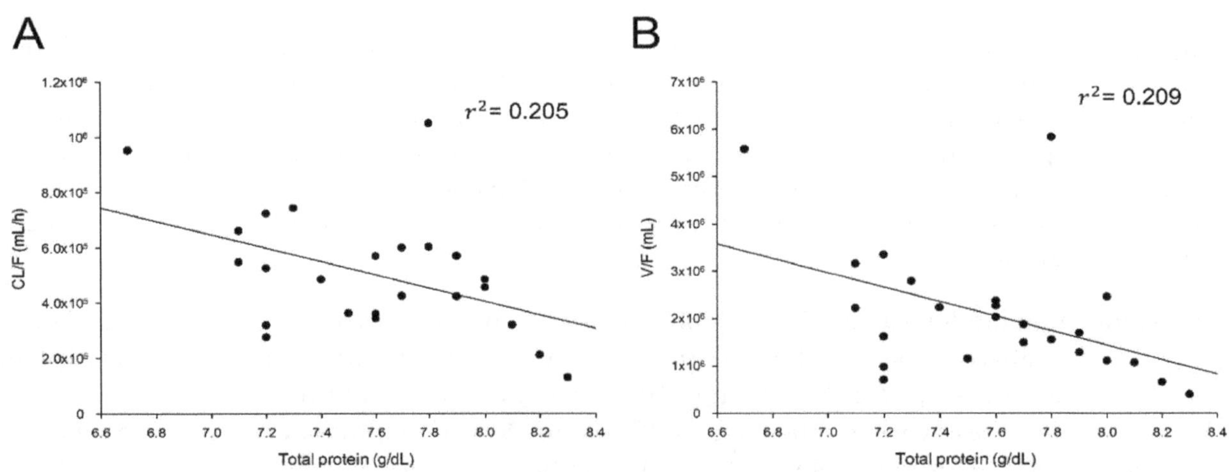

Figure 3. Relationship between subjects' characteristics and individual predicted pharmacokinetic parameters. Clearance (CL/F) of tiropramide according to total protein (**A**). Volume of distribution (V/F) of tiropramide according to total protein (**B**).

When the correlation between the total protein and CL/F was reflected in the PPK model of tiropramide, the ΔOFV was significantly reduced to −9.25 ($p < 0.05$). Furthermore, the addition of total protein and V/F correlation to tiropramide PPK model significantly reduced the ΔOFV to −9.16

($p < 0.05$). However, other covariates including BMI, *PEPT1* 1287G>C, *OCT2* 808G>T, *ABCB1* 1236C>T, *ABCB1* 2677G>T/A, *ABCB1* 3435C>T, and *CYP2D6* (*1 and *10) had no significant effect on model improvement. Even by applying genetic factors (such as *PEPT1* 1287G>C, *OCT2* 808G>T, *ABCB1* 1236C>T, *ABCB1* 2677G>T/A, *ABCB1* 3435C>T, and *CYP2D6* (*1 and *10)) alone to the base model, we examined whether they affected K_{a1}, K_{a2}, CL/F, and V/F, but no significant associations were identified. The final model of tiropramide (reflecting the effects of covariates) is expressed as follows:

$$\begin{gathered}
V/F = tvV/F \cdot (1+ (\text{Totalproteins-7.6}) \cdot dV/Fd\text{Totalproteins}) \cdot \exp(\eta_V) \\
CL/F = tvCL/F \cdot (1+ (\text{Totalproteins-7.6}) \cdot dCL/Fd\text{Totalproteins}) \cdot \exp(\eta_{CL}) \\
T_{lag} = tvT_{lag} \cdot \exp(\eta_{Tlag}) \\
K_{a1} = tvK_{a1} \cdot \exp(\eta_{Ka1}) \\
K_{a2} = tvK_{a2} \cdot \exp(\eta_{Ka2})
\end{gathered} \tag{1}$$

Population estimates of tiropramide were 466,711 mL/h for CL/F and 1,889,250 mL for V/F. CL/F and V/F values by NCA were 482,567 ± 267,433 mL/h and 2,386,871 ± 1,699,847 mL, respectively. As a result, the CL/F and V/F values estimated in the final model were not significantly different from the NCA values. In the final model, the relative standard error (RSE, %) was 9.53–83.51%. The Eta shrinkage values for the estimated PK parameters were suggested as acceptable at 0.02–0.40%. Compared with the base model, the final model (considering total protein effects) of tiropramide reduced the IIV of V/F from 70.70% to 57.12%, and the IIV of CL/F from 50.55% to 39.95%. Table 6 presents the estimated parameter values in the base model and final PPK model of tiropramide. The AUC_{0-t}, $AUC_{0-\infty}$, C_{max}, half-life, and T_{max} estimated values by the final PPK model of tiropramide were 242.73 ± 175.28 h· ng/mL, 260.92 ± 179.08 h· ng/mL, 54.89 ± 46.18 ng/mL, 2.73 ± 0.88 h, and 1.65 ± 0.53 h, respectively.

Table 6. Population pharmacokinetic parameters for tiropramide in base model and final model.

Parameter	Estimate	SE	RSE (%)	Shrinkage (%)	IIV (%)
Base model					
tvK_{a1} (1/h)	3.160	0.511	16.143		
tvK_{a2} (1/h)	3.171	0.510	16.086		
tvV/F (mL)	1,717,060.491	262,434.751	15.284		
tvCL/F (mL/h)	447,163.154	48,667.242	10.884		
tvT_{lag} (h)	0.196	0.021	10.480		
$\omega^2_{V/F}$	0.500	0.170	33.973	0.044	70.701
$\omega^2_{Cl/F}$	0.255	0.103	40.328	0.016	50.546
$\omega^2 T_{lag}$	0.106	0.089	84.320	0.225	32.538
ω^2_{Ka1}	0.608	0.266	43.735	0.399	77.986
ω^2_{Ka2}	0.613	0.261	42.630	0.398	78.269
σ	0.354	0.041	11.673		
Final model					
tvK_{a1} (1/h)	3.187	0.538	16.872		
tvK_{a2} (1/h)	3.183	0.524	16.464		
tvV/F (mL)	1,889,250.002	289,606.633	15.329		
tvCL/F (mL/h)	466,711.101	44,476.962	9.530		
tvT_{lag} (h)	0.196	0.021	10.590		
dCl/FdTotalproteins	−0.804	0.296	36.791		
dV/FdTotalproteins	−1.049	0.232	22.118		
$\omega^2_{V/F}$	0.326	0.158	48.369	0.068	57.118
$\omega^2_{Cl/F}$	0.160	0.067	41.977	0.023	39.947
$\omega^2 T_{lag}$	0.107	0.089	83.508	0.225	32.503
ω^2_{Ka1}	0.557	0.276	49.584	0.405	74.627
ω^2_{Ka2}	0.556	0.269	48.406	0.405	74.566
σ	0.357	0.042	11.895		

3.6. Population Pharmacokinetic Model Evaluation

The developed PPK model of the tiropramide was comprehensively evaluated for GOF, bootstrap analysis, and VPC. Figure 4 shows the GOF plots of the base and the final models of tiropramide.

As shown in Figure 4B, the observed and predicted concentrations of tiropramide showed a relatively good agreement in the final model. CWRES was well distributed symmetrically with respect to zero, and CWRES was included in ±4 at all points. In addition, the residuals in the final model were more improved than in the base model. In other words, without any specific bias, the CWRES was randomly well distributed, and the residuals in the final model showed a significant decrease when compared with the base model (larger than ±4).

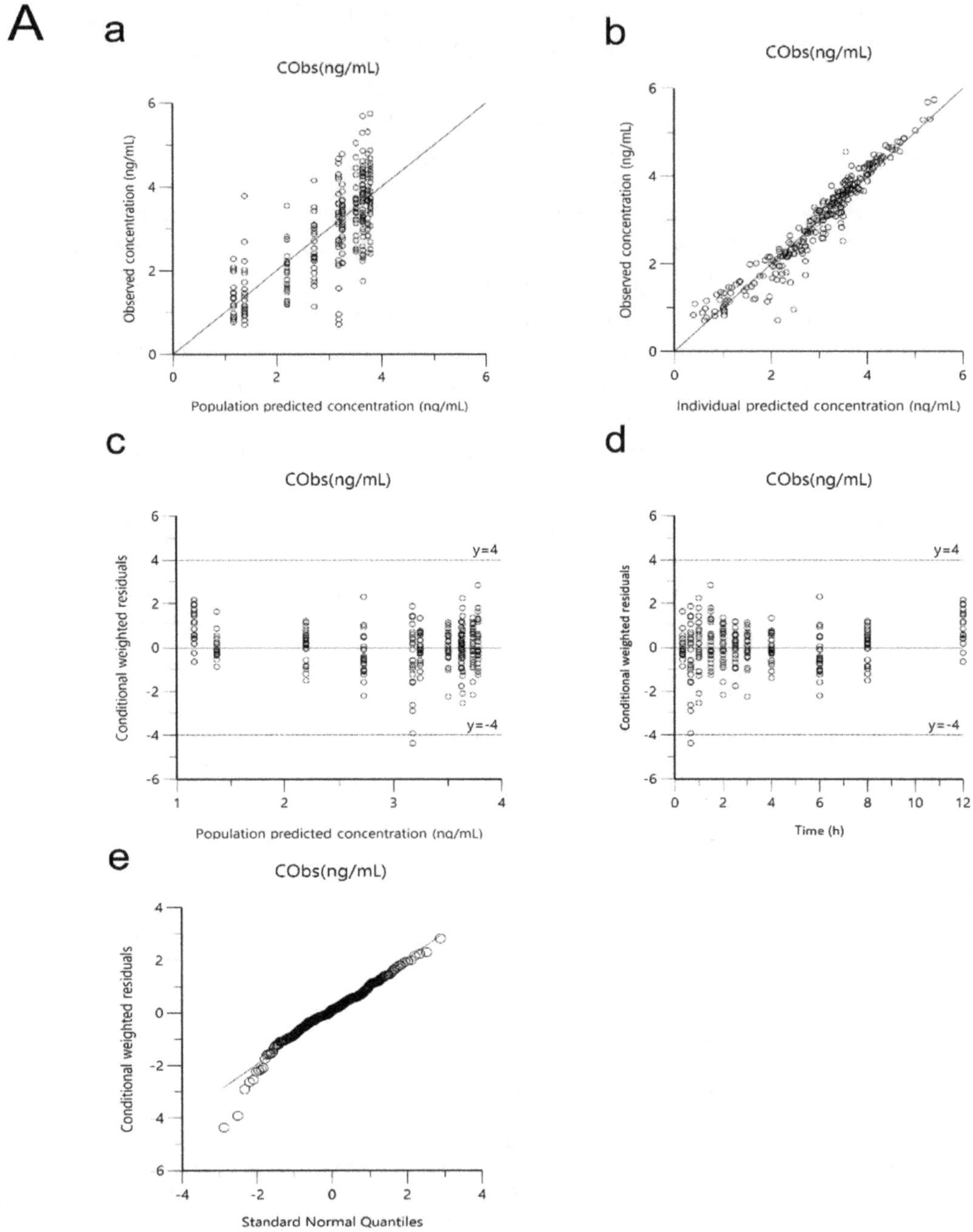

Figure 4. *Cont.*

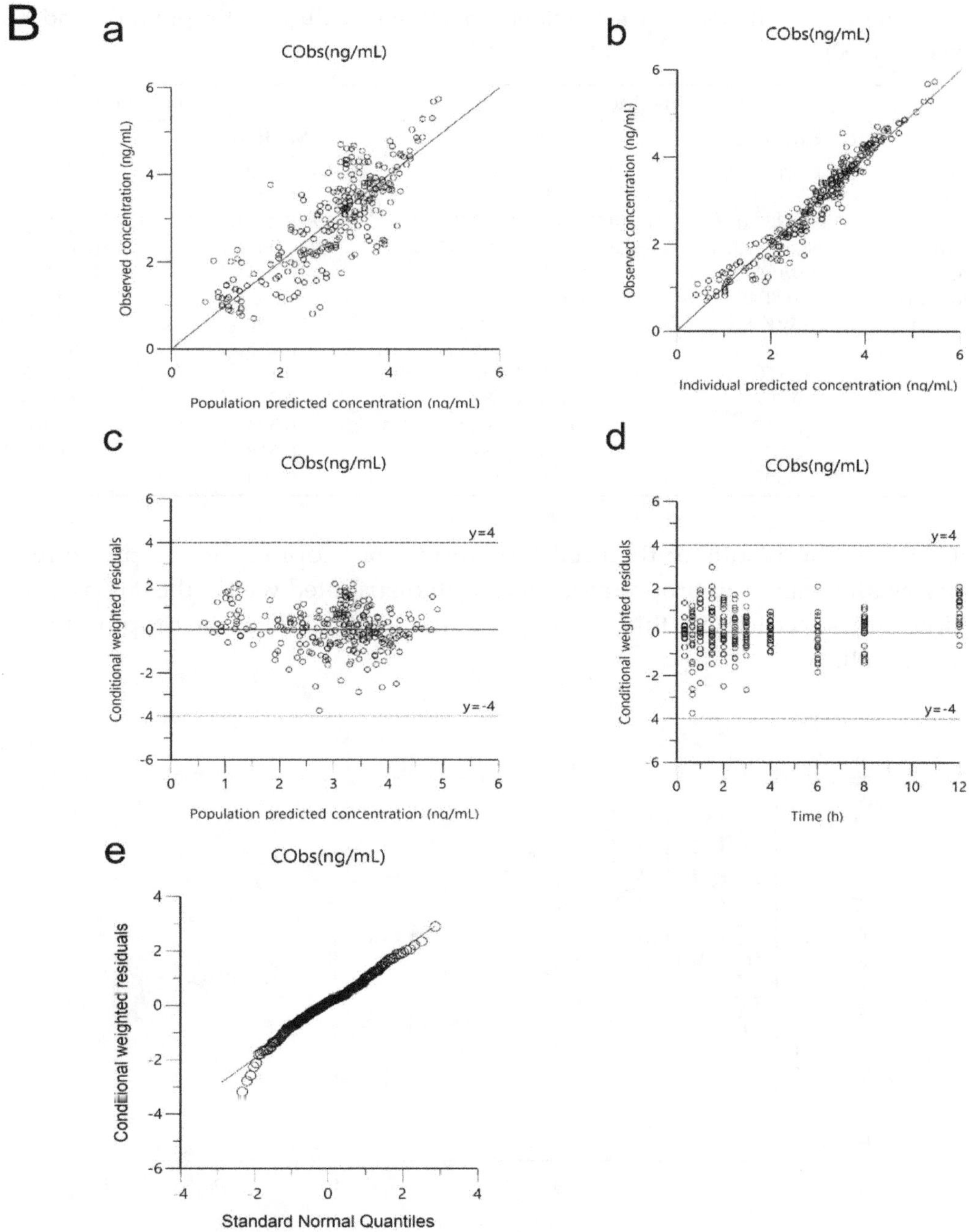

Figure 4. Goodness-of-fit (GOF) plots of base model (**A**) and final model (**B**) for tiropramide. (**a**) Population-predicted concentrations (PRED) against observed plasma concentration (DV), (**b**) individual-predicted concentrations (IPRED) against DV, (**c**) PRED against conditional weighted residuals (CWRES), (**d**) time (IVAR) against CWRES, and (**e**) quantile–quantile plot of components of CWRES.

Bootstrap validation was performed to verify the reproducibility and/or robustness of the final PPK model of tiropramide. Table 7 shows the bootstrapping analysis results. The parameter values estimated in the final model were in the 95% CI range of the bootstrap analysis results, and were similar to the median values of the bootstrap (replicates of 1000).

Table 7. Estimated population pharmacokinetic parameter values of tiropramide and bootstrap validation (n = 1000).

Parameter	Final Model		Bootstrapping	
	Estimate	95% CI	Median	95% CI
tvK_{a1} (1/h)	3.187	2.128–4.246	3.187	2.332–4.733
tvK_{a2} (1/h)	3.183	2.151–4.215	3.183	2.273–4.345
tvV/F (mL)	1,889,250.002	1,318,770.124–2,459,730.256	1,889,250.000	1,397,156.042-2,491,555.125
tvCL/F (mL/h)	466,711.101	379,098.212–554,324.163	466,711.000	374,186.003–550,036.012
tvT_{lag} (h)	0.196	0.155–0.237	0.196	0.144–0.234
dCl/FdTotalproteins	−0.804	−1.387–(−0.221)	−0.804	−1.050–0.082
dV/FdTotalproteins	−1.049	−1.506–(−0.592)	−1.049	−1.222–0.246
$\omega^2_{V/F}$	0.326	0.017–0.636	0.296	0.020–0.572
$\omega^2_{Cl/F}$	0.160	0.028–0.291	0.134	0.023–0.245
$\omega^2 T_{lag}$	0.107	0.068–0.282	0.085	0.045–0.215
ω^2_{Ka1}	0.557	0.016–1.098	0.524	0.016–1.063
ω^2_{Ka2}	0.556	0.028–1.084	0.518	0.013–1.049
σ	0.357	0.273–0.441	0.363	0.276–0.428

The VPC simulation results of the final PPK model of tiropramide are presented in Figure 5. Most of the observation values of tiropramide were well distributed within the 90% prediction interval of the prediction values. As a result, this suggests that the final model of the tiropramide is precise and explains the data well.

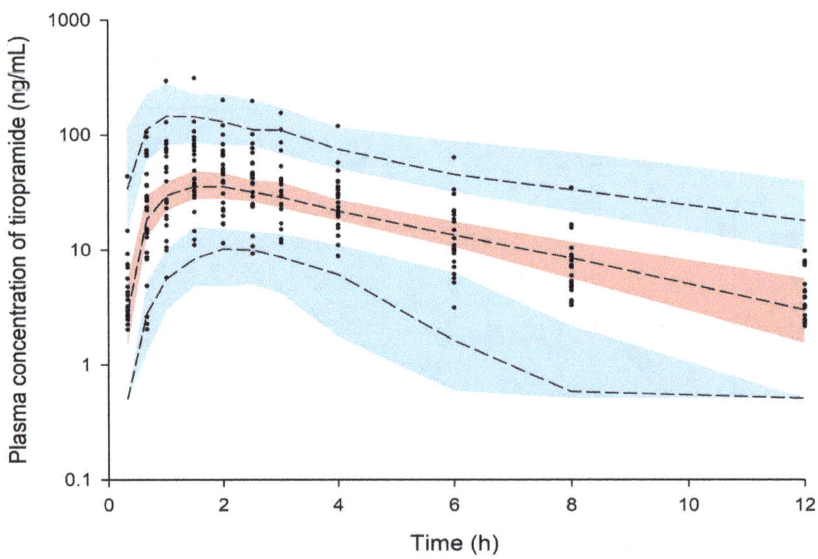

Figure 5. Visual predictive check (VPC) of the final model for tiropramide. Observed concentrations were depicted by the dots. The 95th, 50th, and 5th percentiles of the predicted concentrations are represented by black dashed lines. The 95% confidence intervals (CI) for the predicted 5th and 95th percentiles are represented by the blue shaded regions. The 95% CI for the predicted 50th percentiles are represented by the red shaded regions. The values on the y-axis are logarithms.

The NPDE distribution and histogram are presented in Figure S1. The assumption of a normal distribution for the differences between predictions and observations was acceptable. The quantile–quantile plots and histogram also confirmed the normality of the NPDE (Figure S1).

4. Discussion

The mechanism of action of tiropramide, as mentioned in the Introduction section, has been studied relatively well and has been reported in the past. However, studies on the in vivo PK characteristics (including metabolism and excretion) of tiropramide are still insufficient. Therefore, little data was available regarding the dosage and usage of tiropramide in clinical as well as formulation development.

According to Lee et al., despite the frequent use of tiropramide in clinical practice, studies on safety and efficacy are very poor [4]. We conducted a PPK model development study of tiropramide to explore the effective covariates related to PK diversity of tiropramide and to investigate the characteristics of PK in the population. This study was new and was expected to be useful in the evaluation of the safety and efficacy of tiropramide in clinical use. As mentioned in the Abstract section, although tiropramide has a (relatively) broad margin of safety, this study involving healthy subjects was very important because it could find new covariates in healthy subjects that had not been reported before and/or be used to predict PPK for patients in the clinic by establishing PPK in healthy adults. In addition to this, in patients with abdominal pain and irritable bowel syndrome, it is very likely that the absorption process of tiropramide will change. Therefore, if clinical trials are conducted for patients in the future, it is thought that the PK variation of tiropramide between individuals can be explained more specifically through the application of our PPK model.

In this study, the PK of tiropramide was modelled as a two transit absorption phase-one compartment model with an absorption lag time. Various errors (including residual error and IIV) models and covariate effects were evaluated to establish factors that significantly influence the PK parameters of tiropramide and to explain the PK diversity of the tiropramide in the population. As a result of evaluating the model, the final tiropramide PPK model showed relatively good GOF plots, suggesting that the final PPK model had an acceptable predictive power. In addition, all CWRES values over time or predicted concentrations were in the range of -4 and 4, suggesting that the model is relatively stable. In addition, the bootstrap and VPC simulation results suggested that the final tiropramide PPK model was accurate, stable, and precise. We compared the estimated parameter values (of AUC_{0-t}, $AUC_{0-\infty}$, C_{max}, half-life, and T_{max}) by tiropramide's final PPK model with these values by NCA analysis. As a result, there were no significant differences ($p > 0.05$) between the parameter values predicted by the final PPK model of tiropramide and those calculated by NCA analysis. These results suggest that the final PPK model of tiropramide established in this study explains the experimental data relatively well.

The 24 healthy Korean male PK data used to establish the tiropramide PPK model were similar to the previously reported PK results. In other words, the previously reported PK parameter values of tiropramide were similar to our PK results obtained by NCA analysis. After oral administration of 100 mg of tiropramide in humans, the obtained NCA PK parameters (as previously reported values) were 2.34-6.99 h for $t_{1/2}$, 0.66-1.6 h for T_{max}, 77.4-111 ng/mL for C_{max}, and 267.7-812.7 h·ng/mL for AUC [6,12,18–21]. On the other hand, the NCA PK parameters in this study were 3.41 ± 1.99 h for $t_{1/2}$, 1.74 ± 0.63 h for T_{max}, 69.07 ± 59.74 ng/mL for C_{max}, and 280.34 ± 199.96 h·ng/mL for AUC, which were similar to the previously reported values. Table 8 summarizes these results.

As mentioned above, few studies have been done on the metabolic ratio (including pathway) and excretion of tiropramide in humans (especially patient groups), making it difficult to predict candidate covariates. On the basis of previous reports (as drug information provided by the manufacturer) that tiropramide is metabolized in the liver and excreted into urine (about 10–20% of administered dose), the covariate effects were tested in this study by obtaining the physicochemical information of liver function indicators (such as AST, ALT, and ALP) and genotyping the *CYP2D6* gene related to metabolism in the body. The creatinine clearance and the functional indicator of the kidney were collected for each subject, and the covariate effects related to CL/F were tested. In addition, genotyping of genes (such as *ABCB1*, *OCT2*, and *PEPT1*) associated with various transporters known to be widely involved in the distribution, absorption, excretion, and metabolism of drugs in the body has been performed to identify the effects of the covariate associated with the PK parameters. Despite these efforts, only total protein was found to have a significant effect on V/F and CL/F of tiropramide. As shown in Figure 3, the total protein, and the V/F and CL/F showed a significant negative correlation of 45.72% ($r^2 = 0.209$) and 45.28% ($r^2 = 0.205$), respectively. The correlation values of the total protein to CL/F and V/F were the largest of all the covariates we collected in this study.

Table 8. Previously reported pharmacokinetic (PK) parameter values of tiropramide obtained by non-compartmental analysis (NCA) analysis.

References	Subjects	PK Parameters				
		Half-life (h)	Tmax (h)	Cmax (ng/mL)	$AUC_{0\text{-}\infty}$ (h·ng/mL)	CL/F (L/h)
Kwon et al. (2003) [21]	Human (n = 2, 100 mg dose)	-	0.66–2	87.3–191.3	267.7–812.7	-
Kwon et al. (2003) [20]	Human (n = 16, 100 mg dose)	2.34–2.61	-	96.4 ± 51.6	380.8 ± 239.0	-
Lee et al. (2003) [6]	Human (n = 4, 100 mg dose)	2.7 ± 0.5	1.6 ± 0.6	77.4 ± 33.0	319 ± 147	-
Baek et al. (2003) [12]	Human (n = 14, 100 mg dose)	6.3 ± 2.0	1.6 ± 0.6	111 ± 62	377 ± 220	-
Jhee et al. (2006) [19]	Human (n = 18, 100 mg dose)	6.99 ± 0.83	1.33 ± 0.34	98.77 ± 30.23	434.39 ± 102.35	-
Imran et al. (2007) [18]	Human (n = 12, 100 mg dose)	3.3 ± 1.0	1.5 ± 0.2	105.35 ± 15.7	375.4 ± 76.7	-
In this study	Human (n = 24, 100 mg dose)	3.41 ± 1.99	1.74 ± 0.63	69.07 ± 59.74	280.34 ± 199.96	482.87 ± 267.25

Although the plasma protein binding ratio of tiropramide in humans has not been reported accurately, it has been reported that the plasma protein binding ratio of tiropramide in rats is about 48–51% [22]. This suggests that the amount of plasma protein may affect the in vivo PK properties of tiropramide by binding to the plasma proteins in the blood. According to our tiropramide PPK model, higher total protein levels in the blood mean a smaller distribution of tiropramide in the body and a lower excretion. This can be explained by the fact that tiropramide binds to proteins in the blood and affects the distribution and excretion of substances from the body. Tiropramide combined with proteins in the blood will make it difficult to filter the glomerulus of the kidney and distribute from blood to many organs. The reflection of the total protein covariates in tiropramide PPK model reduced V/F IIV and CL/F IIV by 13.58% and 10.60%, respectively. These results suggested that the variabilities of tiropramide plasma concentrations could be partly explained by individual variances of total protein level related with V/F and CL/F of tiropramide. On the other hand, other candidate covariates (such as AST, ALT, ALP, and creatinine clearance) had no significant effect on the PK parameter values and IIV improvement of tiropramide. Although tiropramide is metabolized in the liver and excreted in the kidney, our results suggest that tiropramide is a drug that does not require dose control depending on the liver and renal function. However, because our PPK model was based on the data from healthy men, further studies (for patient groups) will be needed for further clarification. That is, if PK data significantly different from the normal group (like our study) was obtained from the patient groups, and if the PPK analysis was conducted in the same manner as in this study with our model (from patient groups), other significant covariates may be identified. Therefore, PK studies or PPK analysis of tiropramide in patient groups will need to be performed in the future. Nevertheless, this study was important because it is a PPK model study of tiropramide that has not been previously conducted, and other related studies (such as clinical dose setting, formulation development, and PK comparison with certain other groups) on tiropramide may be possible in the future, on the basis of our findings. In addition, another limitation of our study was that PK analysis and PPK model studies were conducted for limited ages (between 19 and 29 years old). In the future, PK analysis and/or PPK model studies of tiropramide for more diverse age groups will need to be conducted in this regard.

As shown in Table 6, unexplained variability (as IIV) still exists in K_a (74.63% for K_{a1} and 74.57% for K_{a2}) and T_{lag} (32.50%). These results meant that multi-complex gastrointestinal (GI) tract absorption processes of tiropramide including the variabilities of each individual gastric emptying time, GI tract transit time, and other transporters, among others, could considerably affect the variabilities of tiropramide plasma concentrations. This study could not find any significant covariates that could explain K_a IIV and T_{lag} IIV. Perhaps, despite collecting various genetic and demographic information, there was still not enough information to explain the K_a and T_{lag} IIVs of tiropramide. Therefore, further studies are needed to explore significant covariates related to the absorption of tiropramide in the body.

5. Conclusions

A PPK model for tiropramide was developed on the basis of PK data for healthy Korean men in this study. The plasma concentration profiles for tiropramide were described well by a two transit absorption phase-one compartment model with an absorption lag time. The total protein was identified by significant covariates of CL/F and V/F for tiropramide, and their correlation was finally reflected in the PPK model of tiropramide. On the other hand, no significant correlation was found between genetic information such as *ABCB1*, *CYP2D6*, *OCT2*, *PEPT1*, and the PK parameters of tiropramide. To the best of our knowledge, this is the first time a PPK model has been studied for tiropramide, and it is expected to be a valuable resource for future studies (such as in clinical use, as well as dose control and formulation development).

Author Contributions: Research idea planning, S.-H.J., J.-H.J., and Y.-B.L.; method planning, S.-H.J. and J.-H.J.; method and data validation, S.-H.J. and H.-Y.C.; literature search, S.-H.J.; investigation, S.-H.J. and J.-H.J.; data analysis and modeling, S.-H.J. and J.-H.J.; original manuscript writing, S.-H.J. and J.-H.J.; review and editing of manuscript, S.-H.J., J.-H.J., H.-Y.C., and Y.-B.L.; supervision, Y.-B.L. All authors have read and agreed to the published version of the manuscript.

References

1. Setnikar, I.; Makovec, F.; Chiste, R.; Giachetti, C.; Zanolo, G. Tiropramide and metabolites in blood and plasma after intravenous or peroral administration of 14C-tiropramide to the rat. *Arzneim. Forsch.* **1988**, *38*, 1815–1819.
2. Arigoni, R.; Chiste, R.; Drovanti, A.; Makovec, F.; Senin, P.; Setnikar, I. Pharmacokinetics of tiropramide after single doses in man. *Arzneim. Forsch.* **1986**, *36*, 738–744.
3. Arigoni, R.; Chiste, R.; Makovec, F.; Setnikar, I.; Benfenati, E.; Fanelli, R. Identification of metabolites of tiropramide in human urine. *Biomed. Environ. Mass Spectrom.* **1988**, *15*, 205–209. [CrossRef] [PubMed]
4. Lee, K.N.; Lee, O.Y.; Choi, M.-G.; Sohn, C.I.; Huh, K.C.; Park, K.S.; Kwon, J.G.; Kim, N.; Rhee, P.-L.; Myung, S.-J.; et al. Efficacy and safety of tiropramide in the treatment of patients with irritable bowel syndrome: A multicenter, randomized, double-blind, non-inferiority trial, compared with octylonium. *J. Neurogastroenterol. Motil.* **2014**, *20*, 113–121. [CrossRef] [PubMed]
5. Kim, S.-M.; Lee, S.-N.; Yoon, H.; Kang, H.-A.; Cho, H.-Y.; Lee, I.-K.; Lee, Y.-B. Haplotype analysis and single nucleotide polymorphism frequency of organic cation transporter gene (OCT1 and 2) in Korean subjects. *J. Pharm. Investig.* **2009**, *39*, 345–351. [CrossRef]
6. Lee, H.W.; Ji, H.Y.; Kim, H.H.; Cho, H.-Y.; Lee, Y.-B.; Lee, H.S. Determination of tiropramide in human plasma by liquid chromatography–tandem mass spectrometry. *J. Chromatogr. B* **2003**, *796*, 395–400. [CrossRef]
7. Kim, S.-M.; Lee, S.-N.; Kang, H.-A.; Cho, H.-Y.; Lee, I.-K.; Lee, Y.-B. Haplotype analysis and single nucleotide polymorphism frequency of PEPT1 gene (Exon 5 and 16) in Korean. *J. Pharm. Investig.* **2009**, *39*, 411–416. [CrossRef]
8. Kim, S.-M.; Park, S.-A.; Cho, H.-Y.; Lee, Y.-B. Haplotype analysis of MDRI gene (Exon 12, 21 and 26) in Korean. *J. Pharm. Investig.* **2008**, *38*, 365–372.
9. Gaedigk, A.; Simon, S.; Pearce, R.; Bradford, L.; Kennedy, M.; Leeder, J. The CYP2D6 activity score: Translating genotype information into a qualitative measure of phenotype. *Clin. Pharmacol. Ther.* **2008**, *83*, 234–242. [CrossRef]

10. Lee, S.-Y.; Sohn, K.M.; Ryu, J.Y.; Yoon, Y.R.; Shin, J.G.; Kim, J.-W. Sequence-based CYP2D6 genotyping in the Korean population. *Ther. Drug Monit.* **2006**, *28*, 382–387. [CrossRef]
11. Byeon, J.-Y.; Kim, Y.-H.; Lee, C.-M.; Kim, S.-H.; Chae, W.-K.; Jung, E.-H.; Choi, C.-I.; Jang, C.-G.; Lee, S.-Y.; Bae, J.-W. CYP2D6 allele frequencies in Korean population, comparison with East Asian, Caucasian and African populations, and the comparison of metabolic activity of CYP2D6 genotypes. *Arch. Pharm. Res.* **2018**, *41*, 921–930. [CrossRef] [PubMed]
12. Baek, S.K.; Lee, S.S.; Park, E.J.; Sohn, D.H.; Lee, H.S. Semi-micro high-performance liquid chromatographic analysis of tiropramide in human plasma using column-switching. *J. Pharm. Biomed. Anal.* **2003**, *31*, 185–189. [CrossRef]
13. Deurenberg, P.; Weststrate, J.A.; Seidell, J.C. Body mass index as a measure of body fatness: Age-and sex-specific prediction formulas. *Br. J. Nutr.* **1991**, *65*, 105–114. [CrossRef] [PubMed]
14. Mosteller, R. Simplified calculation of body surface area. *N. Engl. J. Med.* **1987**, *317*, 1098.
15. Cockcroft, D.W.; Gault, M.H. Prediction of creatinine clearance from serum creatinine. *Nephron* **1976**, *16*, 31–41. [CrossRef]
16. Comets, E.; Brendel, K.; Mentré, F. Computing normalised prediction distribution errors to evaluate nonlinear mixed-effect models: The npde add-on package for R. *Comput. Methods Programs Biomed.* **2008**, *90*, 154–166. [CrossRef]
17. Deardorff, O.G.; Jenne, V.; Leonard, L.; Ellingrod, V.L. Making sense of CYP2D6 and CYP1A2 genotype vs. phenotype. *Curr. Psychiatry* **2018**, *17*, 41–45.
18. Imran, K.; Punnamchand, L.; Natvarlal, S.M. A simple sample preparation with HPLC–UV method for estimation of tiropramide from plasma: Application to bioequivalence study. *J. Pharm. Biomed. Anal.* **2007**, *43*, 1135–1140. [CrossRef]
19. Jhee, O.H.; Jeon, Y.C.; Choi, H.S.; Lee, M.H.; Om, A.S.; Lee, J.-W.; Hong, J.W.; Kim, Y.S.; Kang, J.C.; Lee, Y.S. Quantitative analysis of tiropramide in human plasma by gas chromatography coupled to mass spectrometry for application to a bioequivalence test. *Clin. Chim. Acta* **2006**, *366*, 179–184. [CrossRef]
20. Kwon, O.-S.; Park, Y.-J.; Chung, Y.-B. Pharmacokinetics and bioequivalence of tiropramide in healthy volunteers. *Arzneim. Forsch.* **2003**, *53*, 578–583. [CrossRef]
21. Kwon, O.-S.; Park, Y.-J.; Ryu, J.-C.; Chung, Y.B. Quantitative analysis of tiropramide in human blood by gas chromatography with nitrogen-phosphorus detector. *Arch. Pharm. Res.* **2003**, *26*, 416–420. [CrossRef] [PubMed]
22. Abe, H.; Inokawa, Y.; Yasuda, E.; Nishioka, Y.; Esumi, Y.; Nemoto, H.; Inaba, A.; Jin, Y.; Ninomiya, S. Pharmacokinetic studies of tiropramide in rats (I). Absorption, distribution, metabolism and excretion after single administration. *Yakuri Chiryo* **1992**, *20*, 113–129.

2

Simultaneous Determination of Chlorogenic Acid Isomers and Metabolites in Rat Plasma Using LC-MS/MS and its Application to a Pharmacokinetic Study Following Oral Administration of *Stauntonia Hexaphylla* Leaf Extract (YRA-1909) to Rats

Won-Gu Choi [1,†], Ju-Hyun Kim [1,2,†], Dong Kyun Kim [1], Yongnam Lee [3], Ji Seok Yoo [3], Dae Hee Shin [3] and Hye Suk Lee [1,*]

1 BK21 PLUS Team for Creative Leader Program for Pharmacomics-based Future Pharmacy and Drug Metabolism and Bioanalysis Laboratory, College of Pharmacy, The Catholic University of Korea, Bucheon 420-743, Korea; cwg0222@catholic.ac.kr (W.-G.C.); noraekajoa@gmail.com (J.-H.K.); kdk3124@catholic.ac.kr (D.K.K.)

2 College of Pharmacy, Yeungnam University, Gyeongsan 38541, Korea

3 Central R&D Institute, YUNGJIN PHARM. CO., LTD., Suwon 16229, Korea; nami0209@yungjin.co.kr (Y.L.); jsyoo@yungjin.co.kr (J.S.Y.); sdh580509@gmail.com (D.H.S.)

* Correspondence: sianalee@catholic.ac.kr

† These authors contributed equally to this work.

Abstract: *Stauntonia hexaphylla* leaf extract (YRA-1909), which is widely used for the antirheumatic properties, has been under phase 2 clinical trials in patients with rheumatoid arthritis since April 2017. Liquid chromatography-tandem mass spectrometric method while using liquid–liquid extraction with ethyl acetate was validated for the simultaneous determination of the major active components of YRA-1909, including chlorogenic acid (CGA), neochlorogenic acid (NCGA), cryptochlorogenic acid (CCGA), and their metabolites (i.e., caffeic acid (CA), caffeic acid 3-*O*-glucuronide (CA-3-G), caffeic acid 4-*O*-glucuronide (CA-4-G), and ferulic acid (FA)) in rat plasma and applied to a pharmacokinetic study of YRA-1909 in rats. Seven analytes were separated on Halo C18 while using gradient elution of formic acid and methanol, and then quantified in selected reaction monitoring mode whle using negative electrospray ionization. Following oral administration of YRA-1909 at doses of 25, 50, and 100 mg/kg to male Sprague-Dawley rats, CGA, NCGA, and CCGA were rapidly absorbed and metabolized to CA, CA-3-G, and CA-4-G. The area under the plasma concentration-time curve (AUC_{last}) of CGA, NCGA, CCGA, and three metabolites linearly increased as the YRA-1909 dose increased. Other pharmacokinetic parameters were comparable among three doses studied. AUC_{last} values for CA, CA-3-G, and CA-4-G exceeded those for CGA, NCGA, and CCGA.

Keywords: *Stauntonia hexaphylla* leaf extract; YRA-1909; pharmacokinetics; chlorogenic acid; neochlorogenic acid; cryptochlorogenic acid; caffeic acid; caffeic acid *O*-glucuronides; LC-MS/MS

1. Introduction

Stauntonia hexaphylla (Lardizabalaceae) is widely distributed throughout Korea, Japan, and China, and is a popular herbal supplement in Korean and Chinese folk medicine due to its analgesic, sedative, and diuretic properties [1,2]. It exhibits anti-osteoporosis [3], antidiabetic activity [4], and anti-inflammatory effects in carrageenan-induced paw edema rats [5]. *Stauntonia hexaphylla* leaf extract, YRA-1909, is associated with the antirheumatic activity [6] and has been undergoing in phase 2 clinical trials in the Republic of Korea since April 2017 to evaluate its safety and efficacy for treating patients suffering from rheumatoid arthritis (ClinicalTrials.gov identifier NCT03275025) [7]. Chlorogenic acid (CGA), neochlorogenic acid (NCGA), and cryptochlorogenic acid (CCGA) have been identified as the active ingredients in *Stauntonia hexaphylla* [4,5] and YRA-1909. CGA and NCGA are associated with various pharmacological properties, including antioxidant [8], anti-cancer [9], anti-virus [10], anti-coagulant, and anti-thrombotic properties [11]. CGA, NCGA, and CCGA are metabolized to caffeic acid (CA) and quinic acid by esterase [12–15]. CA is further metabolized to caffeic acid 3-*O*-glucuronide (CA-3-G) and caffeic acid 4-*O*-glucuronide (CA-4-G) by uridine-5′-diphosphate-glucuronosyltransferase (UGT) 1A1 and 1A9 enzymes, caffeic acid 3- and 4-*O*-sulfate by sulfotransferase (SULT) 1A1 and 1E1 enzymes, and ferulic acid (FA) and isoferulic acid by catechol-*O*-methyltransferase (COMT), which are metabolized to FA 4-*O*-glucuronide, FA 4-*O*-sulfate, and isoferulic acid 3-*O*-sulfate (Figure 1) [12–16]. CA and FA are active metabolites that are associated with various biological activities, including antioxidant [17], anti-mutagenic [18], and anti-cancer [19,20] effects.

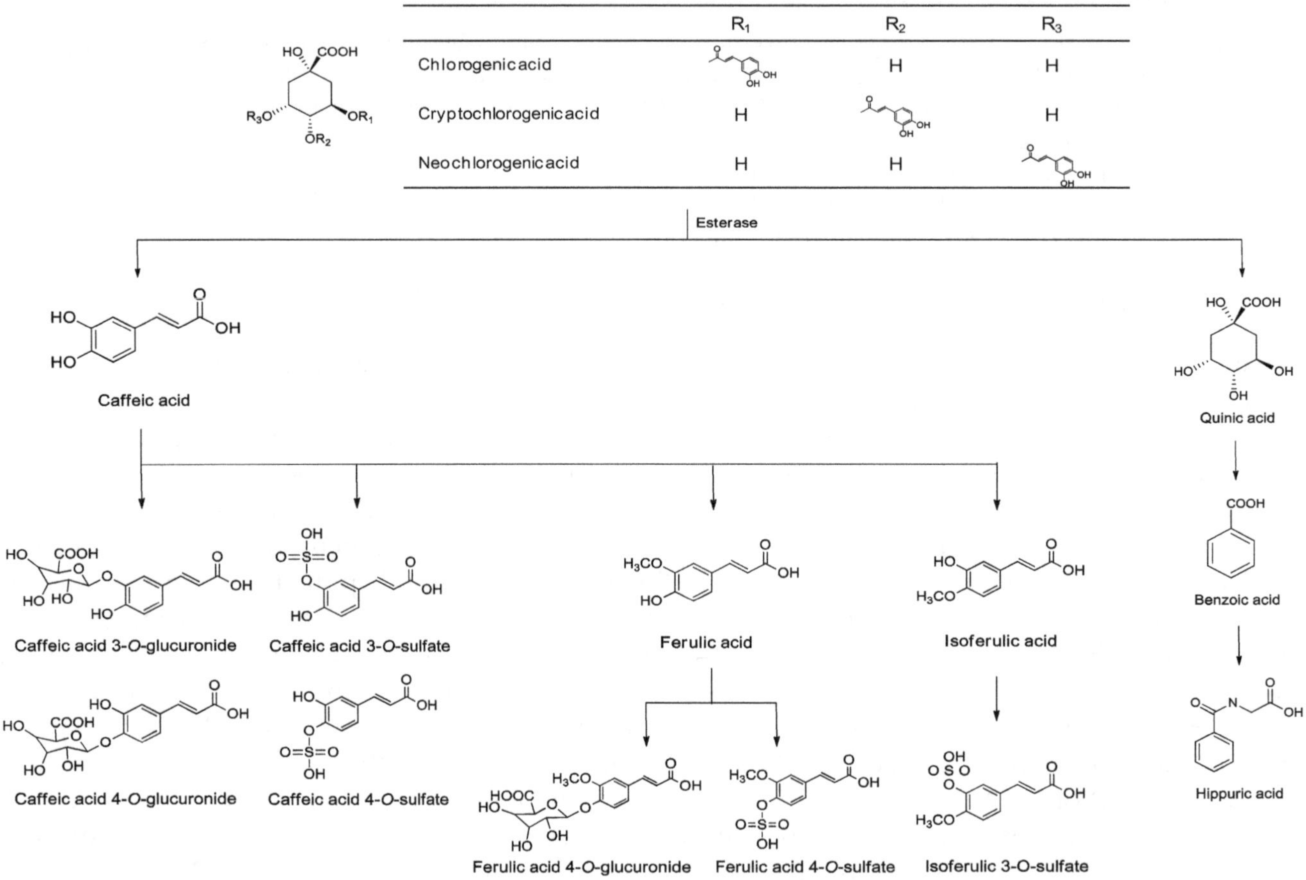

Figure 1. Metabolic pathways of chlorogenic acid, neochlorogenic acid, and cryptochlorogenic acid in rats and humans.

Pharmacokinetic evaluation of herbal drugs is helpful for determining dosage regimens and interpreting the pharmacological effects under clinical conditions. However, typical pharmacokinetic studies can be difficult to apply to herbal drugs that consist of multiple constituents, with frequently unidentified pharmacologically active components. As such, simultaneous determination of the various potential active constituents, major constituents, and/or their metabolites is recommended for the satisfactory pharmacokinetic evaluation of herbal drugs [21–23].

Several studies have applied liquid chromatography-mass spectrometry (LC-MS) or tandem mass spectrometry (LC-MS/MS) methods for the simultaneous determination of CGA, NCGA, CCGA, CA, or FA in human and rat plasma (50–500 μL) while using liquid–liquid extraction [24–27], or solid phase extraction [28], protein precipitation [29], or protein precipitation with disperse solid phase extraction [30]. The LC-MS has also been used in pharmacokinetic studies of these acids following the administration of herbal drugs to rats and humans. For example, one such study used the LC-MS/MS method to simultaneously determine phenolic acids and their metabolites in human plasma following the ingestion of instant coffee containing various chlorogenic and phenolic acids; the study used protein precipitation to prepare samples [31]. The negative [24,26,28–31] and positive [25,27] electrospray ionization (ESI) modes were used for the ionization of phenolic acids in mass spectrometry.

There are currently no reports on the pharmacokinetics of YRA-1909. In this study, we developed a sensitive and selective LC-MS/MS method for evaluating the pharmacokinetics of the active constituents of YRA-1909 (i.e., CGA, NCGA, and CCGA) and their active metabolites (i.e., CA, CA-3-G, CA-4-G, and FA) after the oral administration of YRA-1909 at doses of 25, 50, and 100 mg/kg to the rats.

2. Materials and Methods

2.1. Materials

CGA (purity, 98.1%) was obtained from Hunan Yuanhang Biology Technology Co., Ltd (Changsha, China). CCGA (purity, 99.7%) was obtained from Dailan Meilun Biotech Co., Ltd (Dailan, China). NCGA (purity, 98.0%), CA (purity, 98.0%), FA (purity, 99.0%), dimethyl sulfoxide, and formic acid were purchased from Sigma Aldrich Co. (St. Louis, MO, USA). CA-3-G (purity, 98.1%), CA-4-G (purity, 98.0%), and ferulic acid-d_3 (FA-d_3)(purity, 98.0%; used as an internal standard) were obtained from Toronto Research Chemicals Inc. (Toronto, Canada). Water and methanol (LC-MS grade) were supplied from Burdick and Jackson Inc. (Muskegon, MI, USA). All the other chemicals used were of the highest quality available.

Stauntonia hexaphylla leaves were collected from cultivated fields, in accordance with Good Agricultural Practice guidelines, in Jangheung (Jeonnam, Korea). YRA-1909 was prepared by extracting *Stauntonia hexalphylla* leaves with distilled water, followed by purification using column chromatography. YRA-1909 was produced by KGCYebon (Chungju, Korea) according to the protocol recommended by the International Conference on Harmonization and Good Manufacturing Practice. The contents of CGA, NCGA, and CCGA in YRA-1909 (batch no.: YR-1001) were 4.74, 1.10, and 3.49 mg/g, respectively, as quantified while using high-performance liquid chromatographic method for quality control developed by YUNGJIN PHARM CO., LTD (Suwon, Korea). CA and FA were not detected in YRA-1909.

2.2. Preparation of Clibration Standards and Quality Control Samples

Each standard stock solution was prepared separately by dissolving CGA, NCGA, CCGA, and their four metabolites (1 mg each) in 1 mL dimethyl sulfoxide. A mixed standard stock solution was prepared by mixing each stock solution to final concentrations of 10 μg/mL for CGA and NCGA, 50 μg/mL for CCGA, CA, CA-3-G, and CA-4-G, and 250 μg/mL for FA. Working standard solutions of the seven analytes were prepared by diluting a mixed standard stock solution with methanol. The internal standard working solution (FA-d_3, 20 μg/mL) was prepared by diluting an aliquot of stock solution with methanol. All such standard solutions were stored at 4 °C in darkness for four weeks.

Rat plasma calibration standards were prepared at eight concentration levels by adding 2 μL working standard solution to 50 μL of drug-free rat plasma: 0.5, 1.0, 2.0, 5.0, 10.0, 25.0, 50,0, 100, and 200 ng/mL for CGA and NCGA, 2.5, 5.0, 10.0, 25.0, 50,0, 250, 500, and 1000 ng/mL for CCGA, CA, CA-3-G, and CA-4-G, and 12.5, 25.0, 50.0, 125, 250, 1250, 3750, and 5000 ng/mL for FA, respectively.

5 μL of 5% formic acid was added and vortex-mixed to improve the plasma stability of CGA, CCGA, and NCGA [24,32]. Quality control (QC) samples were prepared at the concentrations of 1.5, 25, and 160 ng/mL for CGA and NCGA, 7.5, 125, and 800 ng/mL for CCGA, CA, CA-3-G, and CA-4-G, and 37.5, 625, and 4000 ng/mL for FA in drug-free rat plasma and then stored at −80 °C until analysis.

2.3. Sample Preparation

50 μL aliquot of blank rat plasma, calibration standards, and QC samples stored on ice were vortex-mixed with 5 μL FA-d_3 in methanol (20 μg/mL), 100 μL 1 M hydrochloric acid, and 600 μL ethyl acetate for 2 min. Following centrifugation at 13000 rpm for 8 min, 475 μL the supernatant was transferred into a new polypropylene tube. The aqueous layer was extracted once more with 600 μL ethyl acetate, and the supernatants were transferred after centrifugation. The organic layer was evaporated to dryness at 35 °C for 20 min while using a vacuum evaporator. The residues were dissolved in 50 μL 10% methanol and centrifuged. An aliquot (3 μL) was injected onto the LC-MS/MS system for analyses.

2.4. LC-MS/MS Analysis

An ultra-performance liquid chromatograph, Agilent 1290, coupled with Agilent 6495 tandem mass spectrometer (Agilent Technologies, Wilmington, DE, USA) was used. Chromatographic separation was performed on a Halo C_{18} column (2.7 μm, 2.1 mm i.d. × 100 mm, Advanced Material Technology, Wilmington, DE, USA) while using a gradient elution of 0.1% formic acid in water (mobile phase A) and 0.1% formic acid in methanol (mobile phase B) at a flow rate of 0.3 mL/min, as follows: 10% mobile phase B for 0.5 min, 10% to 25% mobile phase B for 5.5 min, 25% to 37% mobile phase B for 1 min, 37% mobile phase B for 2 min, 37% to 10% mobile phase B for 0.1 min, and 10% mobile phase B for 2.4 min. The column and autosampler tray were maintained at 35 °C and 4 °C, respectively. The ESI source settings for the ionization of the analytes in negative mode were as follows: gas temperature, 230 °C; gas flow, 19 L/min; Nebulizer, 45 psi; sheath gas temperature, 400 °C; sheath gas flow, 10 L/min; capillary voltage, 3000 V; nozzle voltage, 1000 V. Fragmentation of analytes was performed at collision energy of 14 eV for CGA, NCGA, and CCGA, 8 eV for CA, 20 eV for CA-3-G and CA-4-G, 12 eV for FA, and 10 eV for FA-d_3, respectively, while using nitrogen gas as a collision gas at a pressure of 2 bar on the instrument. Selected reaction monitoring (SRM) mode was employed for the quantification: m/z 352.8 → 191.0 for CGA, NCGA, and CCGA; m/z 179.1 → 135.0 for CA; m/z 355.0 → 178.9 for CA-3-G and CA-4-G; m/z 192.9 → 133.9 for FA; m/z 196.1 → 134.0 for FA-d_3. Mass Hunter software (Agilent Technologies) was used for LC-MS/MS system control and data processing.

2.5. Method Validation

Method validation was performed according to the FDA Guidance on Bioanalytical Method Validation. For the evaluation of intra-and inter-day precision and accuracy, we analyzed batches of calibration standards and QC samples in five replicates on three different days, as follows: 0.5, 1.5, 25, and 160 ng/mL for CGA and NCGA, 2.5, 7.5, 125, and 800 ng/mL for CCGA, CA, CA-3-G, and CA-4-G, and 12.5, 37.5, 625, and 4000 ng/mL for FA were analyzed. Accuracy was defined as relative error (RE, %) of the measured mean value deviated from the nominal value, and precision was defined as the coefficient of variation (CV, %) of the measured concentration.

The stability of each of the seven analytes in rat plasma was evaluated by analyzing low and high QC samples in triplicate: post-preparation sample stability in the autosampler at 4 °C for 24 h, short-term storage stability following storage of plasma samples on ice for 2 h, long-term storage stability following the storage of plasma samples at −80 °C for 28 days, and three freeze-thaw cycles.

The matrix effect for each analyte was assessed by comparing the mean peak areas of the analytes that were spiked after extraction into blank plasma extracts originating from six different rats to mean peak areas for neat solutions of the analytes at 1.5, 25, and 160 ng/mL for CGA and NCGA, 7.5, 125, and 800 ng/mL for CCGA, CA, CA-3-G, and CA-4-G, and 37.5, 625, and 4000 ng/mL for FA.

The recoveries of each analyte were determined by comparing the mean peak areas of the extract of analyte-spiked plasma with those of the analytes spiked post-extraction into six different blank plasma extracts at three concentration levels.

2.6. Pharmacokinetic Study of YRA-1909 in Rats

This validated method was applied to the pharmacokinetic study of CGA, NCGA, CCGA, and their metabolites, such as CA, CA-3-G, CA-4-G, and FA after a single oral administration of YRA-1909 at doses of 25 (n = 6), 50 (n = 12), and 100 mg/kg (n = 6) and repeated oral administration of 50 mg/kg YRA-1909 for seven days (n = 6) to male Sprague-Dawley (SD) rats (body weight, 220–260 g, Samtako Co., Osan, Korea). The effective oral doses of YRA-1909 on preclinical pharmacology studies were 25–100 mg/kg in rats (internal reports of YUNGJIN PHARM CO., LTD). The study protocol was approved by the Institutional Animal Care and Use Committee of The Catholic University of Korea (Approval No. 2015–015). The animals were kept in plastic cages with unlimited access to standard rat diet (Samtako Co.) and water before the experiment. Animals were maintained at a temperature of 23 ± 2 °C with a 12 h light/dark cycle and relative humidity of 50 ± 10%. The rats were anesthetized while using isoflurane and they were cannulated with polyethylene tubing (PE-50, Nastsume Co., Tokyo, Japan) in the jugular vein for blood sampling. Each rat was housed individually in a metabolic cage and permitted a recovery time of one day following anesthesia prior to the study's commencement. During the recovery period, rats were fasted but let free access to water and were not restrained at any time. To prevent blood clotting, each catheter was flushed with heparin in a physiological saline solution (10 U/mL). YRA-1909 was dissolved in purified water and administered to the rats at doses of 25, 50, and 100 mg/kg (equivalent to 1.2, 2.4, and 4.8 mg/kg CGA; 0.275, 0.55, and 1.10 mg/kg NCGA; 0.87, 1.74, and 3.48 mg/kg CCGA). Blood samples (approximately 200 μL) were collected before (control) and 0.083, 0.25, 0.5, 1, 1.5, 2, 3, 4, 6, 8, and 24 h after drug administration. Plasma samples were harvested by centrifugation at 3000 g for 5 min at 4 °C and 50 μL plasma samples were immediately collected and vortex-mixed with 5 μL 5% formic acid. The samples were stored at −80 °C until analyses.

Pharmacokinetic parameters were analyzed while using noncompartment analysis (WinNonlin, Pharsight, Mountain View, CA, USA), including the area under the plasma concentration-time curve during the period of observation (AUC_{last}), the terminal half-life ($t_{1/2}$), and mean residence time (MRT). The peak plasma concentration (C_{max}) and the time to reach C_{max} (T_{max}) were directly obtained from the experimental data. All data are expressed as the means ± standard deviations (S.D.).

3. Results

3.1. LC-MS/MS Analysis

For the simultaneous quantification of CGA, NCGA, CCGA, CA, CA-3-G, CA-4-G, and FA, MS/MS parameters for all analytes were optimized by the flow-injection method to achieve maximum sensitivity, and SRM transitions of the precursor ion ($[M - H]^-$) to the intense product ion were used for data acquisition owing to the high selectivity and sensitivity (Figure 2) [24,28–31].

The retention and base-line separation data are shown in Figure 3B. Analysis of blank plasma samples that were obtained from 30 different rats revealed no significant interference peaks in the retention times across all analytes, which indicates the selectivity of the present method (Figure 3A). Figure 3C illustrates representative SRM chromatograms of a plasma sample obtained 5 min after oral administration of YRA-1909 at a 100 mg/kg dosage in a male SD rat.

3.2. Method Validation

Calibration curves were linear at concentration ranges of 0.5–200 ng/mL for CGA and NCGA, 12.5–5000 ng/mL for FA, and 2.5–1000 ng/mL for CCGA, CA, CA-3-G, and CA-4-G in rat plasma with coefficients of determination ≥0.9959 using linear regression analysis with a weighting of

1/concentration (Table 1). The RE and CV values of the calculated concentrations were less than ±15% and 15%, respectively, for all eight calibration points. The low CV values (≤12.2%) for the regression line slopes of the seven analytes indicated the repeatability of the method.

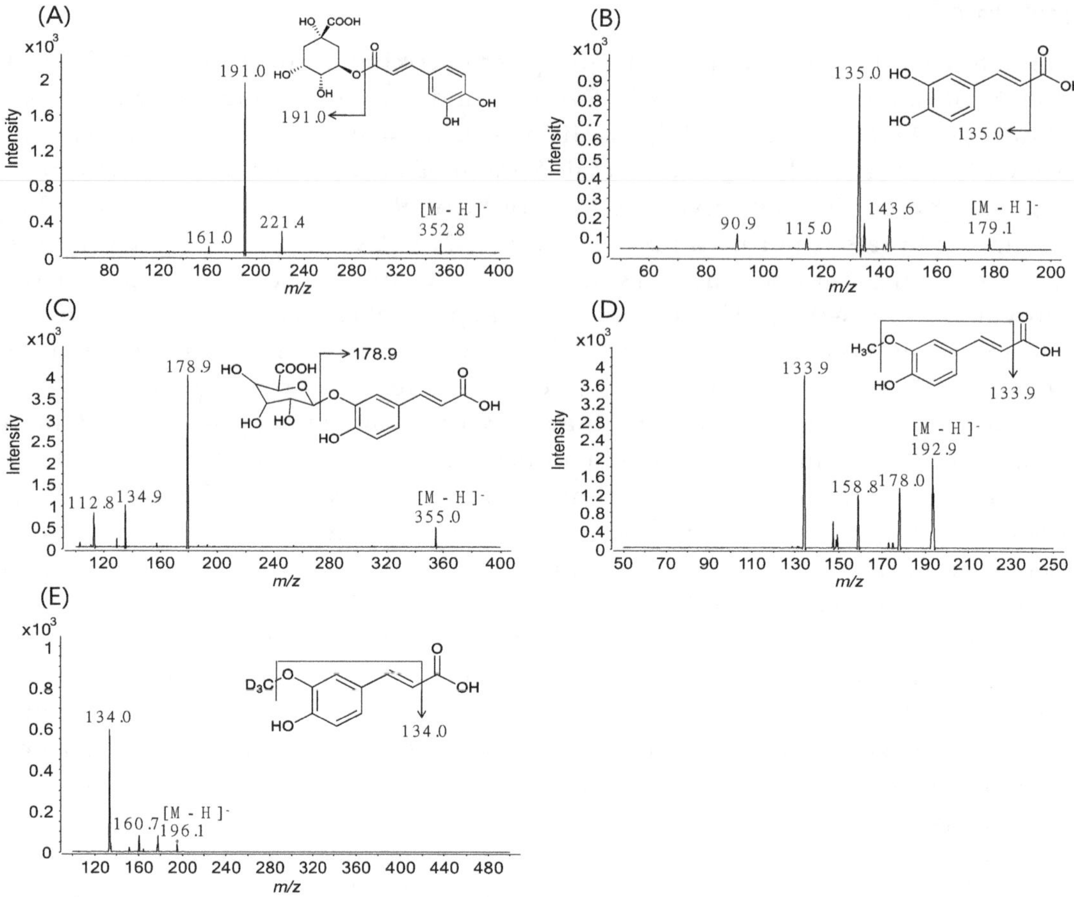

Figure 2. Product ion spectra of (**A**) chlorogenic acid (CGA), (**B**) caffeic acid (CA), (**C**) CA-3-G, (**D**) ferulic acid (FA), and (**E**) FA-d_3 (IS).

The lower limits of quantification (LLOQ), the lowest amounts of the analytes in rat plasma sample that can be quantified with S/N ratio >5 as well as both CV and RE within 20% of nominal concentration, were 0.5 ng/mL for CGA and NCGA, 12.5 ng/mL for FA, and 2.5 ng/mL for CCGA, CA, CA-3-G, and CA-4-G in rat plasma (Table 1).

The intra-day and inter-day precision and accuracy values for QC samples are presented in Table 1. The CV values of the seven analytes ranged from 2.4% to 12.5% at low, medium, and high QC levels and from 4.1% to 18.1% at LLOQ QC levels. The RE values ranged from −10.0% to 10.4% at low, medium, and high QC levels and from −8.8% to 16.0% at LLOQ QC levels. These results confirm the method's acceptable accuracy and precision levels.

A protein precipitation technique while using acetonitrile and methanol was examined as the sample preparation procedure for rat plasma but it was inadequate due to severe matrix effects. The recovery and matrix effects of all analytes in rat plasma were evaluated by extracting acidified rat plasma with ethyl acetate [25], ethyl acetate/ether [24], ethyl acetate/hexane [26], and methyl *ter*-butyl ether. Liquid–liquid extraction using ethyl acetate as the extraction solvent resulted in a higher degree of recovery and fewer matrix effects for all analytes (Table 2): the matrix effects and CV values were 86.5−98.0% and ≤11.8%, respectively. The recovery levels using liquid–liquid extraction at low, medium, and high QC levels are shown in Table 2. Based on the results, liquid–liquid extraction using ethyl acetate after acidification of rat plasma is deemed to be acceptable for the sample preparation procedure.

The processing (freeze-thaw, long-term storage at −80°C, and short-term storage on ice) and post-preparation stabilities of each analyte were evaluated; such processes had negligible effects on the stability of samples (Table 3).

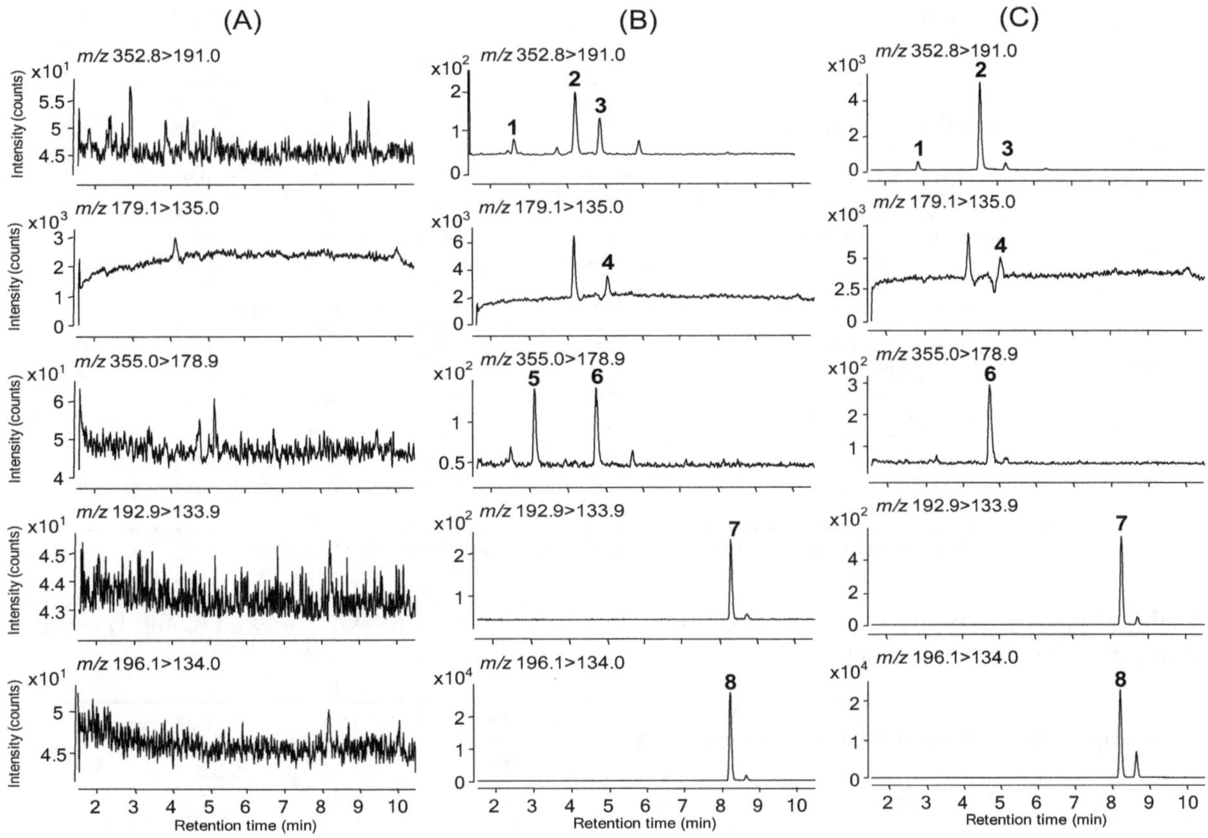

Figure 3. Selected reaction monitoring chromatograms of (**A**) rat blank plasma, (**B**) rat plasma spiked with CGA (0.5 ng/mL), NCGA (0.5 ng/mL), CCGA (2.5 ng/mL), CA (2.5 ng/mL), CA-3-G (2.5 ng/mL), CA-4-G (2.5 ng/mL), and FA (12.5 ng/mL) at lower limits of quantification (LLOQ) level, and (**C**) rat plasma obtained 5 min after oral administration of YRA-1909 at a dose of 100 mg/kg to a male SD rat. 1, NCGA; 2, CGA; 3, CCGA; 4, CA; 5, CA-4-G; 6, CA-3-G; 7, FA; 8, FA-d_3.

Table 1. Linearity, LLOQ, intra-day and inter-day accuracy (RE, %) and precision (CV, %) of CGA, NCGA, CCGA, CA, CA-3-G, CA-4-G, and FA in rat plasma quality control (QC) samples.

Analytes	Concentration Range (ng/mL), Linear Equation [a], Linearity (r^2) [b], LLOQ (ng/mL)	QC Concentration (ng/mL)	Intra-day (n = 5)		Inter-day (n = 15)	
			RE (%)	CV (%)	RE (%)	CV (%)
CGA	0.5–200	0.5	12.0	8.9	2.0	11.8
	$y = 0.01110x - 0.00054$	1.5	−6.7	6.4	−4.7	11.2
	0.9981	25	2.0	3.7	−1.9	10.5
	0.5	160	10.2	2.4	0.1	11.8
NCGA	0.5–200	0.5	−2.0	4.1	−2.0	8.2
	$y = 0.00330x - 0.00039$	1.5	−10.0	3.0	−1.3	10.1
	0.9983	25	0.7	3.1	2.8	8.0
	0.5	160	10.4	2.0	2.0	12.5

Table 1. *Cont.*

Analytes	Concentration Range (ng/mL), Linear Equation [a], Linearity (r^2) [b], LLOQ (ng/mL)	QC Concentration (ng/mL)	Intra-day (n = 5)		Inter-day (n = 15)	
			RE (%)	CV (%)	RE (%)	CV (%)
CCGA	2.5–1000	2.5	16.0	7.2	3.6	11.6
	$y = 0.00149x - 0.00068$	7.5	−6.3	4.8	−3.9	6.7
	0.9974	125	3.0	4.2	2.8	5.6
	2.5	800	−4.4	3.2	−1.9	8.3
CA	2.5–1000	2.5	−8.8	7.9	−2.8	18.1
	$y = 0.03784x - 0.00235$	7.5	−3.9	8.3	−2.8	8.6
	0.9959	125	6.5	5.0	6.5	6.2
	2.5	800	4.1	5.8	0.9	9.2
CA-3-G	2.5–1000	2.5	0.8	7.1	−0.4	8.0
	$y = 0.00174x + 0.00022$	7.5	−8.3	4.2	−5.9	9.6
	0.9981	125	4.3	2.4	2.4	6.2
	2.5	800	8.8	5.1	0.9	10.4
CA-4-G	2.5–1000	2.5	−6.8	10.7	−5.2	9.3
	$y = 0.00140x + 0.00031$	7.5	−7.2	7.0	0.3	11.6
	0.9977	125	10.0	3.5	6.7	6.4
	2.5	800	7.7	4.7	1.2	9.6
FA	12.5–5000	12.5	12.6	8.5	9.0	7.7
	$y = 0.00628x - 0.02194$	37.5	−3.2	7.2	−6.5	7.7
	0.9969	625	−3.0	3.8	−7.4	6.0
	12.5	4000	4.8	3.9	−0.1	9.6

[a] y: peak area ratio, x: concentration; [b] r^2: coefficients of determination.

Table 2. Matrix effects and recoveries of CGA, NCGA, CCGA, CA, CA-3-G, CA-4-G, FA, and FA-d_3 (IS) using six different rat plasma (n = 6).

Compounds	Nominal Concentration (ng/mL)	Matrix Effect [a] (%)		Recovery [b] (Mean ± SD, %)
		Mean	CV (%)	
CGA	1.5	91.6	7.6	63.0 ± 6.3
	25	92.0	11.0	71.7 ± 6.9
	160	87.1	5.4	71.9 ± 9.4
NCGA	1.5	96.1	3.6	41.4 ± 4.0
	25	90.8	3.2	43.4 ± 3.7
	160	89.0	7.1	41.8 ± 1.4
CCGA	7.5	98.0	6.6	61.5 ± 5.2
	125	92.4	2.2	63.0 ± 7.8
	800	89.3	6.2	65.2 ± 5.7
CA	7.5	87.7	7.2	94.0 ± 9.9
	125	93.0	11.8	86.1 ± 10.4
	800	88.6	6.2	91.2 ± 6.3
CA-3-G	7.5	95.9	2.0	46.5 ± 4.3
	125	95.8	7.4	51.2 ± 3.4
	800	88.5	8.5	52.8 ± 4.2
CA-4-G	7.5	92.7	1.7	51.3 ± 6.0
	125	95.6	5.3	53.0 ± 3.4
	800	86.5	9.7	55.8 ± 4.2
FA	37.5	96.8	2.2	93.3 ± 8.7
	625	87.5	8.4	96.9 ± 8.7
	4000	97.5	8.6	97.4 ± 4.2
FA-d3	20	96.0	5.4	100.1 ± 2.0

[a] Matrix effect expressed as the ratio of the mean peak area of an analyte spiked post-extraction to the mean peak area of same analyte standards multiplied by 100. [b] Recovery calculated as the ratio of the mean peak area of an analyte–spiked plasma prior to liquid–liquid extraction to the mean peak of an analyte spiked after liquid-liquid extraction of blank plasma multiplied by 100.

Table 3. Post-preparation, short-term, long-term and freeze-thaw stabilities of CGA, NCGA, CCGA, CA, CA-3-G, CA-4-G, and FA in rat plasma quality control samples (n = 3).

Analytes and Nominal Concentration (ng/mL)		Post-Preparative (24 h at 4 °C)		Short-Term (2 h on ice)		Long-Term (28 days at −80 °C)		Freeze-Thaw 3 Cycles (−80 °C to room temp.)	
		CV, %	RE, %	CV, %	RE, %	CV, %	RE, %	CV, %	RE, %
CGA									
	1.5	8.8	−9.3	2.3	−12.0	7.0	−14.0	6.2	−14.0
	160	2.1	9.4	2.5	−5.4	4.1	−12.3	3.2	−10.0
NCGA									
	1.5	14.4	−2.7	2.3	−12.0	3.7	−9.3	10.1	−14.0
	160	2.7	11.2	4.2	−5.9	5.6	−6.3	5.9	−5.3
CCGA									
	7.5	5.1	−3.2	3.7	−14.3	5.9	−8.9	7.6	−11.9
	800	1.3	5.5	2.9	−4.6	4.4	−14.4	3.0	−9.4
CA									
	7.5	4.1	−0.1	9.0	−12.4	7.3	−6.3	8.3	−7.2
	800	0.9	10.6	2.1	−7.7	7.6	−12.7	2.1	−11.0
CA-3-G									
	7.5	9.9	−10.0	6.1	−14.6	7.3	−7.1	9.1	−10.5
	800	1.1	9.1	2.8	−1.5	2.2	−14.8	4.4	−11.9
CA-4-G									
	7.5	6.2	−9.6	8.1	−9.3	7.9	1.6	4.7	−3.6
	800	1.0	10.9	3.2	−0.4	2.1	−13.9	4.7	−9.4
FA									
	37.5	3.2	−7.0	5.4	−11.2	5.9	−11.0	5.6	−7.7
	4000	4.6	−8.6	2.7	−4.8	6.1	−8.8	3.9	−8.4

3.3. Pharmacokinetics of YRA-1909 in Male SD Rats

Mean plasma concentration-time profiles of CGA, NCGA, CCGA, CA, CA-3-G, and CA-4-G following a single oral administration of YRA-1909 at doses of 25, 50, and 100 mg/kg to male SD rats are shown in Figure 4. Plasma concentrations of CGA, NCGA, CA, CA-3-G, and CA-4-G were below LLOQ 6, 4, 4, 4, and 4 h after oral administration of YRA-1909 at a dosage of 100 mg/kg. Plasma concentrations of CCGA were under LLOQ (2.5 ng/mL) following 25 mg/kg dose (equivalent to 0.87 mg/kg CCGA), and 1 and 3 h after administration of 50 and 100 mg/kg doses of YRA-1909, respectively. Plasma concentrations of FA, which is a metabolite, were under LLOQ (12.5 ng/mL), except in samples taken 0.083 and/or 0.25 h after oral administration of 50 and 100 mg/kg YRA-1909. Therefore, the pharmacokinetic parameters of FA were not calculated. The relevant pharmacokinetic parameters of all other analytes are shown in Table 4.

No significant differences were observed among plasma concentrations and pharmacokinetic parameters of CGA, NCGA, CCGA, CA, CA-3-G, and CA-4-G between single and seven-day repeated administration of 50 mg/kg YRA-1909 (Figure 4, Table 4).

Table 4. Pharmacokinetic parameters of CGA, CCGA, NCGA, CA, CA-3-G, and CA-4-G after a single oral administration of YRA-1909 at doses of 25, 50, and 100 mg/kg (equivalent to 1.2, 2.4, and 4.8 mg/kg CGA; 0.275, 0.55, and 1.10 mg/kg NCGA; 0.87, 1.74 and 3.48 mg/kg CCGA) and repeated administration of 50 mg/kg YRA-1909 for seven days to male rats (mean ± SD).

Compounds	PK Parameters	Dose of YRA-1909 (mg/kg)			
		Single Oral Dosing			7-Day Repeated Oral Dosing
		25 (*n* = 6)	50 (*n* =12)	100 (*n* = 6)	50 (*n* = 6)
CGA	C_{max} (ng/mL)	3.11 ± 0.96	5.59 ± 1.61	8.73 ± 2.83	4.85 ± 1.25
	T_{max} [1] (h)	0.25 (0.083–0.25)	0.25 (0.083–0.5)	0.25	0.25 (0.083–0.5)
	AUC_{last} (ng·h/mL)	4.29 ± 1.92	8.16 ± 3.65	14.38 ± 5.06	7.54 ± 1.86
	$t_{1/2}$ (h)	NC	NC	1.52 ± 0.79	NC
	MRT (h)	1.19 ± 0.22	1.48 ± 0.50	1.67 ± 0.63	1.48 ± 0.18
CCGA	C_{max} (ng/mL)	NC	4.01 ± 0.82	5.64 ± 1.45	3.81 ± 0.72
	T_{max} [1] (h)	NC	0.25 (0.083–0.5)	0.25 (0.083–0.25)	0.25 (0.083–0.5)
	AUC_{last} (ng·h/mL)	NC	4.15 ± 4.10	6.26 ± 4.70	3.35 ± 3.42
	MRT (h)	NC	0.61 ± 0.55	0.84 ± 0.65	0.56 ± 0.57
NCGA	C_{max} (ng/mL)	0.70 ± 0.12	1.18 ± 0.26	1.69 ± 0.43	1.08 ± 0.28
	T_{max} [1] (h)	0.17 (0.083–0.5)	0.25 (0.083–0.5)	0.25 (0.083–0.25)	0.25 (0.083–0.25)
	AUC_{last} (ng·h/mL)	0.81 ± 0.22	1.61 ± 0.90	3.40 ± 1.97	1.60 ± 0.79
	MRT (h)	0.68 ± 0.30	1.00 ± 0.58	1.66 ± 0.91	1.09 ± 0.55
CA	C_{max} (ng/mL)	3.92 ± 1.47	7.31 ± 2.12	16.72 ± 5.45	6.07 ± 0.94
	T_{max} [1] (h)	1.25 (1.0–1.5)	0.25 (0.083–1.0)	0.25 (0.25–2.0)	0.17 (0.083–2.0)
	AUC_{last} (ng·h/mL)	5.60 ± 1.30	12.40 ± 4.03	29.73 ± 15.24	11.75 ± 3.31
	MRT (h)	0.90 ± 0.11	1.29 ± 0.31	1.74 ± 0.87	1.26 ± 0.33
CA-3-G	C_{max} (ng/mL)	69.09 ± 25.06	129.05 ± 30.41	238.55 ± 97.46	132.18 ± 26.70
	T_{max} [1] (h)	0.38 (0.25–1.0)	0.38 (0.25–1.0)	0.25 (0.25–1.0)	0.38 (0.25–1.0)
	AUC_{last} (ng·h/mL)	111.15 ± 37.32	208.77 ± 80.46	405.33 ± 188.56	216.38 ± 25.06
	$t_{1/2}$ (h)	1.05 ± 0.38	0.93 ± 0.23	0.82 ± 0.23	0.88 ± 0.19
	MRT (h)	1.49 ± 0.52	1.33 ± 0.24	1.68 ± 0.69	1.33 ± 0.12
CA-4-G	C_{max} (ng/mL)	3.86 ± 0.94	6.97 ± 1.91	9.38 ± 2.56	7.77 ± 1.85
	T_{max} [1] (h)	1.0 (1.0–1.5)	0.75 (0.25–2.0)	1.0 (0.5–2.0)	1.5 (1.0–2.0)
	AUC_{last} (ng·h/mL)	6.04 ± 0.77	14.95 ± 4.03	25.59 ± 10.84	18.95 ± 3.30
	MRT (h)	1.01 ± 0.18	1.48 ± 0.27	1.77 ± 0.46	± 0.23

[1] T_{max} presented median value with the range in parentheses. NC: Not calculable.

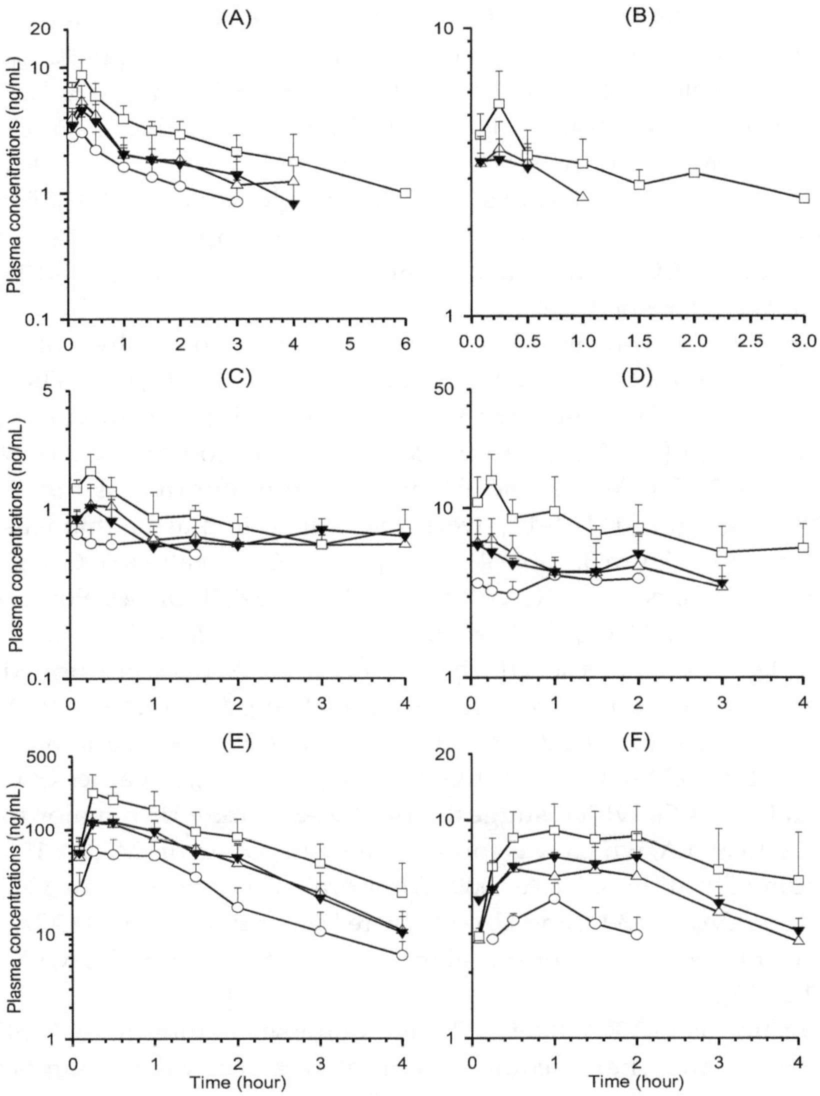

Figure 4. Mean plasma concentration-time profiles of (**A**) CGA, (**B**) CCGA, (**C**) neochlorogenic acid (NCGA), (**D**) CA, (**E**) CA-3-G, and (**F**) CA-4-G after a single oral administration of YRA-1909 at the doses of 25 (○, n = 6), 50 (△, n = 12), and 100 (□, n = 6) mg/kg (equivalent to 1.2, 2.4, and 4.8 mg/kg CGA; 0.275, 0.55, and 1.10 mg/kg NCGA; 0.87, 1.74 and 3.48 mg/kg CCGA) and repeated administration of 50 mg/kg YRA-1909 once/day for seven days (▼, n = 6) in male rats. Each point represents mean ± SD.

4. Discussion

We developed a LC-MS/MS method for the simultaneous determination of CGA, NCGA, CCGA, and their metabolites, such as CA, CA-3-G, CA-4-G, and FA in rat plasma. A gradient elution of formic acid and methanol, as the mobile phase, resulted in less peak tailing and an increase in the ionization efficiency of the seven analytes, when compared to previously reported gradient elution of acetic acid-acetonitrile used as the mobile phase for the analyses of phenolic acids, sulfates, and glucuronides [31]. For sample preparation, liquid–liquid extraction using ethyl acetate at acidic pH resulted in smaller sample volume (50 vs. 100 μL), superior sensitivity (0.5 vs. 1.77 ng/mL for CGA and NCGA), and reduced matrix effects compared to the protein precipitation technique [31]. We successfully applied the present method to study pharmacokinetics of CGA, NCGA, CCGA, and their metabolites after oral administration of YRA-1909 (Figure 4, Table 4).

CGA, NCGA, and CCGA were rapidly absorbed after oral administration of YRA-1909 at doses of 25, 50, and 100 mg/kg; each was detected at the first blood sampling time point (5 min) with rapid T_{max},

0.17–0.25 h for all three doses (Table 4). The AUC_{last} values for CGA and NCGA increased linearly as the oral dose increased. The dose-normalized (based on 25 mg/kg YRA-1909) AUC_{last} of CGA and NCGA were comparable among the doses studied: 4.29 ± 1.92, 4.08 ± 1.82, and 3.60 ± 1.27 ng·h/mL for CGA, respectively, and 0.81 ± 0.22, 0.81 ± 0.45, and 0.85 ± 0.49 ng·h/mL for NCGA in 25, 50, and 100 mg/kg YRA-1909, respectively. Moreover, the slopes between the log AUC_{last} and log dose of CGA and NCGA were close to 1. Plasma concentrations of CCGA were less than LLOQ (2.5 ng/mL) in the group that was administered a 25 mg/kg dose of YRA-1909, but the dose-normalized (based on 50 mg/kg YRA-1909) AUC_{last} values of CCGA were also comparable: 4.15 ± 4.10 and 3.13 ± 2.35 ng·h/mL for 50 and 100 mg/kg YRA-1909, respectively.

CGA, NCGA, and CCGA were absorbed by passive diffusion and hydrolyzed to CA by gastric esterase, and then, CA was metabolized to ferulic acid by COMT [13]. The bioavailability and urinary recovery of CGA or CA were very low after oral administration of CGA or CA in rats due to extensive metabolism [14,15,31]. After oral administration of YRA-1909 at doses of 25, 50, and 100 mg/kg, CA, CA-3-G, CA-4-G, and FA, which were reported as the major metabolites of CGA, CCGA, and NCGA (Figure 1) [12–15], were determined in plasma that was obtained after oral administration of YRA-1909 (Figure 3, Table 4). AUC_{last} and C_{max} values of CA, CA-3-G, and CA-4-G linearly increased with an increase in YRA-1909 dose (Figure 4, Table 4). For CA, dose-normalized (based on 25 mg/kg YRA-1909) AUC_{last} values were 5.60 ± 1.30, 6.20 ± 2.01, and 7.43 ± 3.81 ng·h/mL for 25, 50, and 100 mg/kg YRA-1909, respectively. CA-3-G and CA-4-G were formed from CA, as shown in Figure 1 [12–16] and their dose-normalized (based on 25 mg/kg YRA-1909) AUC_{last} values were 111.15 ± 37.32, 104.39 ± 40.23, and 101.33 ± 47.14 ng·h/mL for CA-3-G and 6.04 ± 0.77, 7.47 ± 2.02, and 6.40 ± 2.71 ng·h/mL for CA-4-G, respectively. AUC_{last} and C_{max} values of CA-3-G were higher than those for CA and CA-4-G, which suggests that CA-3-G may be a major metabolite after oral administration of YRA-1909. FA, which was formed via methylation of CA [12–15], was detected 0.083 or 0.25 h after oral administration of YRA-1909. After oral administration of YRA-1909, the AUC_{last} values of the metabolites, CA, CA-3-G, and CA-4-G were higher than those of CGA, CCGA, and NCGA due to extensive metabolism, which were similar to the metabolism of CGA, CCGA, and NCGA in humans and rats [12,14,15].

Repeated administration of YRA-1909 at 50 mg/kg for seven days to male SD rats did not affect the plasma concentrations and pharmacokinetic parameters of any compounds when compared to those that received single administrations (Figure 4, Table 4).

5. Conclusions

A selective and sensitive LC-MS/MS method using liquid–liquid extraction as sample clean-up procedure was developed and validated for the simultaneous determination of CGA, CCGA, NCGA, and their metabolites, such as CA, CA-3-G, CA-4-G, and FA in rat plasma. The method was successfully applied to characterize the pharmacokinetics of CGA, CCGA, NCGA, CA, CA-3-G, CA-4-G, and FA after oral administration of YRA-1909 at 25, 50, and 100 mg/kg doses to male SD rats. These results constitute useful information for the development of YRA-1909 as a new herbal medicine for the treatment of rheumatoid arthritis, based on the evaluation of the pharmacokinetic properties of its main components (i.e., CGA, CCGA, and NCGA) and their active metabolites (CA, CA-3-G, and CA-4-G).

Author Contributions: Conceptualization, H.S.L. Y.L., J.S.Y, and D.H.S.; Methodology, W.G.C., J.H.K., K.D.K., and H.S.L.; Validation, W.G.C., J.H.K, Y.L., and J.S.Y.; Formal Analysis, W.G.C., J.H.K., D.K.K., and H.S.L.; Investigation, W.G.C., J.H.K. and H.S.L.; Resources, W.G.C., J.H.K, Y.L., and J.S.Y.; Data Curation, W.G.C., J.H.K. and H.S.L.; Writing-Original Draft Preparation, W.G.C., J.H.K., and D.K.K.; Writing-Review & Editing, H.S.L. Y.L., J.S.Y., and D.H.S.; Visualization, W.G.C., J.H.K. and H.S.L; Supervision, H.S.L.; Project Administration, H.S.L.; Funding Acquisition, H.S.L.

References

1. Wang, H.-B.; Mayer, R.; Rücker, G.; Yang, J.-J.; Matteson, D.S. A phenolic glycoside and triterpenoids from *Stauntonia hexaphylla*. *Phytochemistry* **1998**, *47*, 467–470. [CrossRef]

2. Park, Y.J.; Park, Y.S.; Towantakavanit, K.; Park, J.O.; Kim, Y.M.; Jung, K.J.; Cho, J.Y.; Lee, K.D.; Heo, B.G. Chemical components and biological activity of *Stauntonia hexaphylla*. *Korean J. Plant. Resour.* **2009**, *22*, 403–411.
3. Cheon, Y.H.; Baek, J.M.; Park, S.H.; Ahn, S.J.; Lee, M.S.; Oh, J.; Kim, J.Y. *Stauntonia hexaphylla* (Lardizabalaceae) leaf methanol extract inhibits osteoclastogenesis and bone resorption activity via proteasome-mediated degradation of c-Fos protein and suppression of NFATc1 expression. *BMC Complement. Altern. Med.* **2015**, *15*, 280. [CrossRef] [PubMed]
4. Hwang, S.H.; Kwon, S.H.; Kim, S.B.; Lim, S.S. Inhibitory activities of *Stauntonia hexaphylla* leaf constituents on rat lens aldose reductase and formation of advanced glycation end products and antioxidant. *Biomed. Res. Int.* **2017**, *2017*, 4273257. [CrossRef] [PubMed]
5. Kim, J.; Kim, H.; Choi, H.; Jo, A.; Kang, H.; Yun, H.; Im, S.; Choi, C. Anti-inflammatory effects of a *Stauntonia hexaphylla* Fruit Extract in lipopolysaccharide-activated RAW-264.7 macrophages and rats by carrageenan-induced hind paw swelling. *Nutrients* **2018**, *10*, E110. [CrossRef] [PubMed]
6. Yoo, H.J.; Kim, J.Y.; Kang, S.E.; Yoo, J.S.; Lee, Y.; Lee, D.G.; Park, J.S.; Lee, E.B.; Lee, E.Y.; Song, Y.W. YRA-1909 suppresses production of pro-inflammatory mediators and MMPs through downregulating Akt, p38, JNK and NF-κb activation in rheumatoid arthritis fibroblast-like synoviocytes. In Proceedings of the 81st American College of Rheumatology and the 52nd Association of Rheumatology Health Professionals Annual Scientific Meeting, San Diego, CA, USA, 6 November 2017; Abstract Number, 1412.
7. A Phase 2 Study to Evaluate the Safety and Efficacy of YRA-1909 in Patients with Rheumatoid Arthritis. Available online: https://clinicaltrials.gov/ct2/archive/NCT03275025 (accessed on 7 November 2017).
8. Sato, Y.; Itagaki, S.; Kurokawa, T.; Ogura, J.; Kobayashi, M.; Hirano, T.; Sugawara, M.; Lseki, K. In vitro and in vivo antioxidant properties of chlorogenic acid and caffeic acid. *Int. J. Pharm.* **2011**, *403*, 136–138. [CrossRef] [PubMed]
9. Kurata, R.; Adachi, M.; Yamakawa, O.; Yoshimoto, M. Growth suppression of human cancer cells by polyphenolics from sweetpotato (*Ipomoea batatas* L.) leaves. *J. Agric. Food Chem.* **2007**, *55*, 185–190. [CrossRef] [PubMed]
10. Ooi, L.S.; Wang, H.; He, Z.; Ooi, V.E. Antiviral activities of purified compounds from *Youngia japonica* (L.) DC (Asteraceae, Compositae). *J. Ethnopharmacol.* **2006**, *106*, 187–191. [CrossRef] [PubMed]
11. Choi, J.H.; Kim, S. Investigation of the anticoagulant and antithrombotic effects of chlorogenic acid. *J. Biochem. Mol. Toxicol.* **2017**, *31*, e21865. [CrossRef] [PubMed]
12. Del Rio, D.; Stalmach, A.; Calani, L.; Crozier, A. Bioavailability of coffee chlorogenic acids and green tea flavan-3-ols. *Nutrients* **2010**, *2*, 820–833. [CrossRef] [PubMed]
13. Farrell, T.L.; Dew, T.P.; Poquet, L.; Hanson, P.; Williamson, G. Absorption and metabolism of chlorogenic acids in cultured gastric epithelial monolayers. *Drug Metab. Dispos.* **2011**, *39*, 2338–2346. [CrossRef] [PubMed]
14. Omar, M.H.; Mullen, W.; Stalmach, A.; Auger, C.; Rouanet, J.M.; Teissedre, P.L.; Caldwell, S.T.; Hartley, R.C.; Crozier, A. Absorption, disposition, metabolism, and excretion of [3-(14)C] caffeic acid in rats. *J. Agric. Food Chem.* **2012**, *60*, 5205–5214. [CrossRef] [PubMed]
15. Azuma, K.; Ippoushi, K.; Nakayama, M.; Ito, H.; Higashio, H.; Terao, J. Absorption of chlorogenic acid and caffeic acid in rats after oral administration. *J. Agric. Food Chem.* **2000**, *48*, 5496–5500. [CrossRef] [PubMed]
16. Wong, C.C.; Meinl, W.; Glatt, H.R.; Barron, D.; Stalmach, A.; Steiling, H.; Crozier, A.; Williamson, G. In vitro and in vivo conjugation of dietary hydroxycinnamic acids by UDP-glucuronosyltransferases and sulfotransferases in humans. *J. Nutr. Biochem.* **2010**, *21*, 1060–1068. [CrossRef] [PubMed]
17. Piazzon, A.; Vrhovsek, U.; Masuero, D.; Mattivi, F.; Mandoj, F.; Nardini, M. Antioxidant activity of phenolic acids and their metabolites: synthesis and antioxidant properties of the sulfate derivatives of ferulic and caffeic acids and of the acyl glucuronide of ferulic acid. *J. Agric. Food Chem.* **2012**, *60*, 12312–12323. [CrossRef] [PubMed]
18. Yamada, J.; Tomita, Y. Antimutagenic activity of caffeic acid and related compounds. *Biosci. Biotech. Biochem.* **1996**, *60*, 328–329. [CrossRef] [PubMed]
19. Guo, D.; Dou, D.; Ge, L.; Huang, Z.; Wang, L.; Gu, N. A caffeic acid mediated facile synthesis of silver nanoparticles with powerful anti-cancer activity. *Colloids Surf. B Biointerfaces* **2015**, *134*, 229–234. [CrossRef] [PubMed]
20. Yang, G.W.; Jiang, J.S.; Lu, W.Q. Ferulic acid exerts anti-angiogenic and anti-tumor activity by targeting fibroblast growth factor receptor 1-mediated angiogenesis. *Int. J. Mol. Sci.* **2015**, *16*, 24011–24031. [CrossRef] [PubMed]

21. Shi, P.; Lin, X.; Yao, H. A comprehensive review of recent studies on pharmacokinetics of traditional Chinese medicines (2014–2017) and perspectives. *Drug Metab. Rev.* **2018**, *50*, 161–192. [CrossRef] [PubMed]
22. Li, Y.; Wang, Y.; Tai, W.; Yang, L.; Chen, Y.; Chen, C.; Liu, C. Challenges and solutions of pharmacokinetics for efficacy and safety of traditional chinese medicine. *Curr. Drug Metab.* **2015**, *16*, 765–776. [CrossRef] [PubMed]
23. Jeong, J.H.; Kim, D.K.; Ji, H.Y.; Oh, S.R.; Lee, H.K.; Lee, H.S. Liquid chromatography-atmospheric pressure chemical ionization tandem mass spectrometry for the simultaneous determination of dimethoxyaschantin, dimethyllirioresinol, dimethylpinoresinol, epimagnolin A, fargesin and magnolin in rat plasma. *Biomed. Chromatogr.* **2011**, *25*, 879–889. [CrossRef] [PubMed]
24. Wang, X.; Ma, X.; Li, W.; Chu, Y.; Guo, J.; Li, S.; Wang, J.; Zhang, H.; Zhou, S.; Zhu, Y. Simultaneous determination of five phenolic components and paeoniflorin in rat plasma by liquid chromatography-tandem mass spectrometry and pharmacokinetic study after oral administration of Cerebralcare granule. *J. Pharm. Biomed. Anal.* **2013**, *86*, 82–91. [CrossRef] [PubMed]
25. Zhou, W.; Liu, S.; Ju, W.; Shan, J.; Meng, M.; Cai, B.; Di, L. Simultaneous determination of phenolic acids by UPLC-MS/MS in rat plasma and its application in pharmacokinetic study after oral administration of Flos Lonicerae preparations. *J. Pharm. Biomed. Anal.* **2013**, *86*, 189–197. [CrossRef] [PubMed]
26. De Oliveira, D.M.; Pinto, C.B.; Sampaio, G.R.; Yonekura, L.; Catharino, R.R.; Bastos, D.H. Development and validation of methods for the extraction of phenolic acids from plasma, urine, and liver and analysis by UPLC-MS. *J. Agric. Food Chem.* **2013**, *61*, 6113–6121. [CrossRef] [PubMed]
27. Zhou, W.; Shan, J.; Wang, S.; Ju, W.; Meng, M.; Cai, B.; Di, L. Simultaneous determination of caffeic acid derivatives by UPLC-MS/MS in rat plasma and its application in pharmacokinetic study after oral administration of Flos Lonicerae-Fructus Forsythiae herb combination. *J. Chromatogr. B* **2014**, *949–950*, 7–15. [CrossRef] [PubMed]
28. Zeng, L.; Wang, M.; Yuan, Y.; Guo, B.; Zhou, J.; Tan, Z.; Ye, M.; Ding, L.; Chen, B. Simultaneous multi-component quantitation of Chinese herbal injection Yin-zhi-huang in rat plasma by using a single-tube extraction procedure for mass spectrometry-based pharmacokinetic measurement. *J. Chromatogr B* **2014**, *967*, 245–254. [CrossRef] [PubMed]
29. Marmet, C.; Actis-Goretta, L.; Renouf, M.; Giuffrida, F. Quantification of phenolic acids and their methylates, glucuronides, sulfates and lactones metabolites in human plasma by LC-MS/MS after oral ingestion of soluble coffee. *J. Pharm. Biomed. Anal.* **2014**, *88*, 617–625. [CrossRef] [PubMed]
30. Wang, X.; Li, W.; Ma, X.; Chu, Y.; Li, S.; Guo, J.; Jia, Y.; Zhou, S.; Zhu, Y.; Liu, C. Simultaneous determination of caffeic acid and its major pharmacologically active metabolites in rat plasma by LC-MS/MS and its application in pharmacokinetic study. *Biomed. Chromatogr.* **2015**, *29*, 552–559. [CrossRef] [PubMed]
31. Chang, Y.X.; Ge, A.H.; Yu, X.A.; Jiao, X.C.; Li, J.; He, J.; Tian, J.; Liu, W.; Azietaku, J.T.; Zhang, B.L.; et al. Simultaneous determination of four phenolic acids and seven alkaloids in rat plasma after oral administration of traditional Chinese medicinal preparation Jinqi Jiangtang Tablet by LC-ESI-MS/MS. *J. Pharm. Biomed. Anal.* **2016**, *117*, 1–10. [CrossRef] [PubMed]
32. Jung, J.W.; Kim, J.M.; Jeong, J.S.; Son, M.; Lee, H.S.; Lee, M.G.; Kang, H.E. Pharmacokinetics of chlorogenic acid and corydaline in DA-9701, a new botanical gastroprokinetic agent, in rats. *Xenobiotica* **2014**, *44*, 635–643. [CrossRef] [PubMed]

3

Drying Technologies for the Stability and Bioavailability of Biopharmaceuticals

Fakhrossadat Emami [1], Alireza Vatanara [1,*], Eun Ji Park [2] and Dong Hee Na [2,*]

[1] College of Pharmacy, Tehran University of Medical Sciences, Tehran 1417614411, Iran; f-emami@razi.tums.ac.ir

[2] College of Pharmacy, Chung-Ang University, Seoul 06974, Korea; 1978ej@naver.com

[*] Correspondence: vatanara@tums.ac.ir (A.V.); dhna@cau.ac.kr (D.H.N.)

Abstract: Solid dosage forms of biopharmaceuticals such as therapeutic proteins could provide enhanced bioavailability, improved storage stability, as well as expanded alternatives to parenteral administration. Although numerous drying methods have been used for preparing dried protein powders, choosing a suitable drying technique remains a challenge. In this review, the most frequent drying methods, such as freeze drying, spray drying, spray freeze drying, and supercritical fluid drying, for improving the stability and bioavailability of therapeutic proteins, are discussed. These technologies can prepare protein formulations for different applications as they produce particles with different sizes and morphologies. Proper drying methods are chosen, and the critical process parameters are optimized based on the proposed route of drug administration and the required pharmacokinetics. In an optimized drying procedure, the screening of formulations according to their protein properties is performed to prepare a stable protein formulation for various delivery systems, including pulmonary, nasal, and sustained-release applications.

Keywords: biopharmaceuticals; drying technology; protein stability; bioavailability; pharmacokinetics

1. Introduction

The intrinsic instability of protein molecules is currently the predominant challenge for biopharmaceutical scientists [1–3]. Because of their higher molecular weights and diversity of composition, therapeutic proteins have much more complicated structures than conventional chemical drugs [3–5]. Exposure to some environmental stresses, such as pH extremes, high temperatures, freezing, light, agitation, sheer stress, and organic solvents, can cause protein instability [4,5]. Since proteins can be degraded easily during manufacturing and storage, some strategies are suggested to improve protein stability, including the addition of stabilizers, protein modification with biocompatible molecules, nanomedicine, and nano- or micro-particle technology [6–13].

Drying strategies that process and dehydrate proteins to produce more stable protein formulations in the solid state are frequently used for biopharmaceuticals that are insufficiently stable in aqueous solutions [14–16]. Solid dosage forms of proteins are less prone to shear-related denaturation and precipitation during manufacturing and storage [1,15,17,18]. Because water molecules can induce mobilization of therapeutic proteins and other additives, liquid formulations of proteins are more susceptible to unfavorable physicochemical degradation. Consequently, water removal and embedding of proteins in a glassy matrix are good approaches for improved storage against physicochemical protein degradation [1,5,18].

Dried therapeutic protein powders have shown good storage stability at room temperature ($\leq$25 °C), and dehydration is an easy and economical approach [19,20]. Dehydration is not only a drying procedure for improving protein shelf-life, but may also be used for engineering protein particles for various routes of administration. Dried biopharmaceutical powders have gained popularity as inhalation preparations for pulmonary, nasal, and sustained drug-delivery systems [21,22]. Numerous reviews of drying strategies have been published [23,24]. However, most of these reviews focus on small molecules, and reviews of using drying methods to improve stability or pharmacokinetic properties of therapeutic proteins are relatively few [25,26]. Because proteins are sensitive to environmental stresses, the techniques available for producing dried biopharmaceuticals are limited by factors such as production time, temperature, and various process-related stresses [26]. The features and drawbacks of each drying procedure should be considered for rational selection of a drying method to improve the stability of therapeutic proteins for different drug administration applications [27]. In this review, the drying techniques of biopharmaceuticals are discussed, with focus on the selection of appropriate drying methods for improving stability and desired pharmacokinetic properties of biopharmaceuticals. Stabilizers for protein formulations and applications of dried-powder formulations to local or systemic drug delivery are also highlighted.

2. Drying Techniques

Generally, drying involves three steps, which may be operated simultaneously. First, energy is transferred from an external source to water or dispersion medium in the product. The second step is phase transformation of the liquid phase to a vapor or solid phase. Finally, the transfer of vapor generated away from the pharmaceutical product occurs. The characteristics of dried particles can be effectively influenced by process parameters, such as temperature, pressure, relative humidity, and gas feed rate, besides characteristics of protein formulations, such as composition and type of excipients, concentration of solutes, viscosity, and type of solvent [28] (Table 1). Drying based on the mechanism of removing water can be classified into subgroups. Drying can be performed using an evaporation mechanism, such as vacuum dying or foam drying; evaporation and atomization pathways such as spray drying (SD); sublimation mechanisms such as freeze drying (FD) and spray freeze drying; and supercritical fluid drying methods using a precipitation mechanism [27]. The most common drying techniques, namely freeze drying, spray drying, spray freeze drying, and supercritical fluid drying will be discussed in this review.

2.1. Freeze Drying (FD)

The most common drying method for therapeutic proteins is FD [14,26,29], which has been used for many therapeutic proteins, including insulin dry powder for inhalation (Afrezza®, MannKind Corporation, Valencia, CA, USA) [14]. Since water molecules can induce mobilization of protein solution, protein stability can be improved by water removal and embedding of proteins in a glassy matrix through lyophilization [5]. FD is based on sublimation, where solid materials are directly transformed to the gaseous phase. The FD process involves the following three steps: freezing, primary drying, and secondary drying [1,5,18,30,31].

Freeze-dried proteins have greater storage stability than proteins in liquid dosage forms; however, this process applies freezing and dehydration stresses to the proteins, which may result in the alteration of protein structure [31–33]. Upon drying, the hydration shell surrounding the protein, which provides a protective effect, is removed. In addition, the protein solution becomes saturated because of ice crystal formation during the freezing process. The solute concentration, pH change, and ionic strength changes are formulation variables that should be considered for a stable protein formulation (Table 1) [1,33]. Recent infrared spectroscopic analyses have shown that acute freezing and dehydration stresses of lyophilization can induce protein unfolding [29,34]. To develop a successful protein formulation using an FD procedure, physical properties, such as glass transition temperature (T_g) and residual moisture content, and operational parameters, such as pH and cooling rate, should be considered [29].

Furthermore, a hydrophilic molecule can be incorporated into the protein formulation as a lyoprotectant to overcome protein denaturation and preserve stability during lyophilization [1,17]. Stabilizers can protect proteins during freezing (cryoprotectants) and lyophilization (lyoprotectants) through water replacement and hydrogen bond formation (Table 2) [1,18,30,35]. Moreover, excipients have the potential to provide a glassy matrix to decrease protein-protein interactions and reduce protein mobility in a solid dosage form [36]. In summary, optimization of process variables and proper combinations of additives as stabilizers are requirements for stable freeze-dried products [35–37].

Liao et al. investigated the effect of excipients, such as glycerol, sucrose, trehalose, and dextran, on the stability of freeze-dried lysozymes using second derivative Fourier transform infrared (FTIR) spectroscopy [17]. They showed that the combination of trehalose and sucrose could raise the T_g of freeze-dried lysozymes, leading to the stabilization of lysozyme in freeze-dried formulations. This study indicated that the T_g of freeze-dried formulations and the protein stability during lyophilization were dependent on the excipient type and excipient to enzyme mass ratio. A recent study by Tonnis et al. [38] showed the influence of size and molecular flexibility of sugars on the stability of freeze-dried proteins, including insulin, hepatitis B surface antigen, lactate dehydrogenase, and β-galactosidase. Among freeze-dried proteins prepared in the presence or absence of disaccharide (trehalose) or oligosaccharide (inulin, 4 kDa; dextran, 6 kDa; dextran 70 kDa), those prepared in the presence of the smallest sugar (trehalose) showed high stability although trehalose-containing formulations had the lowest T_g. In addition, the flexible oligosaccharide inulin was more stable than the rigid oligosaccharide dextran 6 kDa or 70 kDa. The combination of polysaccharide dextran 70 kDa and trehalose greatly increased the T_g of the formulation and improved the stability of proteins, as compared to formulations containing dextran alone. The flexible oligosaccharide inulin (4 kDa) provided better stabilization than the similarly sized but molecularly rigid oligosaccharide dextran 6 kDa. This study indicated that the combination of trehalose and dextran has an additive effect owing to the interaction potential of trehalose (water replacement) and enhanced T_g of dextran (glassy state).

Table 1. Comparison of characteristics of different drying technologies. Table adopted from [15,21,23,24,39,40].

Drying Procedure	Process Parameters	Stress	Advantages	Limitations	Typical Powder Characteristics
Freeze drying	• Solute concentration • Cooling temperature • Freezing rate • Drying temperature • Drying pressure	• Crystallization • pH changes • Dehydration stress • Ionic strength change • Interfacial stress (ice-liquid) • Ice crystal formation	• Elevated temperature not required for drying • Accurately dosed • Controlled moisture content • Short reconstitution time • Appealing physical form • Homogenous dispersion • Good for materials sensitive to air or O_2	• No particle engineering • Expensive set up • Long processing time • Complex process • Maintenance cost • Exposure to ice-water interface • Few months for large objects	• Intact cake • High surface area • Uniform color • Consistency • Elegant cake appearance • High strength to prevent cracking, powdering, or collapse
Spray drying	• Solute concentration • Feed flow rate • Hot air flow rate (Inlet and outlet) • Additive solubility • Inlet temperature	• Thermal stress • Atomization stress • Mechanical stress • Interfacial stress (air-liquid) • Dehydration stress	• Simple • Convenient system • Cost effectiveness • One step (Short process time) • Scalability • Repeatability • Particle engineering • Good aerosolization	• Yield (50–70%) • Unsuitable for materials sensitive to air • Non-aseptic	• Fine powder • Hollow particle • Shrinkage • Toughening • Spherical, ellipsoid, toroid, or dimpled shape
Spray freeze drying	• Solute concentration • Feed flow rate • Solid content	• Atomization stress • Interfacial stress (air-liquid) • Freezing stress • Interfacial stress (ice-liquid) • Dehydration stress	• Fast freezing • Particle engineering • High yield • Excellent aerosolization • Aseptic drying	• Three steps (Time consuming) • High cost • Fragile particles • Complex • Inconvenient (require liquid N_2)	• Spherical, porous particle • Light weight • Smooth surface • Very low density • High surface area
Supercritical fluid drying	• Solute concentration • Feed flow rate • Co-solvent flow rate • SCF flow rate • Temperature • Pressure • Nozzle size	• Atomization stress • Dehydration stress	• Fast process • Particle engineering • Mild process condition (mild temperature) • Aseptic drying • Scalability	• Exposure to organic solvent • Special set-up • High cost	• Spherical • Smooth surface

2.2. *Spray Drying (SD)*

SD is the most common particle engineering method that generates solid (particulate) proteins for pharmaceutical applications [41]. SD as a single-step process may provide dried protein particles with the required size and morphology [30,42]. SD technology comprises atomization, drying, and separation of particles. Protein solution is sprayed through nozzles into a drying chamber. Droplet formation and subsequent dehydration is performed very rapidly in a hot drying medium. The resulting protein powders are transferred into a cyclone (Figure 1). Owing to the short procedure time, SD is a mild technique for producing stable protein powders for inhalation and other applications [1,42–45].

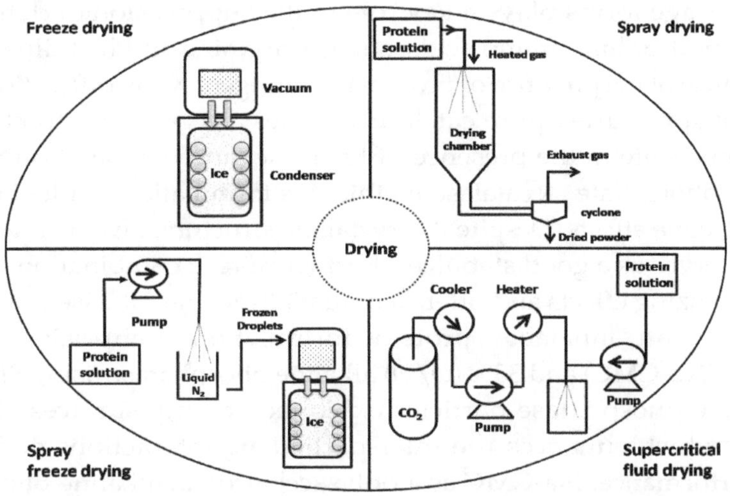

Figure 1. Schematic illustration of drying methods using freeze drying (FD), spray drying (SD), spray freeze drying (SFD), and supercritical fluid drying (SCFD) technologies.

Peclet number (Pe), which is the proportion of droplet evaporation rate and the diffusional motion of solutes in the SD method, can determine the morphology and density of the final particles that are either dense or hollow. The solute concentration, feeding flow rate, flow rate of hot air, solubility of additives through effects on evaporation rate, as well as inlet temperature are adjustable process parameters in the SD method. Large molecules with low diffusional coefficients having low solubility and high density, such as albumin and growth hormone, can prompt surface saturation at high temperatures. In addition, high surface-active agents such as leucine and trileucine would be located on particle surface and saturate the surface rapidly. Thus, for proteins and high surface-active agents, the solutes cannot diffuse to the center of droplets (Pe > 1) and generate hollow particles with low density that are suitable for pulmonary drug delivery [46]. Because of thermo-sensitivity of proteins, the loss of hydration layer in contact with hot air, as well as exposure to air/liquid interface at the droplet surface during atomization may cause degradation. Moreover, this engineering technique may induce shear stress in protein structure during the atomization step (Table 1) [1,2,5,44]. Excipients used as stabilizers may provide a functional shield surrounding the protein and prevent exposure of the protein to the interfacial surface or hot atmosphere [36]. The rational choice of stabilizers and optimization of the process variables are essential approaches to guarantee protein stability and achieve the desired particle properties.

Schule et al. studied the biophysical and conformational stability of spray-dried antibody-mannitol formulations [47] and concluded that antibody formulations during storage stability tests showed some levels of aggregates when measured by size-exclusion chromatography (SEC). FTIR analysis demonstrated that despite antibody aggregation during the SD process, the secondary structure of the antibody was conserved. Furthermore, their data suggested that the unfolding of protein structure was reversible and through reconstitution, the unfolded form of antibody formulation was refolded to a native form.

Ajmera et al. studied the SD of catalase formulations in the presence of some amino acids [1]. The ability of hydrophilic and hydrophobic amino acids to serve as protective agents during the SD of catalase was evaluated. The mean particle size of the spray-dried powder was estimated to be in the range of 3.3–4.8 μm, and amino acids have shown different stabilizing efficacies against the stresses induced by the SD technique. Spray-dried catalase, in comparison with the liquid form, showed greater stability. Arginine and histidine preserved the stability of enzyme formulations during SD. Due to its small size and surface activity, arginine exhibited fast diffusion to the droplet surface during droplet formation. Thus, arginine was localized at the droplet surface and protected the enzyme from air-liquid interface adsorption. Furthermore, hydrogen bond formation between amino acids and proteins in solid dosage forms plays a key role in the suppression of dehydration stress (water replacement). Charged hydrophilic amino acids, such as arginine and histidine, could form hydrogen bonds with catalase because of the presence of protonated nitrogen. X-ray diffraction (XRD) measurements have clearly shown that spray-dried pure catalase assumes a crystalline structure, while the enzyme remains in an amorphous state in the presence of histidine, and combination with arginine shifts its structure to a semi-amorphous state. A catalase-methionine formulation resulted in a crystalline product, which provided no protective effects. Despite its crystalline structure, glycine interacted with proteins as a water substitute and serves as a good stabilizer. Furthermore, a combination of arginine and glycine provides synergistic stabilizing effects and offers a potentially stable catalase powder preparation.

Li et al. prepared an inhalable protein formulation comprising 67% (*w*/*w*) sodium carboxymethylcellulose (Na-CMC) and 33% (*w*/*w*) alkaline phosphatase using SD [48]. They concluded that spray-dried alkaline phosphatase particles exhibited smooth surfaces. Particles with smooth surfaces are cohesive, which enhances the inter-particulate interactions and protein aggregation, causing low aerosol performance. Na-CMC as a polysaccharide in alkaline phosphatase formulations dried by SD may produce wrinkled protein particles. The roughness of protein surfaces may suppress unnecessary interactions and protein degradation. Spray-dried alkaline phosphatase-Na-CMC formulations maintained their stability immediately after preparation or following storage for three months, and subsequent protein powders produced in this manner have shown excellent aerodynamic performance.

2.3. *Spray Freeze Drying (SFD)*

Another effective and versatile technique for transforming protein solution into dried particles is SFD, which is the combination of traditional FD and SD processes. Atomization, fast freezing, and drying by ice sublimation are the three phases of SFD process (Figure 1). SFD is a method for preparing lyophilized protein powders with spherical microparticles [49].

Atmospheric freezing, spray freezing with compressed carbon dioxide, spray freezing into a vapor over a cryogenic liquid, and spray freezing into a liquid are different types of SFD methods [50–52]. SFD involves the atomization of protein solution via a nozzle at extremely low temperatures, and has potential applications for thermo-labile active pharmaceutical ingredients. Because of the critically low temperature, the atomized droplets are rapidly frozen. SFD methods may immobilize the protein and avoid exposure to air-water interface. The frozen micronized droplets are sublimated using a lyophilizer under vacuum to prepare a dried powder.

In SFD, the liquid solution is sprayed into a vapor via a nozzle using a cryogenic fluid, such as liquid nitrogen [43,44,53–55]. The chemical composition, protein solution concentrations, atomization rate, freezing rate, as well as the temperature of cryogenic liquid have key roles in determining the density and particle size distribution of spray freeze-dried powders [50]. Supercooling phenomena using a cryogenic liquid in SFD may reduce the undesirable effects of ice crystallization, pH shift values, as well as phase separation of the drug and excipient that have existence in FD. Moreover, since freezing is very rapid, there is not sufficient time for molecular rearrangements. Biopharmaceuticals are embedded amorphously in the excipients, minimizing the probability of protein crystallization and subsequent phase separation between the active pharmaceutical ingredient and stabilizers [56]. Furthermore,

SFD can create such powders with the required density and particle size distributions for different pharmaceutical applications. Therefore, SFD is more advantageous than traditional FD [4,44,50].

Rogers et al. prepared spray freeze-dried insulin in the presence of tyloxapol and lactose as lyoprotectants [57]. Spray freeze-dried insulin in the presence of surfactant and sugar as lyoprotectants showed improved stability. The concentration of the covalent dimer of insulin in spray freeze-dried pure insulin preparations is only slightly higher than that of the unprocessed bulk insulin. Spray freeze-dried insulin with or without lyoprotectants showed little degradation, indicating that such preparations are as stable as the unprocessed native insulin. Maa et al. showed that SFD powders of influenza vaccines have superior stability compared with liquid formulations [58]. Processing other proteins such as rhDNase, anti-IgE monoclonal antibodies [21], calcitonin [53], and parathyroid hormone [44] using SFD provided stable dried powders with appropriate particle sizes and good flow properties.

Spray freeze-dried powders may be produced for different drug delivery system applications. Specific physical characteristics such as particle size distribution, density, surface area, and volume are required, depending on their application [50]. SFD typically produces highly porous particles with a high percentage of fine particle fraction (FPF) and proper aerodynamic behavior for pulmonary delivery [44]. In addition, spray freeze-dried particles have applications for needle-free intradermal injection system, nasal, colonic, and ophthalmic drug delivery, as well as in processing for microencapsulation platforms [50]. Spray freeze-dried particles with a geometric diameter of 7–42 μm and very low density, representing an aerodynamic diameter of 1–5 μm, could be effective in pulmonary drug delivery systems. However, for nasal delivery and intradermal injection systems, particles with geometric diameters of 25–70 μm and 34–50 μm are required, respectively [50].

2.4. *Supercritical Fluid Drying (SCFD)*

Supercritical fluid drying (SCFD) is an attractive alternative drying method, because dehydration can be rapidly accomplished in the absence of extreme temperatures. SCFD may produce large amounts of dried biopharmaceuticals with adjustable particle sizes and morphology [59]. SCF uses a material such as ethylene, methanol, or carbon dioxide above its critical temperature and pressure. The critical temperature of a liquid is the temperature at which its vapor cannot be liquefied, no matter how much pressure is applied. The pressure that is needed to condense a gas at its critical temperature defines its critical pressure. SCF exhibits the appropriate characteristics of gas and liquid, including penetration of gas and solubility of liquids. Density, viscosity, and diffusivity of SCF above its critical point are in the range of the gas and liquid states of the solvent. SCFD is a versatile process that can adjust the density of SCF and the solubility of a solute through modulation of pressures and temperatures used in the procedure.

Carbon dioxide is a non-toxic, non-inflammable, and relatively cheap fluid, with mild critical temperature (31 °C) and pressure (73 bar) for SCFD processes. Supercritical carbon dioxide ($scCO_2$) may be used as a solvent or non-solvent in several SCFD applications, such as particle formation, chemical extraction, and purification. Rapid expansion of a supercritical solvent (RESS) and particles from a gas-saturated solution (PGSS) are two types of drying using $scCO_2$ as a solvent. Gas anti-solvent (GAS), supercritical anti-solvent process (SAS), and solution-enhanced dispersion system (SEDS) processes are examples of anti-solvent $scCO_2$ drying [15]. In previous studies, two theories explain the use of SCF for drying of protein products. In the first theory, SCFD is based on the anti-solvent and water extraction of SCF for protein formulations. Because of water extraction, the protein would be concentrated and precipitated. The concentrated protein solution is dried through the extraction of remaining water molecules using SFD. In the second theory, SCF is used as a propellant to enhance the atomization rate. In this process, SCF is dissolved at high pressure and the protein solution and SCF pass through a two-fluid nozzle, where the feed solution is atomized by the SCF, allowing a short drying procedure [60]. By monitoring the spraying gas flow rate, solution flow rate, solution concentration, nozzle size, temperature, pressure, and solvent, uniform spherical particles with distinct particle sizes and acceptable flow properties may be achieved [15,22].

Table 2. Studies of solid protein formulations prepared by different drying methods in the presence of stabilizers.

Process	Proteins/Peptides	Stabilizers	Mechanism of Stabilization	Applications		References
				Stability Improvement	Drug Delivery	
Freeze drying	• IgG • Lysozyme • BSA • Anti-IgE antibody	• Trehalose, Sucrose, PEG • PEG, Glycerol, Sucrose, Trehalose, Dextran • Glucose, Sucrose, Maltose, Trehalose, Maltotriose • Histidine, Arginine, Glycine, Aspartic acid	• Glassy state, Water replacement • Water replacement • Glassy state, Water replacement • Glassy state	✓ ✓ ✓ ✓	– – – –	[61,62] [17] [63] [18]
Spray drying	• IgG • Trastuzumab • Anti-IgE Mab, rhDNase • Catalase • Influenza vaccine • Alkaline phosphatase • Erythropoietin	• Trehalose, Sucrose, Leucine, Glycine, Lysine, Phenylalanine • Trehalose, HPβCD, βCD • Mannitol, Trehalose, Sucrose • Arginine, Glycine, Histidine • HEPES buffer, Phosphate buffer • Sodium carboxy methylcellulose • Dextran	• Glassy state, Water replacement • Glassy state, Water replacement • Glassy state, Water replacement • Water replacement, Inhibit interfacial adsorption • Buffer • Glassy state, Water replacement • Glassy state, Water replacement	✓ ✓ – ✓ – ✓ –	• Pulmonary – • Pulmonary – • Pulmonary • Pulmonary • Sustained release	[42,45,47] [2] [21] [1] [64] [48] [65]
Spray freeze drying	• IgG • BSA • Anti-IgE Mab, rhDNase • PTH • Calcitonin • Influenza vaccine • Influenza vaccine • Insulin • Anthrax vaccine	• Leucine, Phenylalanine, Glycine, Trehalose • Ammonium sulfate, Mannitol, Trehalose • Mannitol, Trehalose, Sucrose • Trehalose, HPβCD, Leucine, Citric acid • Trehalose, HPβCD, Maltose, Tween80 • HEPES buffer, Phosphate buffer • Dextran, Mannitol, Trehalose, Arginine • Trehalose, Lactose • Trehalose	• Water replacement • Reduction specific surface area • Glassy state, Water replacement • Water replacement, Inhibit interfacial adsorption • Glassy state, Water replacement, Inhibit interfacial adsorption • Buffer • Glassy state, Water replacement - -	✓ ✓ – ✓ ✓ – ✓ ✓ ✓	– • Sustained release • Pulmonary • Pulmonary • Pulmonary • Pulmonary • Epidermal • Enhance solubility • Nasal	[52] [36] [21] [44] [53] [64] [58] [57] [19]
Supercritical fluid drying	• IgG • Lysozyme • Lysozyme, Myoglobin • Insulin	• Trehalose, HPβCD • Trehalose, Sucrose • Trehalose, Sucrose • TMC, Dextran	- • Glassy state, Water replacement • Glassy state, Water replacement • Carrier	✓ ✓ ✓ ✓	– – – • Pulmonary	[66] [22,59] [67] [68]

Immunoglobulin G (IgG), polyethylene glycol (PEG), hydroxypropyl β cyclodextrin (HPβCD), β cyclodextrin (βCD), bovine serum albumin (BSA), N-trimethyl chitosan (TMC), recombinant human DNase (rhDNase).

2.5. *Comparison of the Physical Characteristics of Dried Powders*

As shown in Figure 2, immunoglobulin G (IgG) formulations prepared using different drying methods with trehalose as a stabilizer represent different particle morphologies. The diversity in the size and morphology of particles in SEM micrographs could be explained by the particle formation procedure used in different drying techniques [64,69].

The most common drying method for proteins and peptides is FD, which produces a dry cake. Intact cakes have very low residual moisture content with great long-term stability. FD powders of protein formulations after reconstitution can be used for parenteral drug delivery [33]. However, the use of FD for particle-based formulations, such as those for pulmonary drug delivery, is limited because it is not a direct particle formation method [37]. For particle formation, additional procedures to break the cake are necessary. Such additional processes may reduce the production yield and lead to poor control of critical particle properties, such as particle size, size distribution, density, and morphology [41].

SD is a well-established particle engineering process producing fine powders with smooth or shrunken surfaces. Generally, SD powders exhibit hollow particles with a dimpled shape. SD methods typically provide small particles between 2–10 μm and an FPF between 20–70%, respectively. Particles with low density have potential for use in pulmonary or nasal drug delivery applications [42,45]. SD processes can be used for microencapsulation of biopharmaceuticals as a controlled-release system [65]. Solid proteins prepared using the SFD method have specific morphological characteristics, namely presence of numerous pores on the surface and within the microparticles. Cross-sections of SFD particles have shown an internal porous structure similar to a honeycomb [59]. Compared with spray-dried particles, SFD particles showed higher sphericity and porosity, resulting in relatively low densities appropriate for inhalation [69]. When atomized with the same combination of feed solution, SFD produced a smaller aerodynamic diameter in comparison with SD particles because of their high porosity and relatively lower density. Small aerodynamic diameter means high FPF and good aerosol performance [50].

Saluja et al. used SD and SFD powders of influenza subunit vaccine with inulin as a stabilizer for inhalation [64]. SD techniques produced particles with a small median volume diameter (<5 μm), but SFD generated particles with a larger volume median diameter (>10 μm). Although these particles have different physical sizes, they have an acceptable aerodynamic size in the range of 1–5 μm for pulmonary drug delivery based on their bulk densities. SFD, rather than SD, is recommended for proteins sensitive to elevated temperatures [50].

Maa et al. reported that the same formulation of rhDNase and anti-IgE antibody prepared by SFD and SD resulted in different particle morphologies [21]. Differing morphologies observed in SEM images of the same protein formulation is indicative of particles with different sizes and densities. Although the diameter of SFD particles is approximately doubled (3.3 μm for SD vs. 7.7 μm for SFD), the FPF increased from 27% to 50%, which reflects an improved aerodynamic performance of SFD powder. These observations suggest that superior aerodynamic behavior by SFD particles is probably correlated with small aerodynamic size. Consequently, SFD powders, in comparison with SD powders, are reported to possess higher FPF and lower aerodynamic diameter, which result in higher aerosolization efficiency [52]. Because of rapid evaporation of water in the drying chamber, SD particles had smaller sizes resulting from particle shrinkage. With the SFD technique, immediately after atomization, droplets were frozen and solid ice crystals were produced throughout the frozen droplet. During lyophilization, the ice crystals sublimate, and particles with an interconnected porous structure are formed. SFD particles can maintain approximately 80% of their droplet size and therefore result in large-sized particles with high sphericity [50,64,69]. Low particle density can compensate for the large geometric diameter. However, particles with low density have lower mechanical strength and are more fragile, and are therefore more susceptible to degradation [70].

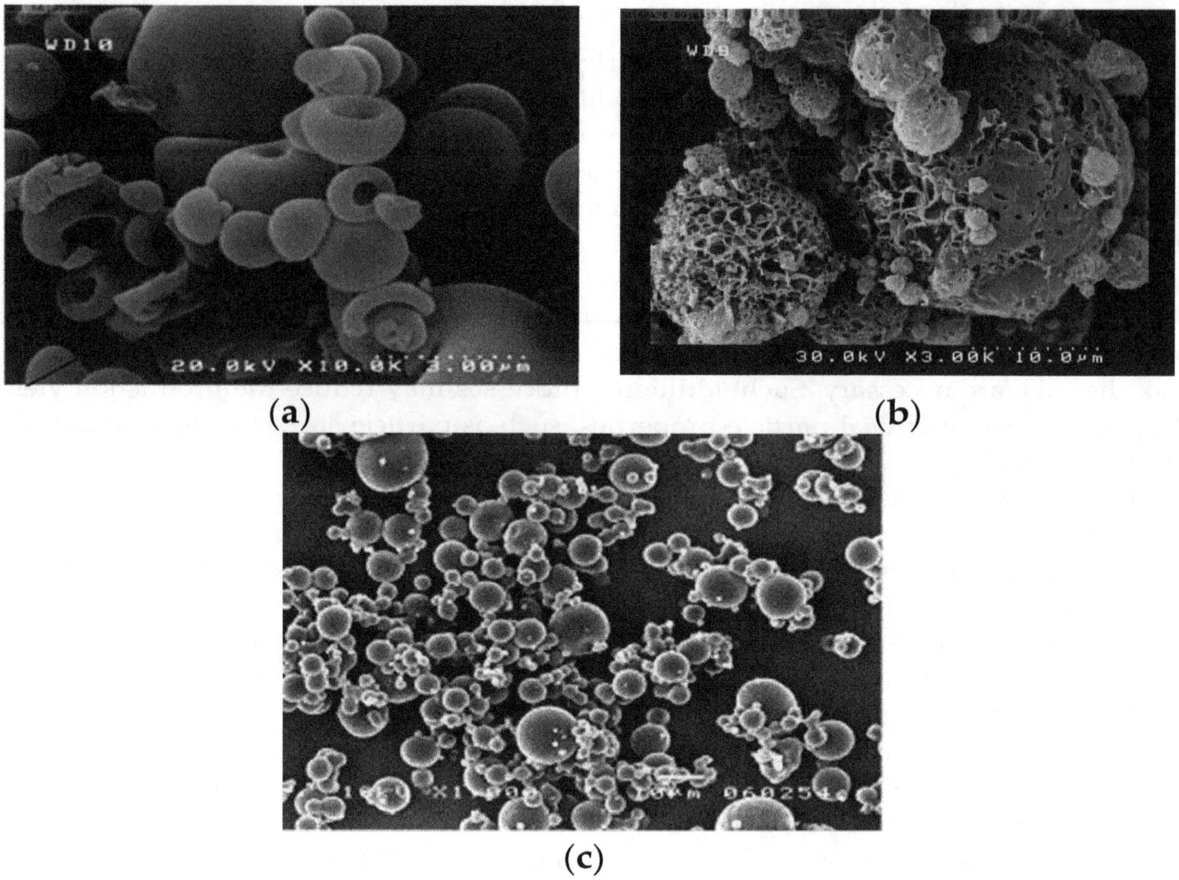

Figure 2. Scanning electron micrographs of dried IgG formulations produced using different drying methods: (**a**) SD [42], (**b**) SFD [52], and (**c**) SCFD methods [66].

Unlike FD, the SFD method can adjust particle size, thereby producing better dispersibility. By managing morphological parameters, dense protein particles may be obtained for intradermal injection applications [58], and low-density particles can be used for nasal [19] and pulmonary drug delivery [44,53]. In addition, supercooling in SFD is advantageous for reducing the unfavorable effects of freezing-induced concentration of proteins that are present in FD. Furthermore, fast freezing during SFD may provide amorphous matrices that can trap proteins in a solid matrix and preserve protein stability [50].

Jovanovic et al. prepared dried IgG powder using an SCFD procedure, in which the product showed decreased aggregation at lower temperature [66]. They evaluated the stability of the antibody using trehalose and hydroxypropyl-β-cyclodextrin (HPβCD) as stabilizers. The occurrence of IgG aggregation in IgG formulations with lower pH values was also reported. Conversely, IgG-sugar formulations in the presence of ethanol as a co-solvent are less stable.

Consequently, all these techniques were useful for improving protein storage stability. These drying methods may be beneficial when the combinining of drying and particle engineering in one process is desired for preparation of dried protein powders.

3. Stabilizers for Dried-Powder Protein Formulations

Although proteins are formulated in a solid dosage form to maintain shelf-life stability, proteins are susceptible to various physicochemical degradations upon drying and in solid form [20]. According to the stress conditions encountered in each drying method, different degradation pathways may occur simultaneously. Various physical instabilities, such as unfolding, adsorption, denaturation, aggregation, and precipitation, may occur during the drying process. Deamination, oxidation, β-elimination, hydrolysis, racemization, isomerization, and disulfide exchange are irreversible reactions that are considered chemical degradations for biopharmaceuticals [71,72]. Physicochemical parameters such as moisture content, temperature, crystallinity of the formulation, and additives have a significant impact on these unfavorable reactions [20]. In addition, the protein sequence, hydrophobicity, isoelectric point (pI), and carbohydrate content play key roles in the susceptibility of proteins to inactivation. Degradation of protein products may result in reduced bioactivity with increased immunogenicity [20,73].

The stresses faced during drying procedures and in solid dosage forms remain a considerable challenge in biopharmaceutical development [18]. Rational selection of stabilizers may help preserve protein stability against stress-induced degradation [20]. The commonly used excipients are listed in five groups, namely proteins (BSA), amino acids (glycine, alanine), polyols (polyethylene glycol), carbohydrates (glucose, lactose, sucrose, trehalose), and others (surfactants, polymers, salts) [35], in Table 3. Cryoprotectants can preserve protein stability in solution and during freezing by preferential exclusion. Higher glass transition temperatures of protein formulations are required to provide stability to protein products. Moreover, lyoprotectants can provide thermodynamic stability of proteins during freeze-drying and dehydration process [17]. In instances where one stabilizer does not act as both a cryoprotectant and lyoprotectant, a combination of stabilizers may be beneficial to protect the proteins against FD-induced stresses [18]. As reported, protective agents can physically preserve protein stability via several mechanisms (Table 3). Among all stabilization pathways, water replacement and the glassy state hypothesis are more prevalent. Addition of excipients for stabilization may be required to stabilize proteins by either a thermodynamic stabilization pathway or by a kinetic mechanism [74].

3.1. *The Water Replacement Hypothesis*

Water plays a critical role in maintaining the native structure of proteins. During dehydration, water is removed and thermodynamic equilibrium between the native and unfolded state of the protein shifts to an unstable form. During drying, some stabilizers in the protein formulation can maintain the native protein conformation. These additives may enhance the free energy of protein unfolding reactions. Stabilizers with functional hydroxyl groups, such as carbohydrate and polyol, have the potential to form hydrogen bonds with bioactive proteins and substitute for the removed water molecules (anhydrobiosis). The hydrogen bonds formed between the carbohydrate and active protein are responsible for ameliorating dehydration stress in the solid state. As mentioned, this pathway can guarantee thermodynamic protein stability during the dying process [20,74].

3.2. *The Glassy Matrix Hypothesis*

The glassy matrix hypothesis is another mechanism that has a considerable effect on the kinetics of protein denaturation reactions. Because of molecular mobility, protein formulations are prone to chemical degradation, including protein aggregation and unfolding reactions. Some excipients, such as high molecular weight carbohydrates, may provide a rigid, glassy matrix that suppresses undesirable degradation reactions (glass dynamic hypothesis). Protein molecules can embed in a solid glassy matrix, which limits global mobility. Since protein mobility in a solid dosage form is restricted, possible protein-protein interactions are slowed, and the stability of proteins are preserved [20,74].

3.3. *Reducing Surface Adsorption*

Surfactants such as polysorbate 20 can localize at the interfacial surface owing to high surface activity. Thus fewer proteins are localized at particle surfaces and inhibit protein degradation [1].

Table 3. Additives used as stabilizers during drying procedures.

Stabilizers		Stabilization		References
		Mechanism	Process	
Proteins	Human or Bovine serum albumin	Water replacement (Hydrogen bonding)		
Amino acids	Glycine, Alanine, Histidine, Leucine Phenylalanine, Arginine, Aspartic acid	Water replacement Bulking agent Buffering agent Prevent protein-protein interactions	Freezing Dehydration Thermal stress	[1,18,52,74]
Polyols	Polyethylene glycol, Mannitol, Sorbitol	Water replacement Glassy state Increase matrix density	Freezing Dehydration	[74]
Carbohydrate (reducing and non-reducing sugar)	Fructose, Glucose, Lactose, Maltose, Maltodextrin Trehalose, Sucrose, Inulin, Dextran	Water replacement Glassy state (reduce global protein mobility) Reduce local protein mobility Protein-sugar interactions	Freezing Dehydration Thermal stress	[20,52,74]
Buffer and Salt	HEPES buffer, Citrate buffer, Phosphate buffer saline, Ammonium sulfate	Buffering agent	Freezing	[64]
Surfactant	Polysorbate 20, 80, Oleic acid, Sodium glycolate	Prevent surface adsorption (Reduce interfacial stress) Prevent protein-protein interactions (Prevent intermolecular interactions) Slow dissolution rate	Shear stress Interfacial stress Freezing Reconstitution	[20,74]
Polymers and Polysaccharides	Cyclodextrin, Dextran, PLGA, Hydroxy propyl β-cyclodextrin, Na-Carboxy methylcellulose	Glassy state	Freezing	[20]
Metals	Zinc	Reduce surface area	Freezing Interfacial stress	[36]

4. Delivery and Pharmacokinetics of Dried-Powder Proteins

4.1. Pulmonary Delivery

The most predominant application of dried-powder protein formulations is for pulmonary delivery. In the pulmonary delivery of proteins, mucocilliary clearance, phagocytosis by macrophages, and alveolar proteolytic enzymes are critical biological barriers to local and systemic delivery. In systemic delivery, passage of the alveolar capillary membrane, proteases in blood circulation, renal clearance, and hepatic clearance are restricting factors that decrease the bioavailability of protein drugs [14].

4.1.1. Local Delivery

Dried protein inhalation has been used as a topical drug delivery method for treating respiratory diseases. Direct drug delivery to the site of action provides high drug concentrations in the lung while reducing systemic blood circulation exposure to the drug, allowing safe therapies with high efficacies. The IL-4/IL-13 antagonist, IgG1, and an anti-IgE monoclonal antibody (Omalizumab®) have been administered as dried powder inhaler preparations for asthma, chronic obstructive pulmonary disease (COPD), or other related lung diseases [75]. For local administration, some important biological barriers should be considered to provide optimal therapeutic efficacy. Alveolar macrophage clearance of inhaled proteins is dependent on particle size, which can be decreased using both nanoparticles (diameter < 0.3 μm) and large particles (geometric diameter > 6 μm) [14]. Using SD method, insulin-loaded phospholipid/chitosan nanoparticles have been incorporated into microspheres in the presence of mannitol. Insulin-loaded microspheres have shown spherical morphology with suitable aerodynamic behavior as an inhalation preparation (aerodynamic diameter: 2–3 μm, density: 0.4–0.5 g/cm^3) [76]. Edwards et al. showed that the in vivo sustained release of insulin in rats was achieved after inhalation of large porous particles (diameter > 5 μm, density < 0.4 g/cm^2) prepared from poly(lactide-co-glycolide) (PLGA) [77]. Large porous insulin particles were inspired deep into the lungs and escaped pulmonary macrophage clearance mechanisms with a decreased immune response. Inhalation of larger porous insulin particles compared with smaller non-porous particles results in higher systemic bioavailability and suppression of systemic glucose levels for a longer period. This study showed that pulmonary protein delivery might provide highly efficient delivery of inhaled drugs into the systemic blood circulation. Additionally, large porous particles present better aerosolization efficiency. Higher aerosolization efficiency results in a decreased possibility of deposition losses before particle entry into the intrapulmonary airways, thereby enhancing the systemic concentration of an inhaled drug. Because of the relatively smaller surface areas of dried powders of large porous particles, less inter-particulate interaction occurs, resulting in decreased aggregation. Large porous particles based on a dipalmitoyl phosphatidylcholine (DPPC) combination as a dried powder inhaler preparation has revealed good characteristics for pulmonary delivery of peptides and proteins, such as parathyroid hormone, insulin, heparin, and human growth hormone. Moreover, in the presence of DPPC, the protein particles might have the potential for sustained release as an inhalant [14]. Among microparticles, hybrid large porous particles that have been prepared by the accumulation of nanoparticles using SD method are advantageous. The drug delivery and release patterns of nanoparticles combined with proper flow properties and aerosolization potential of large porous particles result in greater therapeutic effects of inhaled drugs [78].

Another clearance mechanism is the proteolytic enzymes present in the lung, which can degrade biomacromolecules by proteolysis. The addition of a protease inhibitor such as nafamostat, bacitracin, a trypsin inhibitor, chymostatin, leupeptin, bestatin, or aprotonin to the inhaled protein formulation may be useful for protecting proteins and leads to concentration enhancement [79,80]. When inhalable insulin was co-administered with nafamostat and bacitracin, its relative bioavailability increased, indicating that the proteins escaped from lung protease clearance [81,82].

4.1.2. Systemic Delivery

Besides local inhalation therapies, pulmonary delivery of calcitonin, parathyroid hormone, and insulin (Exubera® and Afrezza®) was developed for the treatment of osteoporosis, growth deficiency, and diabetes, respectively [71]. Systemic protein delivery through inhalation has been suggested to be a very promising alternative to parenteral delivery of proteins, and features the unique combination of a highly dispersed dosage form and an extended surface area to access the blood circulatory system [71]. Specific obstacles must be considered when a therapeutic protein is intended for systemic administration, because a sufficient proportion of drug molecule is required to be absorbed via the alveolar epithelium. For systemic administration of proteins, it is necessary to prevent degradation by blood clearance pathways, such as blood proteolytic enzymes, hepatic metabolism, and renal clearance to achieve an appropriate circulatory drug level leading to sufficient systemic bioavailability [14]. A major challenge to crossing the alveolar capillary membrane is the relative impermeability of the membrane to biomacromolecules. Macromolecule absorption through the double-layered phospholipid membrane by simple diffusion is limited by high molecular weight and hydrophilic nature of proteins. The absorption rates of macromolecules into the blood circulation are usually inversely related to molecular weight, with higher molecular weights leading to a higher T_{max} and lower C_{max} and partition coefficients [83]. There are some strategies to improve protein adsorption through the capillary membrane from the lungs into the blood. Absorption enhancers, such as surfactants, bile salts, cyclodextrins, citric acid, chitosan, and lipid-based carriers (liposomes), are suggested pathways to address the absorption issue [14].

4.2. Nasal Delivery

There is growing interest in the solid dosage forms of vaccines, which eliminate preservatives and the cold chain circulation for shipping and storage, while preserving protein stability at ambient temperature. Nasal delivery of vaccine formulations may be a good alternative to conventional vaccines [19]. Garmise et al. [84] demonstrated that an SFD powder of influenza virus increased local residence time and subsequently enhanced mucosal and systemic antibody production for nasal vaccination. Muco-adhesive compounds were characterized for their effects on the nasal residence time of vaccine powders in rats compared with in vitro data and stimulated immune responses. In vitro studies and in vivo imaging experiments revealed that sodium alginate and carboxy-methyl-cellulose powder combinations could enhance residence time in Brown Norway rats. It was concluded that nasal administration of dry powder influenza vaccine, especially in the presence of sodium alginate, could enhance serum and mucosal antibody responses. Furthermore, nasal delivery is an attractive vaccine platform for inoculating against other mucosal-transmitted diseases. Recently, Cho et al. [85] prepared a nasal powder formulation of salmon calcitonin (sCT) in the presence of a stabilizer (inulin or trehalose) and an absorption enhancer (chitosan, sodium taurocholate, or βCD) to improve its bioavailability. Dried powder inhalers of sCT were prepared by SD and novel SCF-assisted spray drying (SCF-SD). The in vivo absorption test in rats showed that spray-dried and SCF-spray-dried sCT powders increased the bioavailability of the peptide drug when compared with the nasal administration of unprocessed sCT, which was attributed to the absorption enhancer. Among the three absorption enhancers, chitosan-containing formulation showed the highest bioavailability, which was thought to be due to its properties of mucoadhesion or effects on tight junction to decrease mucociliary clearance. In addition, SCF-spray-dried sCT exhibited higher nasal absorption than spray-dried sCT in all formulations owing to the smaller size of particles. This study showed that SCF-SD method would be a promising approach for nasal delivery of dried powder inhaler of sCT.

4.3. Sustained-Release Delivery

Despite the high bioavailability of parenteral protein delivery, frequent injections result in poor patient compliance. Microsphere depot delivery system is designed to release the drug in a sustained manner over an extended period for systemic or local delivery. Spray freeze-dried BSA nanoparticles are encapsulated into PLGA microspheres to allow sustained release and to reduce the burst release pattern. The porous, solid protein particles break up into sub-micrometer particles followed by encapsulation into PLGA microspheres using anhydrous double emulsion techniques. In SFD, because of fast freezing and the absence of interfacial interactions, denaturation and aggregation of BSA were minimized, and the integrity and conformational stability of encapsulated BSA were preserved. The reduced burst release of BSA is attributed to the uniform distribution of protein nanoparticles in PLGA microspheres, which could be used as a sustainable delivery vehicle for biopharmaceuticals. Protein-PEG complexes are prepared by solubilizing BSA and recombinant human growth hormone (rhGH) in the methylene chloride phase. The organic phase containing PLGA and PEG/protein complexes was atomized through SD to prepare PLGA microparticles encapsulating proteins with good stability [86]. They exhibited sustained release profiles of BSA and rhGH and the released protein from the microsphere preserved their stability without aggregation. The protein microencapsulation method may prove to be a good platform for sustained delivery of therapeutic proteins that are not soluble in organic solvents. Cleland et al. [87] prepared PLGA microspheres containing recombinant human vascular endothelial growth factor (rhVEGF). The protein formulation was first sprayed into liquid nitrogen using an ultrasonic atomizer to produce rhVEGF PLGA microspheres. The SFD protein powder was added to a PLGA solution to prepare microspheres with a 9% *w*/*w* loading efficiency. SEC and mitogenic receptor-IgG binding affinity analyses showed that the stability and efficacy of rhVEGF were preserved through the SFD procedure. A study conducted by Al-Qadi et al. [88] presented a dried powder inhaler comprising microencapsulated insulin-loaded chitosan nanoparticles. The developed system was evaluated in rats to evaluate its potential for systemic delivery of insulin. The insulin-loaded chitosan nanoparticles were prepared by ionotropic gelation, followed by co-spray drying of nanoparticles with mannitol. Dried powder inhaler of insulin showed proper aerodynamic behavior for pulmonary delivery. The assessment of plasma glucose levels following intratracheal administration to rats showed that the microencapsulated insulin-loaded chitosan nanoparticles provided a sustained release of insulin with a more pronounced hypoglycemic effect than the insulin solution. This presents a good example of sustained release dried formulations for local or systemic delivery.

4.4. Enhancing Solubility and Bioavailability of Cyclosporine A

Cyclosporine A (CsA) is a cyclic undecapeptide drug used for the prevention of allograft rejection after lung transplantation [37]. As CsA has poor water-solubility, approaches to improve its solubility, bioavailability, and therapeutic efficacy have been designed. The solid dispersion of amorphous CsA in a methylcellulose-based matrix showed higher solubility than the physical mixture of the drug and methylcellulose. Additionally, an inhalable dry-emulsion preparation of CsA in the presence of glycerol monooleate as a surfactant showed better dissolution behavior and improved bioavailability compared with the native drug and its amorphous solid dispersion. The polymer-based amorphous solid dispersion of CsA as a dry powder inhaler revealed improved pharmacodynamic behavior as well as fewer side-effects [37]. Chiou et al. used a liquid impinging jet procedure to precipitate CsA nanoparticles with lecithin and lactose as stabilizing agents, followed by SD to produce nanoparticles for inhalation [89]. The aerosol performance of powders was evaluated using an Aeroliser® dry powder inhaler with multi-stage liquid impinging jets. Nanomatrix powders exhibited appropriate flow properties (with a fine particle fraction of approximately 55%) and corresponding aerosol behavior. They demonstrated that the combination of precipitation with SD procedure has the potential to allow the design of protein particles with improved pharmacokinetics. Yamasaki et al. demonstrated that inhalable CsA nanoparticles in a mannitol-based matrix improved the dissolution of the drug [90]. CsA nanosuspensions were prepared using anti-solvent precipitation and subsequently, the micro aggregates were achieved using an SD procedure. The combination of amorphous CsA and crystalline mannitol showed similar drug content to the theoretical doses. The inclusion of mannitol as a wetting agent improved the dissolution rate of the drug, without significant impact on aerosol performance.

This study indicated that the proper combination of drug and excipients could provide enhanced dissolution rate, with improved bioavailability of hydrophobic drugs, such as CsA.

4.5. Pharmacokinetics of Inhaled Insulins

In 2006, Exubera® (Pfizer Inc., New York, NY, USA; Nektar Therapeutics, San Carlos, CA, USA) became the first inhaled insulin preparation approved by the US Food and Drug Administration (FDA) and European Medicines Evaluation Agency (EMEA). The Exubera® device involves dispersion of insulin dry powder into aerosolized insulin within a large chamber, followed by patient inhalation. Exubera® was delivered in a dry powder formulation containing amorphous insulin, glycine, mannitol, and sodium citrate as stabilizers. The dry powder of matrix particles was prepared using an SD method. The resulting powder, with low moisture content, showed good storage stability at room temperature for two years [91]. The onset of action was more rapid (32 min vs. 48 min, respectively) for Exubera® than for subcutaneously injected (s.c.) insulin, and was comparable to lispro insulin. Furthermore, the duration of action of Exubera® was longer than the duration of lispro (387 min vs. 313 min) and comparable to s.c. insulin [92]. However, after one year of commercialization, Exubera® was withdrawn in 2007 because of its low bioavailability and enhanced treatment-related cost [92,93]. Some previous studies demonstrated the equivalence of Exubera® to regular s.c. insulin in both type I and type II diabetes patients [94,95].

Another inhaled insulin product Afrezza® (MannKind Corporation, Valencia, CA, USA) reached the market in 2014 and is currently the only inhaled insulin available in the market [91]. The formulation is based on Technosphere™ drug carrier technology, in which insulin is trapped and microencapsulated in small precipitated particles during self-assembly [96,97]. The precipitates are freeze-dried, but leaves small residual amounts of water [98]. Afrezza® is a drug–device product containing a Technosphere insulin (TI) inhalation powder in single-use dose cartridges, which are administered with an inhaler. The particle size is 2–3 μm, with an internal porosity of approximately 70%, and once inhaled, it dissolves in the pH-neutral environment of the deep lung and rapidly releases insulin into the systemic blood circulation. TI inhalers mimic rapid-acting s.c. insulin analogs with a C_{max} of 15 min [91,98]. Pfützner and Forst compared the pharmacokinetics of 100 IU of Afrezza®, 10 IU with regular s.c. insulin, and 5 IU of i.v. insulin in healthy subjects [96]. Afrezza® demonstrated very rapid absorption, with a mean T_{max} of 13 min vs. 121 min for regular s.c. insulin. In addition, Afrezza® provided significantly higher bioavailability and faster absorption than Exubera® (bioavailability relative to s.c. regular insulin of 26% and 10% respectively, and T_{max} of 13 min vs. 45 min). Afrezza® still presents a much greater bioavailability than any other inhaled insulin formulations introduced to date. The observed pharmacokinetic profile could be explained by the highly efficient delivery of Afrezza® particles to the deep lung (owing to the smaller particle size of Afrezza®). Because they are very small and porous, particles can be dissolved rapidly and provide high local concentrations of insulin that can be rapidly absorbed in the alveolae [98].

5. Future Perspectives and Conclusions

The development of therapeutic proteins has increased rapidly owing to their high therapeutic efficacy. Since the advent of human insulin in 1982, over hundreds of recombinant proteins have been developed and monoclonal antibody therapeutics market increased exponentially. Structurally modified proteins, such as PEGylated proteins and fusion proteins, and antibody-drug conjugate for cancer therapy have been recently available as therapeutics [99–101]. Biopharmaceuticals are available as liquid or solid dosage forms. In general, proteins have greater stability in the solid state than in the liquid state [33,41]. To achieve the desirable stability of proteins in formulations, solid-state dosage form is preferred to liquid-state dosage form, because it can provide a better shelf-life in storage. Numerous drying technologies, including FD, SD, SFD, and SCFD, have been used for dried protein formulations, and they have become an important method for the manufacture, storage, and delivery of protein-based biopharmaceuticals [14,25,26,37]. However, dried protein formulations still have challenges of stability and further optimization for desirable pharmacokinetic properties [3,83].

Currently, many dried protein powders have been produced through SD methods and other drying methods are still used only at the laboratory scale. In the future, drying methods at the laboratory scale must be scaled up for biopharmaceutical product development. Thus, modification of the existing drying technologies may be required. Achieving higher level of control of drying process parameters and performing under milder conditions may contribute to the improvement of stability and quality of biopharmaceuticals.

Dried powder inhaler preparations have mainly focused on local drug delivery systems for treating pulmonary diseases. However, these dosage forms also have a potential for systemic administration of therapeutic proteins, as demonstrated by the approved inhaled insulin products (Exubera® and Afrezza®) [91]. Inhalation delivery of proteins can be a good choice for systemic delivery of protein drugs because pulmonary administration generally leads to higher bioavailability of protein drugs than other nonparenteral administrations, such as nasal or transdermal delivery [14]. Pulmonary route leads to rapid drug absorption owing to large surface area, low thickness of the epithelium, and rich blood supply, and avoids hepatic first-pass metabolism [83].

Since the development of pulmonary protein administration has shown significant progress, it can be predicted that soon the inhalation of proteins may become the first practical alternative to parenteral delivery. Clinical trials, as well as experimental studies have demonstrated that insulin as an inhaler possesses similar pharmacokinetic properties to that of s.c. injection of regular insulin, and even better properties than those observed with s.c. administration of rapid-acting insulin analogs. Substitution of injection with inhalation would be preferred by patients. However, there is no improvement with respective developments. If inhaled insulin becomes successful for diabetic therapy in terms of bioavailability and treatment cost, it will most probably create opportunities for the use of other biopharmaceuticals as inhalation preparations. Recently, other proteins and peptides have been studied for treating diabetes through the pulmonary route [100,102]. The major concerns regarding the long-term application of protein inhalers, such as insulin, are the development of insulin-antibodies and lung safety issues, which should be considered in future studies. Additionally, there are not sufficient studies considering the economic aspects of healthcare systems.

In conclusion, the successful solid dosage form of protein formulations in the presence of stabilizing agents could be achieved using several drying technologies. Cryoprotectants and lyoprotectants can maintain the stability and bioactivity of biopharmaceuticals. In each drying method, critical process parameters should first be optimized. Finally, screening of formulations based on protein properties is performed to determine the optimal stable protein/stabilizer combinations for a sustained-release, pulmonary, or nasal formulation.

Author Contributions: F.E. wrote the paper as the primary author. E.J.P. contributed to part of the text. D.H.N. and A.V. conceived the design of the article, supervised its writing, and had editorial responsibility. All the authors approved the final manuscript.

Acknowledgments: This work was supported by the National Research Foundation of Korea (NRF) grants funded by the Ministry of Science and ICT (NRF-2018R1A2B3004266) and by the Technology Innovation Program (20000265, Stabilization platform of high concentration and stable liquid injection based on physical properties of biomaterials) funded by the Ministry of Trade, Industry & Energy (MOTIE, Korea).

References

1. Ajmera, A.; Scherliess, R. Stabilisation of proteins via mixtures of amino acids during spray drying. *Int. J. Pharm.* **2014**, *463*, 98–107. [CrossRef] [PubMed]
2. Ramezani, V.; Vatanara, A.; Najafabadi, A.R.; Shokrgozar, M.A.; Khabiri, A.; Seyedabadi, M. A comparative study on the physicochemical and biological stability of IgG 1 and monoclonal antibodies during spray drying process. *DARU J. Pharm. Sci.* **2014**, *22*, 31. [CrossRef] [PubMed]
3. Cicerone, M.T.; Pikal, M.J.; Qian, K.K. Stabilization of proteins in solid form. *Adv. Drug Deliv. Rev.* **2015**, *93*, 14–24. [CrossRef] [PubMed]

4. Daugherty, A.L.; Mrsny, R.J. Formulation and delivery issues for monoclonal antibody therapeutics. *Adv. Drug Deliv. Rev.* **2006**, *58*, 686–706. [CrossRef] [PubMed]
5. Kumar, V.; Sharma, V.K.; Kalonia, D.S. In situ precipitation and vacuum drying of interferon alpha-2a: Development of a single-step process for obtaining dry, stable protein formulation. *Int. J. Pharm.* **2009**, *366*, 88–98. [CrossRef] [PubMed]
6. Na, D.H.; Youn, Y.S.; Lee, I.B.; Park, E.J.; Park, C.J.; Lee, K.C. Effect of molecular size of pegylated recombinant human epidermal growth factor on the biological activity and stability in rat wound tissue. *Pharm. Dev. Technol.* **2006**, *11*, 513–519. [CrossRef] [PubMed]
7. Lee, W.; Park, E.J.; Kwak, S.; Lee, K.C.; Na, D.H.; Bae, J.-S. Trimeric peg-conjugated exendin-4 for the treatment of sepsis. *Biomacromolecules* **2016**, *17*, 1160–1169. [CrossRef] [PubMed]
8. Park, E.J.; Tak, T.H.; Na, D.H.; Lee, K.C. Effect of PEGylation on stability of peptide in poly(lactide-*co*-glycolide) microispheres. *Arch. Pharm. Res.* **2010**, *33*, 1111–1116. [CrossRef] [PubMed]
9. Na, D.H.; DeLuca, P.P. PEGylation of octreotide: I. Separation of positional isomers and stability against acylation by poly(D,L-lactide-*co*-gycolide). *Pharm. Res.* **2005**, *22*, 736–742. [CrossRef] [PubMed]
10. Kim, Y.; Park, E.J.; Na, D.H. Recent progress in dendrimer-based nanomedicine. *Arch. Pharm. Res.* **2018**, *41*, 571–582. [CrossRef] [PubMed]
11. Szlachcic, A.; Zakrzewska, M.; Otlewski, J. Longer action means better drug: Tuning up protein therapeutics. *Biotechnol. Adv.* **2011**, *29*, 436–441. [CrossRef] [PubMed]
12. Mohtashamian, S.; Boddohi, S. Nanostructured polysaccharide-based carriers for antimicrobial peptide delivery. *J. Pharm. Investig.* **2017**, *47*, 85–94. [CrossRef]
13. Kim, C.H.; Lee, S.G.; Kang, M.J.; Lee, S.; Choi, Y.W. Surface modification of lipid-based nanocarriers for cancer cell-specific drug targeting. *J. Pharm. Investig.* **2017**, *47*, 203–227. [CrossRef]
14. Depreter, F.; Pilcer, G.; Amighi, K. Inhaled proteins: Challenges and perspectives. *Int. J. Pharm.* **2013**, *447*, 251–280. [CrossRef] [PubMed]
15. Maltesen, M.J.; Van De Weert, M. Drying methods for protein pharmaceuticals. *Drug Discov. Today Technol.* **2008**, *5*, e81–e88. [CrossRef] [PubMed]
16. Smales, C.M.; James, D.C. *Therapeutic Proteins: Methods and Protocols*; Springer: Berlin, Germany, 2005; Volume 308.
17. Liao, Y.H.; Brown, M.B.; Martin, G.P. Investigation of the stabilisation of freeze-dried lysozyme and the physical properties of the formulations. *Eur. J. Pharm. Biopharm.* **2004**, *58*, 15–24. [CrossRef] [PubMed]
18. Tian, F.; Sane, S.; Rytting, J.H. Calorimetric investigation of protein/amino acid interactions in the solid state. *Int. J. Pharm.* **2006**, *310*, 175–186. [CrossRef] [PubMed]
19. Wang, S.H.; Kirwan, S.M.; Abraham, S.N.; Staats, H.F.; Hickey, A.J. Stable dry powder formulation for nasal delivery of anthrax vaccine. *J. Pharm. Sci.* **2012**, *101*, 31–47. [CrossRef] [PubMed]
20. Mensink, M.A.; Frijlink, H.W.; van der Voort Maarschalk, K.; Hinrichs, W.L. How sugars protect proteins in the solid state and during drying (review): Mechanisms of stabilization in relation to stress conditions. *Eur. J. Pharm. Biopharm.* **2017**, *114*, 288–295. [CrossRef] [PubMed]
21. Maa, Y.-F.; Nguyen, P.-A.; Sweeney, T.; Shire, S.J.; Hsu, C.C. Protein inhalation powders: Spray drying vs. spray freeze drying. *Pharm. Res.* **1999**, *16*, 249–254. [CrossRef] [PubMed]
22. Nuchuchua, O.; Every, H.A.; Hofland, G.W.; Jiskoot, W. Scalable organic solvent free supercritical fluid spray drying process for producing dry protein formulations. *Eur. J. Pharm. Biopharm.* **2014**, *88*, 919–930. [CrossRef] [PubMed]
23. Walters, R.H.; Bhatnagar, B.; Tchessalov, S.; Izutsu, K.; Tsumoto, K.; Ohtake, S. Next generation drying technologies for pharmaceutical applications. *J. Pharm. Sci.* **2014**, *103*, 2673–2695. [CrossRef] [PubMed]
24. Weers, J.G.; Miller, D.P. Formulation design of dry powders for inhalation. *J. Pharm. Sci.* **2015**, *104*, 3259–3288. [CrossRef] [PubMed]
25. Langford, A.; Bhatnagar, B.; Walters, R.; Tchessalov, S.; Ohtake, S. Drying of biopharmaceuticals: Recent developments, new technologies and future direction. *Jpn. J. Food Eng.* **2018**, *19*, 15–24.
26. Langford, A.; Bhatnagar, B.; Walters, R.; Tchessalov, S.; Ohtake, S. Drying technologies for biopharmaceutical applications: Recent developments and future direction. *Dry. Technol.* **2018**, *36*, 677–684. [CrossRef]
27. Abdul-Fattah, A.M.; Kalonia, D.S.; Pikal, M.J. The challenge of drying method selection for protein pharmaceuticals: Product quality implications. *J. Pharm. Sci.* **2007**, *96*, 1886–1916. [CrossRef] [PubMed]

28. Guerrero, M.; Albet, C.; Palomer, A.; Guglietta, A. Drying in pharmaceutical and biotechnological industries. *Food Sci. Technol. Int.* **2003**, *9*, 237–243. [CrossRef]
29. Shukla, S. Freeze drying process: A review. *Int. J. Pharm. Sci. Res.* **2011**, *2*, 3061.
30. Faghihi, H.; Khalili, F.; Amini, M.; Vatanara, A. The effect of freeze-dried antibody concentrations on its stability in the presence of trehalose and hydroxypropyl-β-cyclodextrin: A box–behnken statistical design. *Pharm. Dev. Technol.* **2017**, *22*, 724–732. [CrossRef] [PubMed]
31. Roy, I.; Gupta, M.N. Freeze-drying of proteins: Some emerging concerns. *Biotechnol. Appl. Biochem.* **2004**, *39*, 165–177. [CrossRef] [PubMed]
32. Tang, X.; Pikal, M.J. Design of freeze-drying processes for pharmaceuticals: Practical advice. *Pharm. Res.* **2004**, *21*, 191–200. [CrossRef] [PubMed]
33. Lim, J.Y.; Kim, N.A.; Lim, D.G.; Kim, K.H.; Choi, D.H.; Jeong, S.H. Process cycle development of freeze drying for therapeutic proteins with stability evaluation. *J. Pharm. Investig.* **2016**, *46*, 519–536. [CrossRef]
34. Pieters, S.; De Beer, T.; Kasper, J.C.; Boulpaep, D.; Waszkiewicz, O.; Goodarzi, M.; Tistaert, C.; Friess, W.; Remon, J.P.; Vervaet, C.; et al. Near-infrared spectroscopy for in-line monitoring of protein unfolding and its interactions with lyoprotectants during freeze-drying. *Anal. Chem.* **2012**, *84*, 947–955. [CrossRef] [PubMed]
35. Oetjen, G.W. *Freeze-Drying*; Wiley: Hoboken, NJ, USA, 2004.
36. Costantino, H.R.; Firouzabadian, L.; Wu, C.; Carrasquillo, K.G.; Griebenow, K.; Zale, S.E.; Tracy, M.A. Protein spray freeze drying. 2. Effect of formulation variables on particle size and stability. *J. Pharm. Sci.* **2002**, *91*, 388–395. [CrossRef] [PubMed]
37. Chen, L.; Okuda, T.; Lu, X.-Y.; Chan, H.-K. Amorphous powders for inhalation drug delivery. *Adv. Drug Deliv. Rev.* **2016**, *100*, 102–115. [CrossRef] [PubMed]
38. Tonnis, W.; Mensink, M.; De Jager, A.; Van Der Voort Maarschalk, K.; Frijlink, H.; Hinrichs, W. Size and molecular flexibility of sugars determine the storage stability of freeze-dried proteins. *Mol. Pharm.* **2015**, *12*, 684–694. [CrossRef] [PubMed]
39. Pilcer, G.; Amighi, K. Formulation strategy and use of excipients in pulmonary drug delivery. *Int. J. Pharm.* **2010**, *392*, 1–19. [CrossRef] [PubMed]
40. Sosnik, A.; Seremeta, K.P. Advantages and challenges of the spray-drying technology for the production of pure drug particles and drug-loaded polymeric carriers. *Adv. Colloid Interface Sci.* **2015**, *223*, 40–54. [CrossRef] [PubMed]
41. Ameri, M.; Maa, Y.-F. Spray drying of biopharmaceuticals: Stability and process considerations. *Dry. Technol.* **2006**, *24*, 763–768. [CrossRef]
42. Faghihi, H.; Vatanara, A.; Najafabadi, A.R.; Ramezani, V.; Gilani, K. The use of amino acids to prepare physically and conformationally stable spray-dried IgG with enhanced aerosol performance. *Int. J. Pharm.* **2014**, *466*, 163–171. [CrossRef] [PubMed]
43. Maa, Y.-F.; Sellers, S.P. Solid-state protein formulation. In *Therapeutic Proteins Methods Protocols*; Humana Press: New York, NY, USA, 2005; pp. 265–285.
44. Poursina, N.; Vatanara, A.; Rouini, M.R.; Gilani, K.; Rouholamini Najafabadi, A. Systemic delivery of parathyroid hormone (1–34) using spray freeze-dried inhalable particles. *Pharm. Dev. Technol.* **2017**, *22*, 733–739. [CrossRef] [PubMed]
45. Ramezani, V.; Vatanara, A.; Najafabadi, A.R.; Gilani, K.; Nabi-Meybodi, M. Screening and evaluation of variables in the formation of antibody particles by spray drying. *Powder Technol.* **2013**, *233*, 341–346. [CrossRef]
46. Vehring, R. Pharmaceutical particle engineering via spray drying. *Pharm. Res.* **2008**, *25*, 999–1022. [CrossRef] [PubMed]
47. Schüle, S.; Frieß, W.; Bechtold-Peters, K.; Garidel, P. Conformational analysis of protein secondary structure during spray-drying of antibody/mannitol formulations. *Eur. J. Pharm. Biopharm.* **2007**, *65*, 1–9. [CrossRef] [PubMed]
48. Li, H.Y.; Song, X.; Seville, P.C. The use of sodium carboxymethylcellulose in the preparation of spray-dried proteins for pulmonary drug delivery. *Eur. J. Pharm. Sci.* **2010**, *40*, 56–61. [CrossRef] [PubMed]
49. Wanning, S.; Suverkrup, R.; Lamprecht, A. Jet-vortex spray freeze drying for the production of inhalable lyophilisate powders. *Eur. J. Pharm. Sci.* **2017**, *96*, 1–7. [CrossRef] [PubMed]
50. Wanning, S.; Süverkrüp, R.; Lamprecht, A. Pharmaceutical spray freeze drying. *Int. J. Pharm.* **2015**, *488*, 136–153. [CrossRef] [PubMed]

51. Rogers, T.L.; Johnston, K.P.; Williams, R.O., 3rd. Solution-based particle formation of pharmaceutical powders by supercritical or compressed fluid CO_2 and cryogenic spray-freezing technologies. *Drug Dev. Ind. Pharm.* **2001**, *27*, 1003–1015. [CrossRef] [PubMed]
52. Emami, F.; Vatanara, A.; Najafabadi, A.R.; Kim, Y.; Park, E.J.; Sardari, S.; Na, D.H. Effect of amino acids on the stability of spray freeze-dried immunoglobulin G in sugar-based matrices. *Eur. J. Pharm. Sci.* **2018**, *119*, 39–48. [CrossRef] [PubMed]
53. Poursina, N.; Vatanara, A.; Rouini, M.R.; Gilani, K.; Najafabadi, A.R. The effect of excipients on the stability and aerosol performance of salmon calcitonin dry powder inhalers prepared via spray freeze drying process. *Acta Pharm.* **2016**, *66*, 207–218. [CrossRef] [PubMed]
54. Rahmati, M.R.; Vatanara, A.; Parsian, A.R.; Gilani, K.; Khosravi, K.M.; Darabi, M.; Najafabadi, A.R. Effect of formulation ingredients on the physical characteristics of salmeterol xinafoate microparticles tailored by spray freeze drying. *Adv. Powder Technol.* **2013**, *24*, 36–42. [CrossRef]
55. Parsian, A.R.; Vatanara, A.; Rahmati, M.R.; Gilani, K.; Khosravi, K.M.; Najafabadi, A.R. Inhalable budesonide porous microparticles tailored by spray freeze drying technique. *Powder Technol.* **2014**, *260*, 36–41. [CrossRef]
56. Rogers, T.L.; Nelsen, A.C.; Hu, J.; Brown, J.N.; Sarkari, M.; Young, T.J.; Johnston, K.P.; Williams, R.O. A novel particle engineering technology to enhance dissolution of poorly water soluble drugs: Spray-freezing into liquid. *Eur. J. Pharm. Biopharm.* **2002**, *54*, 271–280. [CrossRef]
57. Rogers, T.L.; Hu, J.; Yu, Z.; Johnston, K.P.; Williams, R.O. A novel particle engineering technology: Spray-freezing into liquid. *Int. J. Pharm.* **2002**, *242*, 93–100. [CrossRef]
58. Maa, Y.F.; Ameri, M.; Shu, C.; Payne, L.G.; Chen, D. Influenza vaccine powder formulation development: Spray-freeze-drying and stability evaluation. *J. Pharm. Sci.* **2004**, *93*, 1912–1923. [CrossRef] [PubMed]
59. Jovanovic, N.; Bouchard, A.; Sutter, M.; Van Speybroeck, M.; Hofland, G.W.; Witkamp, G.J.; Crommelin, D.J.; Jiskoot, W. Stable sugar-based protein formulations by supercritical fluid drying. *Int. J. Pharm.* **2008**, *346*, 102–108. [CrossRef] [PubMed]
60. Jovanović, N.; Bouchard, A.; Hofland, G.W.; Witkamp, G.-J.; Crommelin, D.J.; Jiskoot, W. Stabilization of proteins in dry powder formulations using supercritical fluid technology. *Pharm. Res.* **2004**, *21*, 1955–1969. [CrossRef] [PubMed]
61. Garidel, P.; Pevestorf, B.; Bahrenburg, S. Stability of buffer-free freeze-dried formulations: A feasibility study of a monoclonal antibody at high protein concentrations. *Eur. J. Pharm. Biopharm.* **2015**, *97*, 125–139. [CrossRef] [PubMed]
62. Mohammad Zadeh, A.H.; Rouholamini Najafabadi, A.; Vatanara, A.; Faghihi, H.; Gilani, K. Effect of molecular weight and ratio of poly ethylene glycols' derivatives in combination with trehalose on stability of freeze-dried IgG. *Drug Dev. Ind. Pharm.* **2017**, *43*, 1945–1951. [CrossRef] [PubMed]
63. Imamura, K.; Ogawa, T.; Sakiyama, T.; Nakanishi, K. Effects of types of sugar on the stabilization of protein in the dried state. *J. Pharm. Sci.* **2003**, *92*, 266–274. [CrossRef] [PubMed]
64. Saluja, V.; Amorij, J.P.; Kapteyn, J.C.; de Boer, A.H.; Frijlink, H.W.; Hinrichs, W.L. A comparison between spray drying and spray freeze drying to produce an influenza subunit vaccine powder for inhalation. *J. Control. Release* **2010**, *144*, 127–133. [CrossRef] [PubMed]
65. Bittner, B.; Morlock, M.; Koll, H.; Winter, G.; Kissel, T. Recombinant human erythropoietin (rhEPO) loaded poly (lactide-*co*-glycolide) microspheres: Influence of the encapsulation technique and polymer purity on microsphere characteristics. *Eur. J. Pharm. Biopharm.* **1998**, *45*, 295–305. [CrossRef]
66. Jovanovic, N.; Bouchard, A.; Hofland, G.W.; Witkamp, G.J.; Crommelin, D.J.; Jiskoot, W. Stabilization of IgG by supercritical fluid drying: Optimization of formulation and process parameters. *Eur. J. Pharm. Biopharm.* **2008**, *68*, 183–190. [CrossRef] [PubMed]
67. Jovanovic, N.; Bouchard, A.; Hofland, G.W.; Witkamp, G.J.; Crommelin, D.J.; Jiskoot, W. Distinct effects of sucrose and trehalose on protein stability during supercritical fluid drying and freeze-drying. *Eur. J. Pharm. Sci.* **2006**, *27*, 336–345. [CrossRef] [PubMed]
68. Amidi, M.; Pellikaan, H.C.; de Boer, A.H.; Crommelin, D.J.; Hennink, W.E.; Jiskoot, W. Preparation and physicochemical characterization of supercritically dried insulin-loaded microparticles for pulmonary delivery. *Eur. J. Pharm. Biopharm.* **2008**, *68*, 191–200. [CrossRef] [PubMed]
69. Ali, M.E.; Lamprecht, A. Spray freeze drying for dry powder inhalation of nanoparticles. *Eur. J. Pharm. Biopharm.* **2014**, *87*, 510–517. [CrossRef] [PubMed]

70. Mueannoom, W.; Srisongphan, A.; Taylor, K.M.; Hauschild, S.; Gaisford, S. Thermal ink-jet spray freeze-drying for preparation of excipient-free salbutamol sulphate for inhalation. *Eur. J. Pharm. Biopharm.* **2012**, *80*, 149–155. [CrossRef] [PubMed]
71. Filipe, V.; Hawe, A.; Carpenter, J.F.; Jiskoot, W. Analytical approaches to assess the degradation of therapeutic proteins. *TrAC Trends Anal. Chem.* **2013**, *49*, 118–125. [CrossRef]
72. Song, J.G.; Lee, S.H.; Han, H.-K. The stabilization of biopharmaceuticals: Current understanding and future perspectives. *J. Pharm. Investig.* **2017**, *47*, 475–496. [CrossRef]
73. Wang, W.; Singh, S.; Zeng, D.L.; King, K.; Nema, S. Antibody structure, instability, and formulation. *J. Pharm. Sci.* **2007**, *96*, 1–26. [CrossRef] [PubMed]
74. Chang, L.L.; Pikal, M.J. Mechanisms of protein stabilization in the solid state. *J. Pharm. Sci.* **2009**, *98*, 2886–2908. [CrossRef] [PubMed]
75. Hertel, S.P.; Winter, G.; Friess, W. Protein stability in pulmonary drug delivery via nebulization. *Adv. Drug Deliv. Rev.* **2015**, *93*, 79–94. [CrossRef] [PubMed]
76. Grenha, A.; Remuñán-López, C.; Carvalho, E.L.; Seijo, B. Microspheres containing lipid/chitosan nanoparticles complexes for pulmonary delivery of therapeutic proteins. *Eur. J. Pharm. Biopharm.* **2008**, *69*, 83–93. [CrossRef] [PubMed]
77. Edwards, D.A.; Hanes, J.; Caponetti, G.; Hrkach, J.; Ben-Jebria, A.; Eskew, M.L.; Mintzes, J.; Deaver, D.; Lotan, N.; Langer, R. Large porous particles for pulmonary drug delivery. *Science* **1997**, *276*, 1868–1872. [CrossRef] [PubMed]
78. Tsapis, N.; Bennett, D.; Jackson, B.; Weitz, D.A.; Edwards, D. Trojan particles: Large porous carriers of nanoparticles for drug delivery. *Proc. Natl. Acad. Sci. USA* **2002**, *99*, 12001–12005. [CrossRef] [PubMed]
79. Hussain, A.; Arnold, J.J.; Khan, M.A.; Ahsan, F. Absorption enhancers in pulmonary protein delivery. *J. Control. Release* **2004**, *94*, 15–24. [CrossRef] [PubMed]
80. Siekmeier, R.; Scheuch, G. Treatment of systemic diseases by inhalation of biomolecule aerosols. *J. Physiol. Pharmacol.* **2009**, *60*, 15–26. [PubMed]
81. Okumura, K.; Iwakawa, S.; Yoshida, T.; Seki, T.; Komada, F. Intratracheal delivery of insulin absorption from solution and aerosol by rat lung. *Int. J. Pharm.* **1992**, *88*, 63–73. [CrossRef]
82. Todo, H.; Okamoto, H.; Iida, K.; Danjo, K. Improvement of stability and absorbability of dry insulin powder for inhalation by powder-combination technique. *Int. J. Pharm.* **2004**, *271*, 41–52. [CrossRef] [PubMed]
83. Hu, X.; Yang, F.F.; Liao, Y.H. Pharmacokinetic Considerations of inhaled pharmaceuticals for systemic delivery. *Curr. Pharm. Des.* **2016**, *22*, 2532–2548. [CrossRef] [PubMed]
84. Garmise, R.J.; Staats, H.F.; Hickey, A.J. Novel dry powder preparations of whole inactivated influenza virus for nasal vaccination. *AAPS PharmSciTech* **2007**, *8*, 2–10. [CrossRef] [PubMed]
85. Cho, W.; Kim, M.-S.; Jung, M.-S.; Park, J.; Cha, K.-H.; Kim, J.-S.; Park, H.J.; Alhalaweh, A.; Velaga, S.P.; Hwang, S.-J. Design of salmon calcitonin particles for nasal delivery using spray-drying and novel supercritical fluid-assisted spray-drying processes. *Int. J. Pharm.* **2015**, *478*, 288–296. [CrossRef] [PubMed]
86. Mok, H.; Park, T.G. Water-free microencapsulation of proteins within PLGA microparticles by spray drying using PEG-assisted protein solubilization technique in organic solvent. *Eur. J. Pharm. Biopharm.* **2008**, *70*, 137–144. [CrossRef] [PubMed]
87. Cleland, J.L.; Duenas, E.T.; Park, A.; Daugherty, A.; Kahn, J.; Kowalski, J.; Cuthbertson, A. Development of poly-(D,L-lactide-coglycolide) microsphere formulations containing recombinant human vascular endothelial growth factor to promote local angiogenesis. *J. Control. Release* **2001**, *72*, 13–24. [CrossRef]
88. Al-Qadi, S.; Grenha, A.; Carrión-Recio, D.; Seijo, B.; Remuñán-López, C. Microencapsulated chitosan nanoparticles for pulmonary protein delivery: In vivo evaluation of insulin-loaded formulations. *J. Control. Release* **2012**, *157*, 383–390. [CrossRef] [PubMed]
89. Chiou, H.; Chan, H.-K.; Heng, D.; Prud'homme, R.K.; Raper, J.A. A novel production method for inhalable cyclosporine a powders by confined liquid impinging jet precipitation. *J. Aerosol Sci.* **2008**, *39*, 500–509. [CrossRef]
90. Yamasaki, K.; Kwok, P.C.L.; Fukushige, K.; Prud'homme, R.K.; Chan, H.-K. Enhanced dissolution of inhalable cyclosporine nano-matrix particles with mannitol as matrix former. *Int. J. Pharm.* **2011**, *420*, 34–42. [CrossRef] [PubMed]
91. Cavaiola, T.S.; Edelman, S. Inhaled insulin: A breath of fresh air? A review of inhaled insulin. *Clin. Ther.* **2014**, *36*, 1275–1289. [CrossRef] [PubMed]

92. Rave, K.; Bott, S.; Heinemann, L.; Sha, S.; Becker, R.H.; Willavize, S.A.; Heise, T. Time-action profile of inhaled insulin in comparison with subcutaneously injected insulin lispro and regular human insulin. *Diabetes Care* **2005**, *28*, 1077–1082. [CrossRef] [PubMed]
93. Bailey, C.J.; Barnett, A.H. Inhaled insulin: New formulation, new trial. *Lancet* **2010**, *375*, 2199–2201. [CrossRef]
94. Quattrin, T.; Bélanger, A.; Bohannon, N.J.; Schwartz, S.L. Efficacy and safety of inhaled insulin (Exubera) compared with subcutaneous insulin therapy in patients with type 1 diabetes: Results of a 6-month, randomized, comparative trial. *Diabetes Care* **2004**, *27*, 2622–2627. [CrossRef] [PubMed]
95. Skyler, J.S.; Weinstock, R.S.; Raskin, P.; Yale, J.-F.; Barrett, E.; Gerich, J.E.; Gerstein, H.C. Use of inhaled insulin in a basal/bolus insulin regimen in type 1 diabetic subjects: A 6-month, randomized, comparative trial. *Diabetes Care* **2005**, *28*, 1630–1635. [CrossRef] [PubMed]
96. Pfützner, A.; Forst, T. Pulmonary insulin delivery by means of the technosphere™ drug carrier mechanism. *Expert Opin. Drug Deliv.* **2005**, *2*, 1097–1106. [CrossRef] [PubMed]
97. Cassidy, J.P.; Amin, N.; Marino, M.; Gotfried, M.; Meyer, T.; Sommerer, K.; Baughman, R.A. Insulin lung deposition and clearance following technosphere® insulin inhalation powder administration. *Pharm. Res.* **2011**, *28*, 2157–2164. [CrossRef] [PubMed]
98. Angelo, R.; Rousseau, K.; Grant, M.; Leone-Bay, A.; Richardson, P. Technosphere® insulin: Defining the role of technosphere particles at the cellular level. *J. Diabetes Sci. Technol.* **2009**, *3*, 545–554. [CrossRef] [PubMed]
99. Swierczewska, M.; Lee, K.C.; Lee, S. What is the future of PEGylated therapies? *Expert Opin. Emerg. Drugs* **2015**, *20*, 531–536. [CrossRef] [PubMed]
100. Park, E.J.; Lim, S.M.; Lee, K.C.; Na, D.H. Exendins and exendin analogs for diabetic therapy: A patent review (2012–2015). *Expert Opin. Ther. Pat.* **2016**, *26*, 833–842. [CrossRef] [PubMed]
101. Kim, Y.; Park, E.J.; Na, D.H. Antibody-drug conjugates for targeted anticancer drug delivery. *J. Pharm. Investig.* **2016**, *46*, 341–349. [CrossRef]
102. Li, X.; Huang, Y.; Huang, Z.; Ma, X.; Dong, N.; Chen, W.; Pan, X.; Wu, C. Enhancing stability of exenatide-containing pressurized metered-dose inhaler via reverse microemulsion system. *AAPS PharmSciTech* **2018**, *19*, 2499–2508. [CrossRef] [PubMed]

4

Species Differences in Stereoselective Pharmacokinetics of HSG4112: A New Anti-Obesity Agent

In Yong Bae [1,†], Min Sun Choi [1,†], Young Seok Ji [1], Sang-Ku Yoo [2], Kyungil Kim [2] and Hye Hyun Yoo [1,*]

1 Institute of Pharmaceutical Science and Technology and College of Pharmacy, Hanyang University, Ansan, Gyeonggi-do 15588, Korea; iybae722@naver.com (I.Y.B.); chm2456@hanyang.ac.kr (M.S.C.); wldudtjr23@hanyang.ac.kr (Y.S.J.)

2 Glaceum Inc., Yeongtong-gu, Suwon, Gyeonggi-do 16675, Korea; skyoo@glaceum.com (S.-K.Y.); kikim@glaceum.com (K.K.)

* Correspondence: yoohh@hanyang.ac.kr

† These authors contributed equally to this work.

Abstract: HSG4112, a racemic drug, is a new anti-obesity agent. In this study, the stereoselective pharmacokinetics of HSG4112 were investigated in rats and dogs, and the underlying mechanism was investigated. The plasma concentrations of HSG4112(S) and HSG4112(R) were quantitated in plasma from rats and beagle dogs after IV and/or oral administration of racemic HSG4112. The concentration of HSG4112(S) was significantly higher than that of HSG4112(R) in rat plasma. Contrarily, the concentration of HSG4112(R) was significantly higher than HSG4112(S) in dog plasma. A metabolic stability test with liver microsomes showed that HSG4112(S) was more stable than HSG4112(R) in rat liver microsomes, but the difference between stereoisomers did not appear in dog liver microsomes. However, the stereoselectivity was observed in dog liver and intestinal microsomes after uridine 5′-diphospho-glucuronic acid was added. Thus, stereoselective metabolism by uridine 5′-diphospho-glucuronosyltransferases is mainly responsible for the stereoselective pharmacokinetics in dogs. These results suggest that the species difference in the stereoselective plasma pharmacokinetics of HSG4112 is due to the stereoselective metabolism.

Keywords: HSG4112; anti-obesity agent; stereoselectivity; pharmacokinetics

---

1. Introduction

HSG4112 is a new drug candidate which has been developed as a treatment for obesity. Its chemical structure is derived from glabridin. Glabridin is an isoflavane, which is found in *Glycyrrhiza glabra* extract [1–3]. It is known to have whitening activity by suppressing the activity of tyrosinase during the synthesis of melanin and to help alleviate gastroenteric disorders. Recently, it was confirmed that glabridin is effective in metabolic syndromes, including hyperlipidemia, fatty liver, impaired glucose metabolism, diabetes, and obesity and has anti-inflammatory actions, anticancer actions, and the like [4]. However, in spite of useful medicinal efficacy, glabridin is easily broken down by sunlight, moisture, acidity, basicity, oxygen, heat, and the like due to low chemical stability, so it is very difficult to develop a product actually utilizing glabridin [4]. For these reasons, we synthesized a new pyranochromenylphenol derivative, HSG4112, by modifying the structure of glabridin. HSG4112 is stable under various physical conditions, while maintaining or improving its medicinal efficacy [4]. HSG4112 is a racemic compound with a chiral carbon. Thus, glabridin has the structure of R-enantiomer whereas HSG4112 is a mixture of S and R enantiomers (Figure 1).

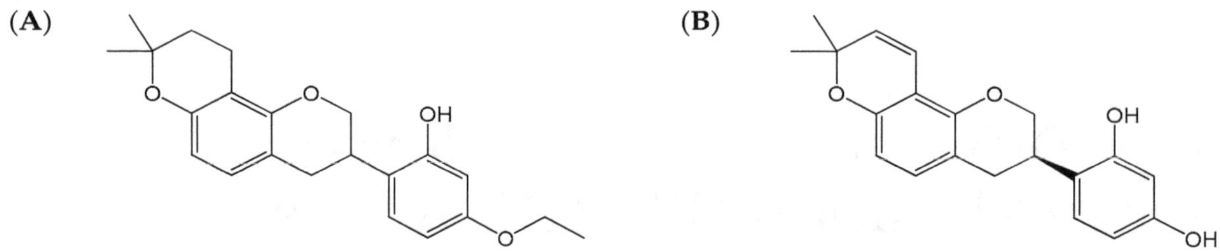

Figure 1. Chemical structures of (**A**) HSG4112 and (**B**) glabridin.

In many cases with chiral drugs, one of the two enantiomers is active and the other is either non-active or even harmful [5–7]. This is because the interaction between a drug molecule and its target is dependent on its three-dimensional environment. The most famous example is thalidomide, which was sold in the 1950s; the drug was introduced as a racemic mixture for use as a sedative but was later withdrawn from the market following the occurrence of birth defects in the children of mothers who took it to treat morning sickness. It was later found that the inactive enantiomer was the cause of the teratogenicity. This disaster was a driving force behind the requirement to strictly test drugs before making them available to the public [8]. In particular, for racemate candidates, both enantiomers should be studied separately as early as possible to assess the relevance of stereoisomerism to effects and fate. Accordingly, a pharmacokinetic evaluation should be provided for each enantiomer [9,10].

In this study, the stereoselective pharmacokinetics of HSG4112 were investigated in rats and beagle dogs. In addition, the metabolic stability was investigated in liver and intestinal microsomes from five different species (rat, mouse, dog, monkey, and human) to evaluate the role of metabolism in the species differences in its stereoselective pharmacokinetic behavior.

2. Materials and Methods

2.1. Chemicals and Materials

HSG4112(S) and HSG4112(R) were given from Glaceum Incorporation (Suwon, Korea). Pooled rat liver microsome (RLM), mouse liver microsome (MLM), dog liver microsome (DLM), and human liver microsome (HLM) were obtained from Gentest (Woburn, MA, USA). Pooled rat intestinal microsome (RIM), mouse intestinal microsome (MIM), dog intestinal microsome (DIM), and human intestinal microsome (HIM) were obtained from Sekisui Xenotech (Kansas City, KS, USA). Glucose 6-phosphate, β-NADP+, glucose 6-phosphate dehydrogenase and alamethicin were obtained from Sigma-Aldrich (St. Louis, MO, USA). HPLC-grade acetonitrile (ACN) and formic acid were purchased from J.T. Baker (Phillipsburg, NJ, USA). Distilled water (DW) was prepared using a Milli-Q purification system (Millipore, Bedford, MA, USA).

2.2. Preparation of Calibration and Quality Control (QC) Standards

HSG4112(S) 10 mg, HSG4112(R) 10 mg, and HSG4112-d5 (internal standard; IS) 5 mg were weighted and transferred to a 10 mL volumetric flask and ACN was added to the marking line to completely dissolve and store in a refrigerator (4 °C). The standard stock solutions of HSG4112(S) and HSG4112(R) were serially diluted to the designated concentrations to prepare the working standard solutions. The IS stock solution was diluted to 100 ng/mL with ACN and used for plasma sample preparation. Working standard solutions (5 μL) were added to plasma (95 μL) to yield calibration standards of 5, 20, 50, 100, 500, 1000, 2000, and 5000 ng/mL. QC samples were prepared at final concentrations of 5(LOQ), 15(low), 400(mid), and 4000(high) ng/mL in the same manner as the calibration standards.

2.3. Animal Plasma Samples

Rat and dog plasma samples were obtained from Biotoxtech Co. Ltd. (Cheongju, Korea). Plasma samples for oral pharmacokinetic study were obtained from the 4-week repeated oral toxicity study. The information on the plasma samples were provided in the Supplementary data. Briefly, for the pharmacokinetic analysis in rats, HSG4112 was orally administered HSG4112 at a dose of 100 mg/kg/day for 4 weeks and the plasma samples were collected on the 28th day. The blood drain time point was 0, 0.5, 1, 2, 4, 6, 10, and 24 h ($n = 3$; Table S1). In addition, rats were intravenously administrated HSG4112 at a dose of 10 mg/kg and blood was collected at 0, 0.083, 0.25, 0.5, 0.75, 1, 2, 3, 6, 12, and 24 h ($n = 3$). For the pharmacokinetic analysis in dogs, HSG4112 was orally administered at a dose of 100 mg/kg/day for 4 weeks ($n = 3$), and the plasma samples were collected on the 28th day. Blood samples were taken at 0, 1, 2, 4, 6, 10, 12, and 24 h. In addition, dogs were administrated HSG4112 intravenously at a dose of 2 mg/kg ($n = 2$) and blood was collected at 0, 0.083, 0.25, 0.5, 1, 2, 3, 4, 6, 12, and 24 h. All animal studies were performed according to the guidelines of the Ethics Committee for Use of Experimental Animals and approved by the Institutional Animal Care and Use Committee of Biotoxtech Co. Ltd. (Approval ID and date: 2016-05-160252, 2016-05-160276).

2.4. Sample Preparation

The plasma (30 μL) sample was put into a 1.5 mL tube and added with 60 μL IS solution. The tube was vortexed and centrifuged at 13,200 rpm for 5 min at room temperature. The supernatant was transferred to an LC vial for LC-MS/MS analysis.

2.5. In Vitro Metabolic Stability

Incubation mixture containing liver or intestinal microsomes (1 mg/mL), and HSG4112 (10 μM) in potassium phosphate buffer (0.1 M, pH 7.4) were preincubated at 37 °C for 5 min. The reactions were initiated by the addition of an NADPH-generation solution in a final incubation volume of 100 μL ($n = 3$). For glucuronide conjugate formation, incubation mixture containing microsomes (1 mg/mL), magnesium chloride (2.5 mM), UDPGA (2 mM), alamethicin (25 μg/mL), and drug (10 μM) in potassium phosphate buffer (0.1 M, pH 7.4) were preincubated at 37 °C for 5 min. The reactions were initiated by the addition of the NADPH-generation solution in a final incubation volume of 200 μL ($n = 3$). After the incubation for 0, 30, 60, and 120 min, the reaction was stopped by the addition of 200 μL ACN with IS. The samples were vortex-mixed and centrifuged at 13,200 rpm for 5 min. The supernatant (5 μL) was injected on to ultra-performance liquid chromatographic (UPLC) column for LC-MS/MS analysis. The experiment was performed in triplicate.

2.6. LC-MS/MS

In order to quantify HSG4112(S) and HSG4112(R), the Acquity UPLC-MS/MS system (Waters, Milford, MA, USA) was used with an electrospray ionization source. Mass detection was performed in the negative ion mode, and the column temperature was maintained at 40 °C using a thermostatically controlled column oven. The column used for the separation was a CHIRALPAK® IC-U (1.6 μm, 3.0 × 100 mm; DAICEL, New York, NY, USA). The mobile phases consisted of D.W (solvent A) and ACN (solvent B). For quantification of the analytes, isocratic elution was performed at a flow rate of 0.5 mL/min. Solvent B was maintained at 60%. For multiple reaction monitoring (MRM) analyses, the target ions used were m/z 353.3→137.1 for HSG4112(S) and HSG4112(R) and m/z 358.3→142.0 for HSG4112-d5. The capillary voltage was 3 kV and cone voltage was 50 V. Collision energy was 23 V. Nitrogen was used as the desolvation gas at a flow rate of 650 L/h and at 450 °C. The representative chromatograms of HSG4112(S) and HSG4112(R) in rat and dog plasma are provided in Supplementary data (Figure S1). The validation for the quantitation method was conducted and the resulting data were satisfactory (Supplementary data). For metabolite profiling, an ACQUITY UPLC BEH C18 column (2.1 × 150 mm, 1.7 μm; Waters, Milford, MA, USA) was used and a gradient elution program was used as follows: 30%B to 75% B at 10 min, to 30% B at 10.1 min, and held at 30% B for 3 min. The metabolite levels were measured using selected ion monitoring based on the *m/z* values of the deprotonated ions of metabolites. Other mass spectrometer conditions were the same as above.

2.7. LC-QTOF/MS for Metabolite Analysis

The high performance liquid chromatography quadruple time of the flight mass spectrometer (LC-QTOF/MS) system consisted of an Agilent 1260 series binary pump HPLC system and an Agilent 6530 Q-TOF/MS/MS equipped with an electrospray ionization source (Agilent Technologies, Palo Alto, CA, USA). The column used for the separation was a Thermo Hypersil Gold column (2.1 × 150 mm, 3 µm; Thermo Fisher Scientific Inc., Waltham, MA, USA). Column temperature was maintained at 40 °C using a thermostatically controlled column oven. The HPLC mobile phases consisted of 0.1% formic acid in distilled water (A) and 90% acetonitrile in 0.1% formic acid (B). A gradient program was used for the HPLC separation with a flow rate of 0.2 mL/min. The initial composition of the mobile phase was 30% B and it was changed to 90% B over 13 min and followed by a 7 min re-equilibration to the initial condition. The entire column eluent was directly introduced into the mass spectrometer. Nitrogen was used both as the nebulizing gas at 20 psi and as the drying gas at a flow rate of 10 L/min at 300 °C. The mass spectrometer was operated in the negative ion mode in *m/z* 50–400.

2.8. Pharmacokinetic and Data Analysis

All data were expressed as mean ± SD. Pharmacokinetic parameters were calculated by non-compartmental analysis using Pheonix WinNonlin (Ver. 6.2, Pharsight-A Certara Company, USA). The area under the concentration–time curve from time zero to the last measurable concentration (AUC_{last}), area under the plasma concentration–time curve to the infinite time (AUC_{inf}), maximum plasma concentration (C_{max}), time to reach C_{max} (T_{max}), terminal elimination half-life ($t_{1/2}$), total body clearance (C_l), apparent volume of distribution (V_z), apparent volume of distribution at steady state (V_{ss}), and equation for the mean residence time (MRT) were estimated by non-compartmental analysis of the plasma concentration versus time. The significance of the pharmacokinetic parameters was assessed using the paired Student's *t*-test. The analysis was performed on log-transformed data. When p value was less than 0.05, it was judged to be significant.

3. Results

3.1. Analysis of HSG4112(S) and HSG4112(R) in Rat Plasma

The time–plasma concentration plots of HSG4112(S) and HSG4112(R) are presented in Figure 2A, and the pharmacokinetic parameters are described in Table 1. The plasma concentration levels of HSG4112(S) were significantly higher than those of HSG4112(R) throughout all time points. The C_{max} of HSG4112(S) and HSG4112(R) were 2904.9 ng·h/mL and 984.6 ng/mL, respectively. The area under the curve (AUC) of HSG4112(S) and HSG4112(R) were 45,733.3 and 12,190.6 ng·h/mL, respectively. The pharmacokinetics of HSG4112(S) and HSG4112(R) after IV administration of HSG4112 were also investigated. The plasma concentration profiles of HSG4112(S) and HSG4112(R) after IV injection of HSG4112 at a dose of 10 mg/kg are presented in Figure 2B, and the pharmacokinetic parameters are described in Table 2. The stereoselective differences in plasma concentration were also observed in the IV administration. The AUC of HSG4112(S) and HSG4112(R) were 3806.7 ± 894.6 ng·h/mL and 1390.4 ± 92.7 ng·h/mL, respectively. Validation Data are presented in Tables S2–S5.

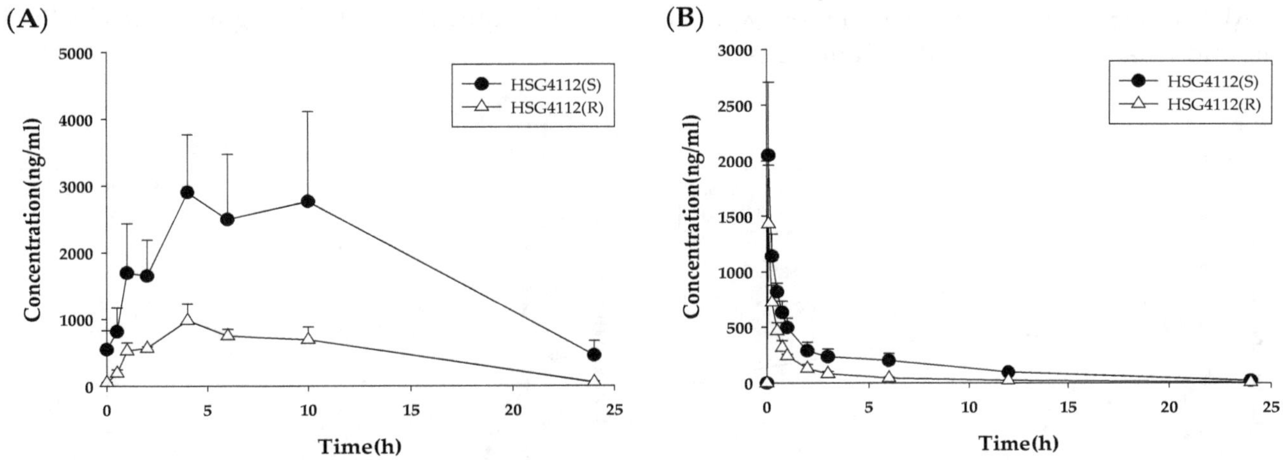

Figure 2. Plot for time-plasma concentration of HSG4112 after (**A**) oral (100 mg/kg/day, 28th day, $n = 3$) and (**B**) iv (10 mg/kg, single dose, $n = 3$) administration in rats.

Table 1. Pharmacokinetic parameters of HSG4112(S) and HSG4112(R) after PO administration at a repeated dose of 100 mg/kg/day to rats.

PK Parameter [a]	Rat 100 mg/kg (PO, 28th Day)	
	HSG4112(S)	HSG4112(R)
T_{max} (h)	4	4
C_{max} (ng/mL)	2904.9	984.6
AUC_{last} (ng·h/mL)	45,733.3	12,190.6
$T_{1/2}$ (h)	7.3	4.7
AUC_{inf} (ng·h/mL)	50,555.8	12,558.1
MRT (h)	8.8	7.8

[a] The blood samples were collected by a sparse sampling method from six rats (Table S1). Accordingly, the pharmacokinetic parameters were calculated from the mean plasma concentration data.

Table 2. Pharmacokinetic parameters of HSG4112(S) and HSG4112(R) after IV administration at a single dose of 10 mg/kg to rats.

PK Parameter	Rat 10 mg/kg (IV, $n = 3$)	
	HSG4112(S)	HSG4112(R)
C_{max} (ng/mL)	2049.7 ± 654.0	1431.7 ± 530.5 ***
AUC_{last} (ng·h/mL)	3806.7 ± 894.6	1390.4 ± 92.7 **
$T_{1/2}$(h)	5.3 ± 1.0	5.9 ± 0.4
AUC_{inf} (ng·h/mL)	3976.5 ± 1027.7	1436 ± 98.7 **
V_z (mL/kg)	9667.6 ± 697.8	29,483.8 ± 393.6 ***
C_l (mL/h/kg)	1318.8 ± 360.1	3493.4 ± 247.2 **
MRT (h)	5.4 ± 0.9	3.9 ± 0.4 *
V_{ss} (mL/kg)	16374 ± 1281	33,462 ± 4228 ***

*: $p < 0.05$, **: $p < 0.01$, ***: $p < 0.005$ versus HSG4112(S).

3.2. *Analysis of HSG4112(S) and HSG4112(R) in Dog Plasma*

The time–plasma concentration plots of HSG4112(S) and HSG4112(R) are presented in Figure 3A, and the pharmacokinetic parameters are described in Table 3. The C_{max} of HSG4112(S) and HSG4112(R) were 102.6 ± 69.6 and 707.6 ± 442.7, respectively. The AUC of HSG4112(S) and HSG4112(R) were 1408.4 ± 1418.0 and 12,324.8 ± 9715.7, respectively. The plasma concentration profiles of HSG4112(S) and HSG4112(R) after IV injection of HSG4112 at a dose of 2 mg/kg are presented in Figure 3B, and the pharmacokinetic parameters are described in Table 4. After IV injection of 2 mg/kg to beagle dogs, the AUC of HSG4112(S) and HSG4112(R) were 1002.6 ± 163.6 and 1837.4 ± 20.4 ng·h/mL, respectively. Validation Data are presented in Tables S6–S9.

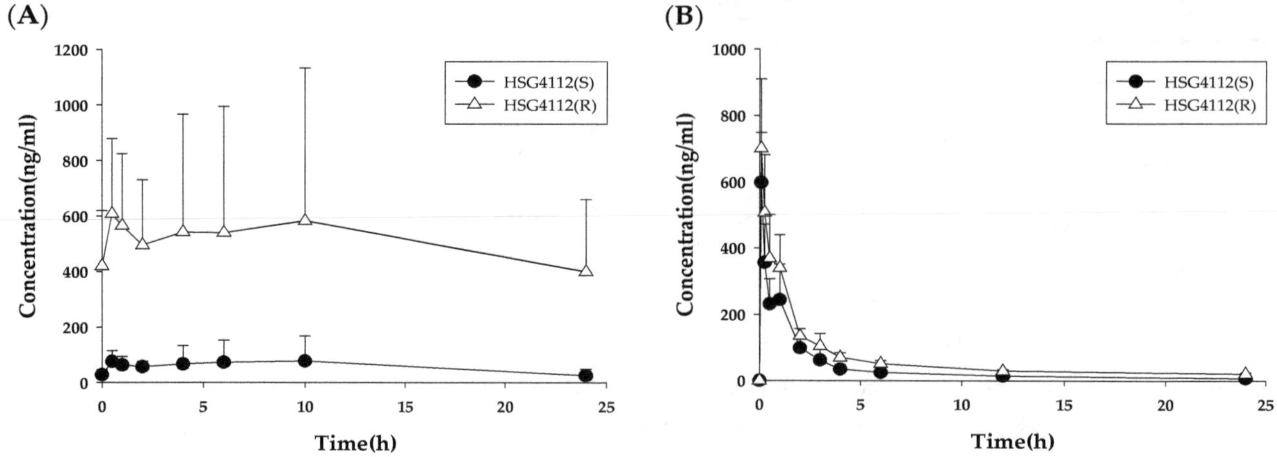

Figure 3. Plot for time–plasma concentration of HSG4112 after (**A**) oral (100 mg/kg/day, 28th day, $n = 3$) and (**B**) iv (2 mg/kg, single dose, $n = 2$) administration in dogs.

Table 3. Pharmacokinetic parameters of HSG4112(S) and HSG4112(R) after PO administration at a repeated dose of 100 mg/kg/day to dogs.

PK Parameter	**Dog 100 mg/kg (PO, 28th day, n = 3)**	
	HSG4112(S)	**HSG4112(R)**
T_{max} (h)	4.2 ± 5.1	3.7 ± 5.5
C_{max} (ng/mL)	102.6 ± 69.6	707.6 ± 442.7 ***
AUC_{last} (ng·h/mL)	1408.4 ± 1418.0	12324.8 ± 9715.7 ***
$T_{1/2}$ (h)	17.5 ± 4.5	49.4 ± 19.1
AUC_{inf} (ng·h/mL)	NA	24329.9 ± 6226.4 **
MRT (h)	9.2 ± 0.4	11.1 ± 0.2 *

*: $p < 0.05$, **: $p < 0.01$, ***: $p < 0.005$ versus HSG4112(S). NA: not available.

Table 4. Pharmacokinetic parameters of HSG4112(S) and HSG4112(R) after IV administration at a single dose of 2 mg/kg to dogs.

PK Parameter	**Dog 2 mg/kg (IV, n = 2)**	
	HSG4112(S)	**HSG4112(R)**
C_{max} (ng/mL)	598.8 ± 149.2	700.9 ± 208.7
AUC_{last} (ng·h/mL)	902.7 ± 165.2	1519.0 ± 95.1
$T_{1/2}$(h)	10.3 ± 1.5	12.0 ± 1.6
AUC_{inf} (ng·h/mL)	1002.6 ± 163.6	1837.4 ± 20.4
V_z (mL/kg)	15180.7 ± 4635.6	9437.1 ± 1333.6
C_l (mL/h/kg)	1008.6 ± 164.5	533.1 ± 5.2
MRT (h)	4.4 ± 0.3	5.7 ± 0.1
V_{ss} (mL/kg)	8047.5 ± 1885.4	6500.5 ± 1157.4

3.3. Metabolic Stability

The results for the metabolic stability of HSG4112(S) and HSG4112(R) in rat (RLM), mouse (MLM), dog (DLM), and human liver microsomes (HLM) is shown in Figure 4 (left). The remaining amounts of HSG4112(S) at 120 min were 9.1 ± 3.2%, 6.9 ± 1.5%, 84.1 ± 6%, and 78.4 ± 0.5% in the RLM, MLM, DLM, and HLM, respectively. The half-life of HSG4112(S) was 15.5, 14.2, 664.8, and 424.6 min in the RLM, MLM, DLM, and HLM, respectively. The remaining amounts of HSG4112(R) at 120 min were 4.9 ± 3%,

23.9 ± 1.1%, 77.9 ± 2.9%, and 54.5 ± 1.1% in the RLM, MLM, DLM, and HLM, respectively. The half-life of HSG4112(R) was 8.2, 28.0, 376.8, and 133.9 min in the RLM, MLM, DLM, and HLM, respectively.

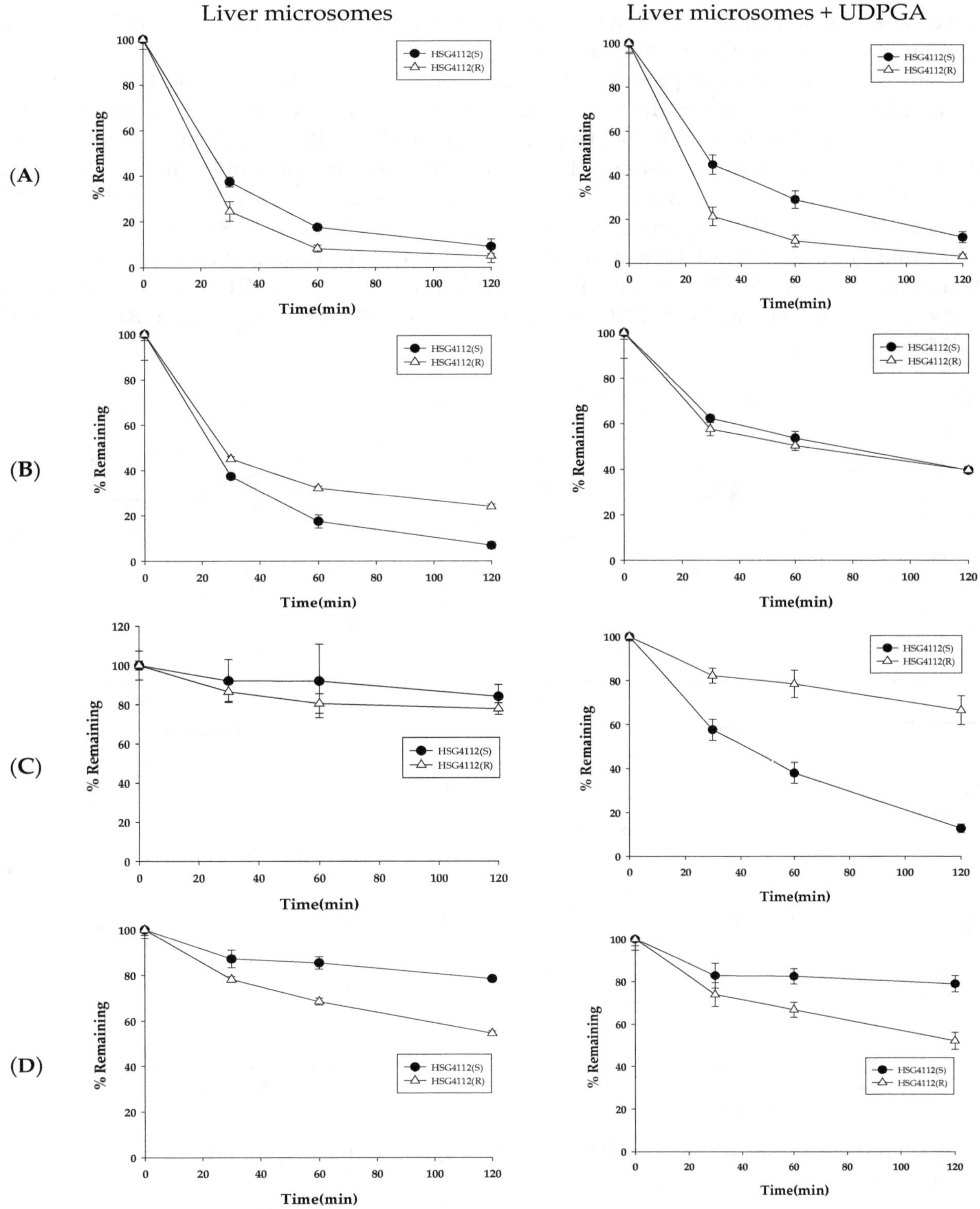

Figure 4. Metabolic stability of HSG4112 in (**A**) rat, (**B**) mouse, (**C**) dog, and (**D**) human liver microsomes ($n = 3$). UDPGA, uridine 5′-diphosphoglucuronic acid.

To investigate the effects of the phase II metabolism by glucuronidation, metabolic stability was tested after adding the glucuronidation cofactor, UDPGA. The results for the metabolic stability of HSG4112(S) and HSG4112(R) in rat, mouse, dog, and human liver microsomes with UDPGA are shown in Figure 4 (right). The remaining amounts of HSG4112(S) at 120 min were 11.9 ± 2.5%, 39.6 ± 1.5%,

12.8 ± 2%, and 78.9 ± 3.8% in the RLM, MLM, DLM, and HLM, respectively. The half-life of HSG4112(S) was 25.6, 64.3, 40.0, and 419.6 min in the RLM, MLM, DLM, and HLM, respectively. The remaining amounts of HSG4112(R) at 120 min were 3.2 ± 1.1%, 39.7 ± 0.9%, 66.5 ± 6.6%, and 52.2 ± 4% in the RLM, MLM, DLM, and HLM, respectively. The half-life values of HSG4112(R) were 9.1, 52.4, 226.8, and 150.5 min in the RLM, MLM, DLM, and HLM, respectively.

As glucuronidases are also predominantly distributed in the intestine, HSG4112 was tested in intestinal microsomes to confirm the metabolic stability results while considering glucuronidation. The results for the metabolic stability of HSG4112(S) and HSG4112(R) in rat (RIM), mouse (MIM), dog (DIM), and human intestinal microsomes (HIM) with UDPGA are shown in Figure 5. The remaining amounts of HSG4112(S) at 120 min were 87.9 ± 2.3%, 70.1 ± 6.1%, 37.9 ± 1.8%, and 76.7 ± 2.1% in RIM, MIM, DIM, and HIM, respectively. The half-life values of HSG4112(S) were 733.9, 247.9, 78.1, and 368.1 min in the RIM, MIM, DIM, and HIM, respectively. The remaining amounts of HSG4112(R) at 120 min were 95.8 ± 5.6%, 59.4 ± 6.3%, 65.9 ± 1.8%, and 75.5 ± 3.6% in RIM, MIM, DIM, and HIM, respectively. The half-life of HSG4112(R) was 1943.9, 136.7, 215.3, and 351.1 min in RIM, MIM, DIM, and HIM, respectively.

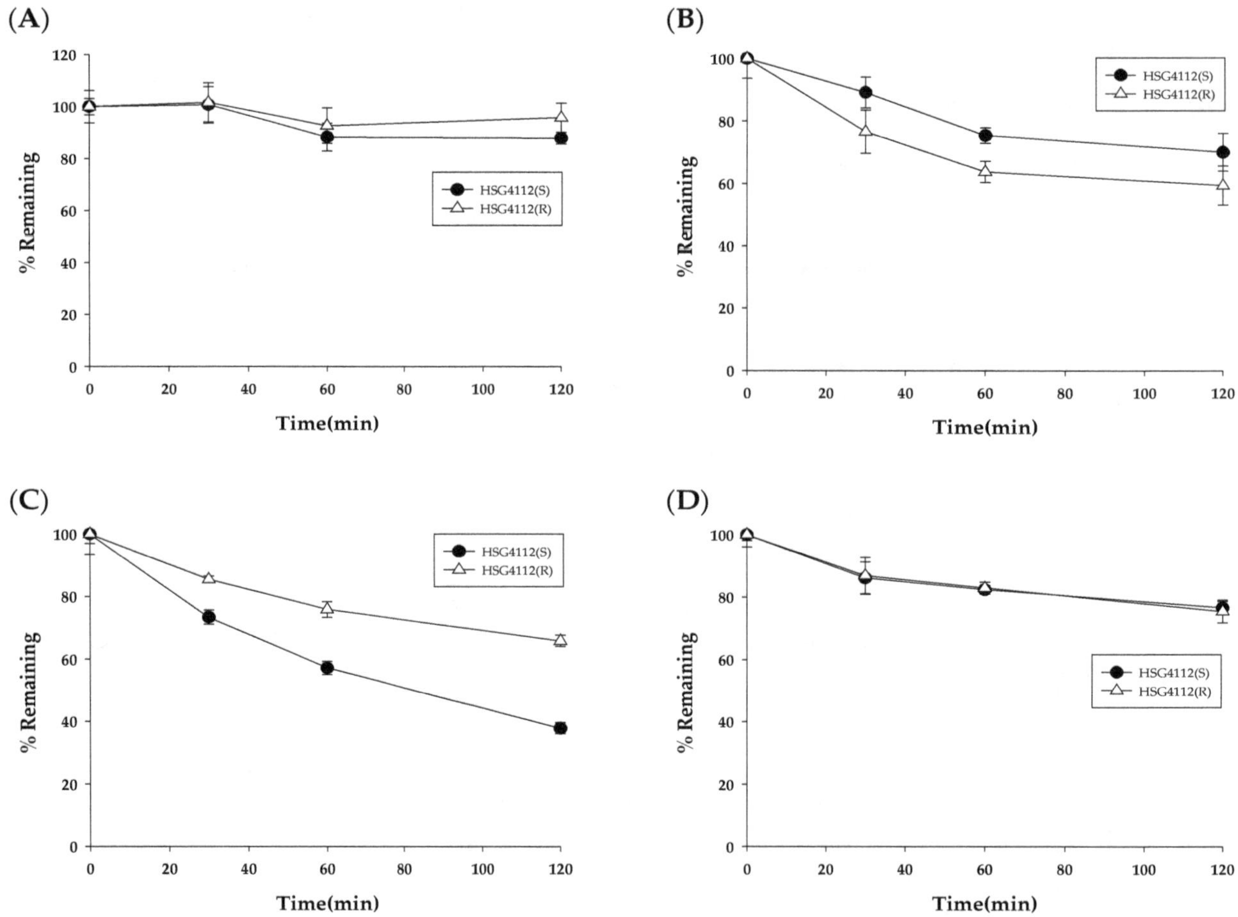

Figure 5. Metabolic stability of HSG4112 in (**A**) rat, (**B**) mouse, (**C**) dog, and (**D**) human intestinal microsomes (n = 3).

3.4. Metabolite Profile

To elucidate the main factor responsible for the stereospecific pharmacokinetic properties in rats, the metabolite profiles of HSG4112(S) and HSG4112(R) were investigated. When HSG4112(S) and HSG4112(R) were incubated in the rat liver microsomes for 60 min, the remaining amounts of HSG4112(S) and HSG4112(R) were 36.2% and 17.6%, respectively (Figure 6A). HSG4112(S) and HSG4112(R) were metabolized to yield metabolites by oxidation (M1a ~ M2b). M1c-1 and M1c-2 were detected as one peak on a general C18 column but they were separated on a chiral column. Thus, M1c-1 and M1c-2 were supposed to be stereoisomers. The types of metabolites produced from the two isomers were similar, but the amounts produced were different. The predominant metabolites of HSG4112(S) were M1a and M2b, whereas those of HSG4112(R) were M1c-2 and M1a (Figure 6B). Subsequently, the metabolite profile was investigated in the rat plasma samples (on the 28th day of an oral dose of 100 mg/kg/day). A total of seven metabolites were detected (Figure 7); a metabolite with hydroxyl and carbonyl groups (M3a) and glucuronide conjugate (M4) were additionally detected besides the metabolites observed in liver microsomes. Their peak area values were plotted according to the time (Figure 8A), and the concentration of the parent (as racemate), M1c-1, and M1c-2 were quantitated (Figure 8B). M1c-2 was shown to be the predominant metabolite (Figure 8C). The accurate mass data for each postulated metabolite is tabulated in Table 5. The tentative structures of HSG4112 metabolites are provided as Supplementary data (Figure S2).

Table 5. Accurate mass data for HSG4112 and its postulated metabolites in rats.

Metabolites	ΔM	Theoretical Mass [M-H]$^-$	Measured Mass [M-H]$^-$	Error (ppm)
HSG4112	-	353.1758	353.1756	−0.57
M1a	+16	369.1707	369.1712	1.35
M1c-1	+16	369.1707	369.1718	2.98
M1c-2	+16	369.1707	369.1718	2.98
M2a	+30	383.1500	383.1499	−0.26
M2b	+30	383.1500	383.1531	8.09
M3a	+30	385.1657	385.1662	1.30
M4	+30	529.2079	529.2071	−1.51

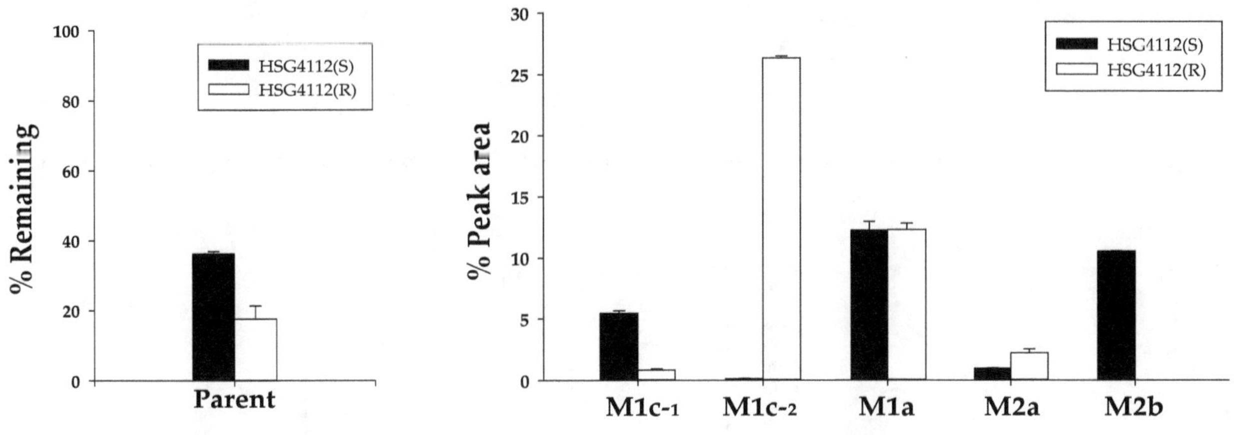

Figure 6. Metabolic profiles of HSG4112(S) and HSG4112(R) in rat liver microsomes. (**A**) Percent remaining amounts of HSG4112(S) and HSG4112(R). (**B**) Relative peak areas of the metabolites generated from HSG4112(S) and HSG4112(R). HSG4112(S) and HSG4112(R) were incubated separately in rat liver microsomes for 60 min and the resulting amount of the parent drug and its metabolites was measured based on peak area.

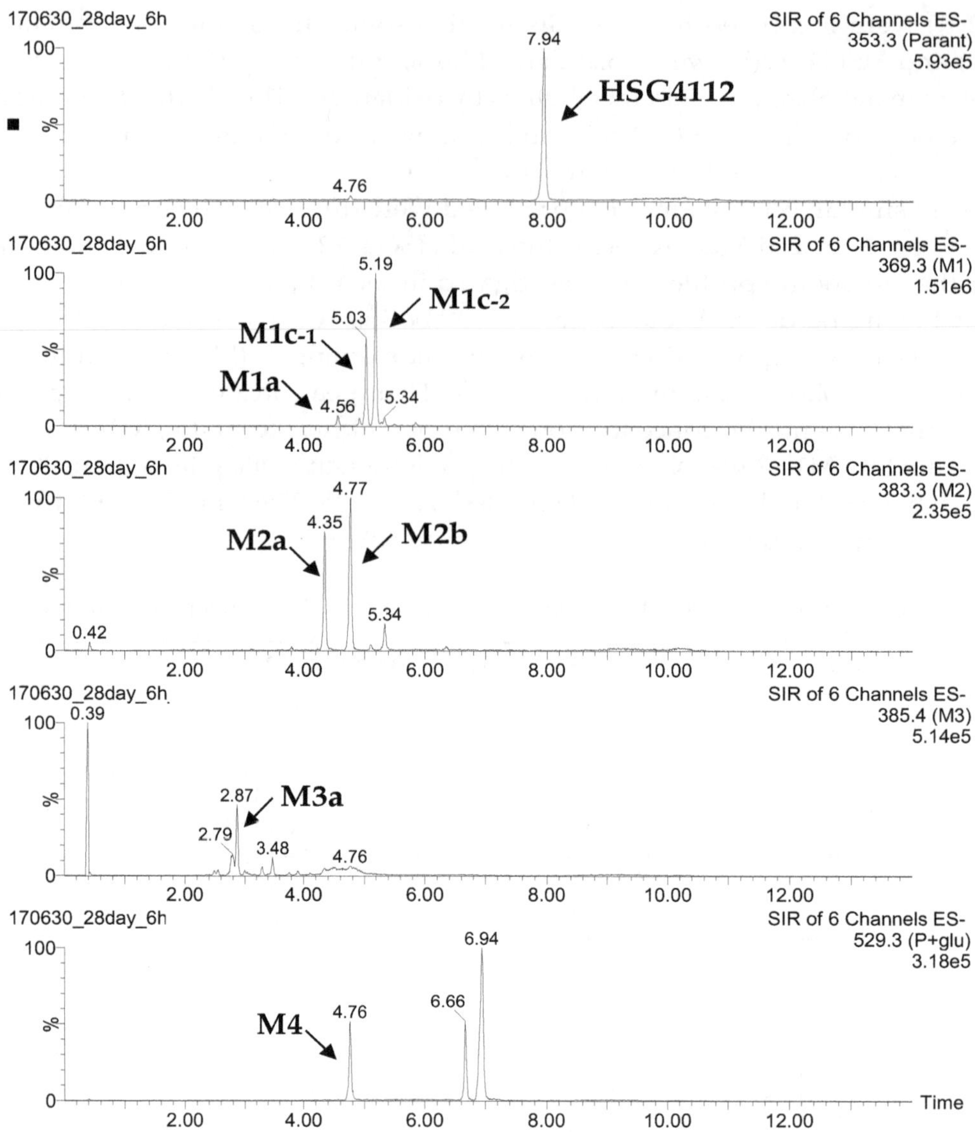

Figure 7. Representative extracted ion chromatograms of HSG4112 and its metabolites in rat plasma.

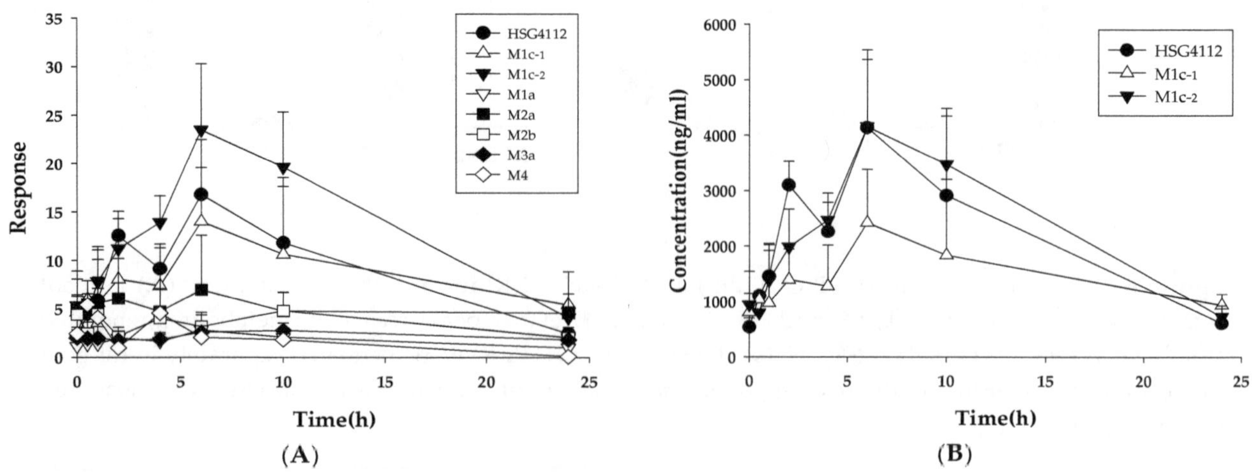

Figure 8. *Cont.*

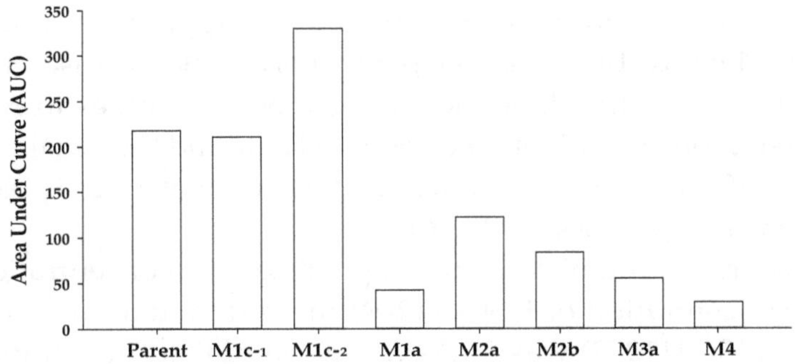

(C)

Figure 8. Metabolic profiles of HSG4112 in rat plasma after oral administration (100 mg/kg/day, 28th day, $n = 3$). (**A**) Plot for time-peak area of HSG4112 and its metabolites. (**B**) Plot for time-plasma concentration of HSG4112, M1c-1 and M1c-2. (**C**) Area under curve values of HSG4112 and its metabolites calculated from (**A**).

Meanwhile, the dog plasma sample showed only two metabolites (M1d and M4); M4, the glucuronide metabolite, was the predominant metabolite (Figure 9). Due to the unavailability of the sample and reference standards, the time–plasma concentration profile could not be obtained.

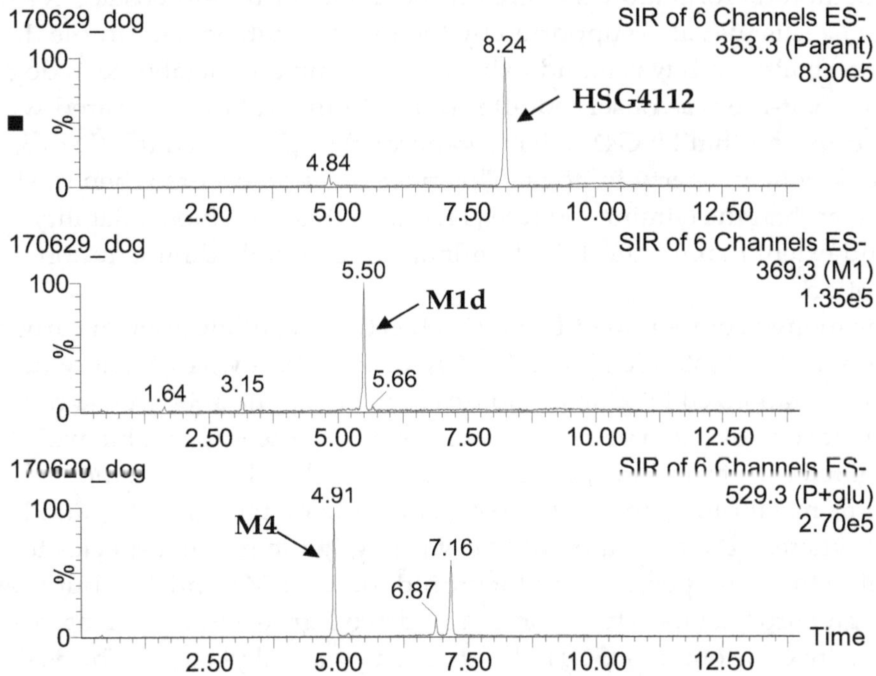

Figure 9. Representative extracted ion chromatograms of HSG4112 and its metabolites in dog plasma.

4. Discussion

In this study, concentration profiles of HSG4112(S) and HSG4112(R) after intravenous and/or oral administration of HSG4112 were investigated in rats and dogs, and the stereoselectivity in the metabolism of HSG4112 was investigated in vitro and in vivo. The resulting data showed a characteristic stereoselective pharmacokinetic pattern depending on the species.

When HSG4112(S) and HSG4112(R) were quantified in rat plasma, the concentration of HSG4112(S) generally measured higher, and, consequently, the AUC of HSG4112(S) was 4.9–7.8 times higher than that of HSG4112(R). This trend was also observed in the plasma samples from rats administered intravenously; the concentration ratio (S/R) over time was 1.4–4.8, and the AUC of HSG4112(S) was 2.7 times higher than that of HSG4112(R). Therefore, the systemic exposure of HSG4112(S) was significantly higher than that of HSG4112(R) in rats, indicating stereospecificity in the pharmacokinetics.

This stereoselective pharmacokinetic property in rats is supposedly due to the stereoselective metabolism of HSG4112. The possible metabolic pathways of HSG4112 isomers in rats are presented in Figure S3. The metabolic stability data and the metabolite profiles in rat plasma showed that HSG4112(R) is metabolized more extensively than HSG4112(S), and their main metabolic pathways are different. The metabolic profile data suggested that the formation of M1c is predominantly responsible for the stereoselective pharmacokinetics of HSG4112.

When HSG4112 was orally administered to beagle dogs, the concentration ratio (S/R) over time was 0.06–0.24, and the concentration of HSG4112(R) measured at a much higher level. The AUC ratio of HSG4112(S) and HSG4112(R) was 0.12–0.13 in the oral administration group. In addition, when HSG4112 was intravenously administered to beagle dogs, the concentration ratio (S/R) over time was 0.3–0.9, and the AUC ratio of HSG4112(S) and HSG4112(R) was 0.5. Therefore, the systemic exposure of HSG4112(R) was significantly higher than HSG4112(S) in beagle dogs, indicating stereospecificity in the pharmacokinetics. Interestingly, the predominant isomer form in dogs was opposite to that of rats. The metabolic stability data for phase I metabolism did not exhibit any difference between HSG4112(S) and HSG4112(R). However, the metabolic stability data including glucuronide formation showed significant differences between HSG4112(S) and HSG4112(R); the metabolic rate of HSG4112(S) was much higher than that of HSG4112(R). This metabolism pattern was also obviously observed in dog intestinal microsomes, which also have high glucuronidase activities. This revealed that the stereoselective glucuronide formation is mainly responsible for the stereoselective pharmacokinetics of HSG4112 in dogs. This was also supported by the in vivo metabolism profile data of dog plasma; the glucuronide metabolite (M4) was found to be the predominant metabolite in dog plasma. Notably, the longer terminal half-life was observed after oral administration compared with IV injection in dogs. Thus, it is supposed that HSG4112 has a general-case pharmacokinetic property in rats but a flip-flop pharmacokinetic property in dogs. This phenomenon occurs when the absorption rate of drugs is much slower than the elimination rate [11,12]. In this case, bioavailability factors such as the absorption rate and extent mainly affect the terminal slope of oral administration than clearance and volume of distribution.

Glabridin, the motive compound of HSG4112, has the R configuration at carbon C-3. According to the previous report, the systemic bioavailability of glabridin was very low (about 7.5% in rats). Glabridin is mainly metabolized by glucuronidases in the intestine and liver, and the first-pass effects of glucuronidation are one of the main factors responsible for the low oral bioavailability of glabridin. Guo et al. investigated the tissue and species differences in the glucuronidation of glabridin. In their study, glabridin was metabolized to yield two glucuronide metabolites: M1 and M2. M2 formation was predominant whereas the formation of M1 was negligible in most species tested. The authors could not determine the exact position of glucuronidation for M1 and M2, but they suggested that M2 might have a glucuronide moiety at the C-4 hydroxyl group in the B ring based on the earlier reports. The C-4 hydroxyl group of HSG4112 is masked by an alkyl chain. This is the reason why the glucuronidation was not the main metabolic pathway in humans and rats in our study with HSG4112. It is notable that dog liver microsomes showed the highest value of the intrinsic clearance by M1 formation (glucuronidation at the C-2 hydroxyl group) in glabridin. This result agrees with our finding that the formation of the glucuronide metabolite predominantly occurred in dog liver and intestinal microsomes. The results by Guo et al. showed that the metabolic clearance by glucuronidation both for M1 and M2 was negligible in humans. This is also consistent with our data that the contribution of glucuronidation to the metabolic clearance of HSG4112 was minimal.

Stereoselectivity for HSG 4112 metabolism was also shown in human liver microsomes. The metabolism pattern in human liver microsomes is somewhat close to that in rat liver microsomes. Thus, this is supposedly due to CYP-mediated metabolism rather than glucuronidation. Although the metabolic rate in humans is lower than that in other species, the present data suggests that stereoselective pharmacokinetics by stereoselective metabolism (i.e., higher exposure of the (S)-isomer) could be shown in the clinical trial of HSG4112. Another factor that should be considered regarding stereoselective pharmacokinetics is the possibility of interconversion between the isomers. To address this issue, HSG4112 isomers were analyzed after oral administration of each isomer to rats. When one isomer was administered, the other isomer was not detected (data not shown). This suggests that interconversion between isomers does not occur at least in rats. Further investigation should be followed in humans.

In conclusion, the present study demonstrates that HSG4112 showed species-specific stereoselective pharmacokinetics. Notably, the pharmacokinetic stereoselectivity of HSG4112 isomers showed opposing patterns between rats and dogs. This is because the major metabolic pathways involved in the clearance of HSG4112 are different in rats and dogs. Each metabolic enzyme may have different stereoselectivity. We presented the possible mechanisms for these stereoselective pharmacokinetic patterns by the metabolite profiling data in vitro and in vivo. These results will provide helpful information for understanding the pharmacological and toxicological effects of HSG4112, depending on its configurations. In addition, caution should be taken in extrapolating preclinical data with different experimental animal models to clinical data for humans.

Supplementary Materials:
Figure S1: Representative chromatograms of HSG4112(S) and HSG4112(R) in (A) rat (oral, 100 mg/kg, 6h) and (B) dog (oral, 100 mg/kg, 6h) plasma, Figure S2: Proposed chemical structures of HSG4112 metabolites, Figure S3: Postulated metabolic pathways of HSG4112 isomers, Table S1: Blood drain time points for oral pharmacokinetic analysis in rats (repeated dose, 100 mg/kg/day, 28th day), Table S2: Linearity of HSG4112(S) and HSG4112(R) in rat plasma (n = 3), Table S3: Intra-day and inter-day accuracy and coefficient of variation for determination of HSG4112(S) and HSG4112(R) in rat plasma, Table S4: Matrix effect, recovery and process efficiency data for HSG4112(S) and HSG4112(R) in rat plasma (n = 3), Table S5: Stability of HSG4112(S) and HSG4112(R) in rat plasma, Table S6: Linearity of HSG4112(S) and HSG4112(R) in dog plasma, Table S7: Intra-day and inter-day accuracy and coefficient of variation for determination of HSG4112(S) and HSG4112(R) in dog plasma, Table S8: Matrix effect, recovery and process efficiency data for HSG4112(S) and HSG4112(R) in dog plasma (n = 3), Table S9: Stability of HSG4112(S) and HSG4112(R) in dog plasma.

Author Contributions: Contributed to the research design: H.H.Y., S.-K.Y., K.K.; Conducted experiments: I.Y.B, Y.S.J.; Contributed to data analysis and interpretation: M.S.C.; Contributed to the preparation of the manuscript: I.Y.B., M.S.C., H.H.Y. All authors have read and agreed to the published version of the manuscript.

References

1. Simmler, C.; Pauli, G.F.; Chen, S.N. Phytochemistry and biological properties of glabridin. *Fitoterapia* **2013**, *90*, 160–184. [CrossRef] [PubMed]
2. Cui, Y.M.; Ao, M.Z.; Li, W.; Yu, L.J. Effect of glabridin from Glycyrrhiza glabra on learning and memory in mice. *Planta Med.* **2008**, *74*, 377–380. [CrossRef] [PubMed]
3. Ito, C.; Oi, N.; Hashimoto, T.; Nakabayashi, H.; Aoki, F.; Tominaga, Y.; Yokota, S.; Hosoe, K.; Kanazawa, K. Absorption of dietary licorice isoflavan glabridin to blood circulation in rats. *J. Nutr. Sci. Vitaminol. (Tokyo)* **2007**, *53*, 358–365. [CrossRef] [PubMed]
4. Guo, B.; Fang, Z.; Yang, L.; Xiao, L.; Xia, Y.; Gonzalez, F.J.; Zhu, L.; Cao, Y.; Ge, G.; Yang, L.; et al. Tissue and species differences in the glucuronidation of glabridin with UDP-glucuronosyltransferases. *Chem. Biol. Interact.* **2015**, *231*, 90–97. [CrossRef] [PubMed]
5. Kasprzyk-Hordern, B. Pharmacologically active compounds in the environment and their chirality. *Chem. Soc. Rev.* **2010**, *39*, 4466–4503. [CrossRef] [PubMed]
6. Eriksson, T.; Bjorkman, S.; Roth, B.; Fyge, A.; Hoglund, P. Stereospecific determination, chiral inversion in vitro and pharmacokinetics in humans of the enantiomers of thalidomide. *Chirality* **1995**, *7*, 44–52. [CrossRef] [PubMed]
7. Agranat, I.; Wainschtein, S.R. The strategy of enantiomer patents of drugs. *Drug Discov. Today* **2010**, *15*, 163–170. [CrossRef] [PubMed]
8. Stephens, T.D.; Bunde, C.J.; Fillmore, B.J. Mechanism of action in thalidomide teratogenesis. *Biochem. Pharmacol.* **2000**, *59*, 1489–1499. [CrossRef]
9. Williams, K.; Lee, E. Importance of drug enantiomers in clinical pharmacology. *Drugs* **1985**, *30*, 333–354. [CrossRef] [PubMed]

10. Chu, D.T.; Nordeen, C.W.; Hardy, D.J.; Swanson, R.N.; Giardina, W.J.; Pernet, A.G.; Plattner, J.J. Synthesis, antibacterial activities, and pharmacological properties of enantiomers of temafloxacin hydrochloride. *J. Med. Chem.* **1991**, *34*, 168–174. [CrossRef] [PubMed]
11. Toutain, P.L.; Bousquet-Mélou, A. Plasma terminal half-life. *J. Vet. Pharmacol. Ther.* **2004**, *27*, 427–439. [CrossRef] [PubMed]
12. Kim, H.; Ji, Y.S.; Rehman, S.U.; Choi, M.S.; Gye, M.C.; Yoo, H.H. Pharmacokinetics and Metabolism of Acetyl Triethyl Citrate, a Water-Soluble Plasticizer for Pharmaceutical Polymers in Rats. *Pharmaceutics* **2019**, *11*, 162. [CrossRef] [PubMed]

Altered Protein Expression of Cardiac CYP2J and Hepatic CYP2C, CYP4A and CYP4F in a Mouse Model of Type II Diabetes—A Link in the Onset and Development of Cardiovascular Disease?

Benoit Drolet [1,2,*], Sylvie Pilote [2], Carolanne Gélinas [1], Alida-Douce Kamaliza [1], Audrey Blais-Boilard [1], Jessica Virgili [1,2], Dany Patoine [2] and Chantale Simard [1,2]

1 Faculté de Pharmacie, Université Laval, 1050 Avenue de la Médecine, Québec, QC G1V 0A6, Canada; carolanne.gelinas.1@ulaval.ca (C.G.); lovedk90@hotmail.com (A.-D.K.); audrey.blais-boilard.1@ulaval.ca (A.B.-B.); jessica.virgili.1@ulaval.ca (J.V.); chantale.simard@pha.ulaval.ca (C.S.)

2 Centre de Recherche, Institut Universitaire de Cardiologie et de Pneumologie de Québec, 2725 Chemin Sainte-Foy, Québec, QC G1V 4G5, Canada; sylvie.pilote@criucpq.ulaval.ca (S.P.); dany.patoine@criucpq.ulaval.ca (D.P.)

* Correspondence: benoit.drolet@pha.ulaval.ca

Abstract: Arachidonic acid can be metabolized by cytochrome P450 (CYP450) enzymes in a tissue- and cell-specific manner to generate vasoactive products such as epoxyeicosatrienoic acids (EETs-cardioprotective) and hydroxyeicosatetraenoic acids (HETEs-cardiotoxic). Type II diabetes is a well-recognized risk factor for developing cardiovascular disease. A mouse model of Type II diabetes (C57BLKS/J-*db/db*) was used. After sacrifice, livers and hearts were collected, washed, and snap frozen. Total proteins were extracted. Western blots were performed to assess cardiac CYP2J and hepatic CYP2C, CYP4A, and CYP4F protein expression, respectively. Significant decreases in relative protein expression of cardiac CYP2J and hepatic CYP2C were observed in Type II diabetes animals compared to controls (CYP2J: 0.80 ± 0.03 vs. 1.05 ± 0.06, $n = 20$, $p < 0.001$); (CYP2C: 1.56 ± 0.17 vs. 2.21 ± 0.19, $n = 19$, $p < 0.01$). In contrast, significant increases in relative protein expression of both hepatic CYP4A and CYP4F were noted in Type II diabetes mice compared to controls (CYP4A: 1.06 ± 0.09 vs. 0.18 ± 0.01, $n = 19$, $p < 0.001$); (CYP4F: 2.53 ± 0.22 vs. 1.10 ± 0.07, $n = 19$, $p < 0.001$). These alterations induced by Type II diabetes in the endogenous pathway (CYP450) of arachidonic acid metabolism may increase the risk for cardiovascular disease by disrupting the fine equilibrium between cardioprotective (CYP2J/CYP2C-generated) and cardiotoxic (CYP4A/CYP4F-generated) metabolites of arachidonic acid.

Keywords: arachidonic acid; CYP450 enzymes; Type II diabetes; cardiovascular disease

1. Introduction

Arachidonic acid (AA) is an essential polyunsaturated fatty acid notably found in cell membrane phospholipids. It has an important role in a number of cell signaling and regulation pathways upon its cleavage from membranes via a sequence of tightly regulated events [1]. The cleavage sequence is initiated by the activation of a calcium-dependent type IV phospholipase A2 in response to a stimulus, such as ischemia [2]. The released non-esterified AA acts as a substrate for oxidation by cyclooxygenases (COX), lipoxygenases (LOX), and cytochrome P450 (CYP450) enzymes in the heart and elsewhere, thereby generating a cascade of lipid second messengers, orchestrating a broad range of critical physiological processes, including hemodynamic functions [1–3]. Both the lipoxygenase [4] and the cyclooxygenase [5] pathways have been thoroughly studied and described. Briefly, via the LOX pathway, AA is converted into a large number of lipid mediators with vasoactive and immunomodulatory effects such as lipoxins, leukotrienes, hepoxilins, eoxins, resolvins, protectins, and others [4]. On the other hand, cyclooxygenase (COX), with both its COX-1 and COX-2 isoforms, transforms AA in either prostaglandins, prostacyclins, or thromboxane; other products are known for their vasoactive, immunomodulatory, and platelet-aggregating effects [5]. In contrast, the CYP450 pathway, also known as the third pathway, was far less understood [1,6]. However, this pathway is increasingly recognized as a 'yin and yang' in relation to its potential opposing effects on the cardiac function, depending on which subfamily of the CYP enzyme is metabolizing AA. Indeed, when it is transformed by epoxidation, AA generates a number of products known as epoxyeicosatrienoic acids (EETs) that promote vasodilation, angiogenesis, and thrombolysis. It then also inhibits inflammation, smooth muscle cell migration, and apoptosis, which together lead to a preserved cardiac function [7]. In contrast, when AA is hydroxylated, it produces compounds such as hydroxyeicosatetraenoic acids (HETEs) that promote vasoconstriction, inflammation, smooth muscle cell migration, and apoptosis, all leading to cardiac dysfunction [7]. In fact, CYP450 enzymes can metabolize AA in a tissue- and cell-specific manner to generate major and highly relevant derivatives, such as cardioprotective EETs and cardiotoxic HETEs. These epoxygenated and hydroxylated lipid derivatives are known to have various biological functions, such as regulating the vascular tone and reactivity, renal and pulmonary functions, ion transport, and growth response [8]. The epoxygenases (CYP2C and CYP2J) generate EETs, while the ω-hydroxylases (CYP4A and CYP4F) generate HETEs [2,6,9]. The human CYP2C subfamily consists of four members (CYP2C8, CYP2C9, CYP2C18, and CYP2C19) and they account for approximately 20% of the P450 enzymes in the human liver. Moreover, they are expressed to variable extents in a number of tissues such as liver, kidney, gut, brain, lungs, aorta, and importantly, in the heart [10,11]. The human CYP2J subfamily has only a single gene, CYP2J2 metabolizing AA [12]. CYP2J2 was detected in tissues such as lung, intestine, liver, pancreas, and seminal vesicles, and is particularly abundant in the cardiovascular tissue [13–17]. Enzymes of the CYP4A subfamily have been identified in virtually all mammalian species. In human, CYP4A11 and CYP4A12 have been identified. The CYP4A fatty acid ω-hydroxylases are ubiquitously expressed and consistently found in strong levels in the kidney, liver, lung, intestine, skeletal muscle, and heart [18]. The mammalian CYP4F subfamily consists of seven human forms: CYP4F2 (liver and kidney), CYP4F3A (bone marrow and neutrophiles), CYP4F3B (liver and kidney), CYP4F8 (prostate), CYP4F11 (liver, kidney, heart, and skeletal muscle), CYP4F12 (gastrointestinal tract, heart, and kidney), and CYP4F22 (skin). Therefore, both CYP2 and CYP4 families are present in the heart.

CYP-derived HETEs have deleterious effects in the heart during ischemia. These include a significant pro-inflammatory effect during reperfusion and potent vasoconstriction in the coronary arteries [2]. In contrast, epoxidation of AA generates 5,6-, 8,9-, 11,12-, and 14,15-EET that have been shown to limit ischemia-reperfusion injury, to have potent anti-inflammatory effects within the vasculature, and to be potent vasodilators of the coronary arteries [2]. Once formed, EETs undergo hydrolysis by soluble epoxide hydrolase (sEH) to less biologically active dihydroeicosatrienoic acids (DHETs) [2]. Soluble epoxide hydrolase (sEH) is widely distributed in mammalian tissues. Indeed, it is present in vascular endothelia [19] and in vascular smooth muscle cells [20]. Dysregulation of lipid metabolism has frequently been associated with disorders such as inflammation, neoplasia, diabetes, and neurodegeneration, as well as cardiovascular disease [8]. In line with this, a probable link between CYP450 expression/activity and cardiovascular disease (CVD), such as high blood pressure, coronary artery disease, myocardial ischemia and infarction, congestive heart failure, stroke, dilated cardiomyopathies, and rhythm disturbances has been established [21]. It is therefore suggested that alterations in the expression and/or activity of specific CYP450 epoxygenase/hydroxylase and sEH enzymes are likely to affect the delicate balance between the cardiovascular effects of EETs, HETEs, and DHETs [2]. As a consequence, abnormalities in these pathways may contribute to and/or promote the pathogenesis of CVD [22].

Well-known to be a major contributor to the onset and development of CVD [23], Type II diabetes (T2D) is therefore thought to perturbate the fine equilibrium between cardioprotective and cardiotoxic CYP-generated metabolites of AA by contributing to the cardiotoxic side. Indeed, this modulation of AA metabolism is suggested to be associated with the onset of coronary vasoconstriction leading to endothelial dysfunction, atherosclerosis, and CVD in general [24]. Of note, while both COX- and LOX-associated cardiovascular alterations have been demonstrated in the *db/db* mouse model of T2 [25,26], such demonstration is far less clear when considering the CYP pathway.

It was therefore our objective to evaluate the T2D-induced disturbances in the CYP450 pathway of AA metabolism that may contribute to the observed increase in the risk of CVD.

2. Materials and Methods

2.1. Animal Model

Male 7-weeks old BKS.Cg-m +/+ $Lepr^{db}$/J mice (*db/db*: T2D) and control C57BLKS/J wild-type mice were purchased from The Jackson Laboratory (Bar Harbor, ME, USA). The animals were fed with standard chow and water ad libitum. At 12 weeks-old, blood drawns were performed by using the submandibular vein, and, thereafter, the animals were killed by cervical dislocation. Livers and hearts were quickly harvested, washed with ice-cold PBS, snap-frozen in liquid nitrogen, and further kept at −80 °C. These experiments were carried out in accordance with the Guide to the Care and Use of Experimental Animals of the Canadian Council on Animal Care. The research protocol was approved by the Comité de protection des animaux de l'Université Laval (CPAUL; Authorization # 2009140-3, on 20 December 2011).

2.2. Western Blots of Liver Proteins

Western blotting experiments were performed as previously described [27] to assess CYP2C, CYP4A, and CYP4F protein expression. Briefly, samples of frozen liver were homogenized in an ice-cold lysis buffer (in mmol/L): Tris-HCl (pH 7.4) 10, sucrose 320, EDTA 1, dithiothreitol 1, and a protease inhibitor cocktail 0.1% from Sigma-Aldrich (St. Louis, MO, USA). Total protein content was evaluated with the DC protein assay kit (Bio-Rad, Mississauga, ON, Canada). Western blot analysis of 10 μg (CYP2C), 12 μg (CYP4A), and 20 μg (CYP4F) of proteins were used to evaluate the levels of these three CYPs in the livers. The Mini-Protean TGX Stain-Free Precast Gel (Bio-Rad) or standard SDS-PAGE gel was used. The membrane was incubated overnight at 4 °C with either anti-CYP2C9 (Ab48558), anti-CYP4A (Ab3573), or anti-CYP4F12 (Ab71565) polyclonal primary antibodies (all three 1:1000; Abcam, Toronto, ON, Canada). The membrane was washed and then incubated with a goat anti-rabbit IgG HRP-linked secondary antibody (SC2004; 1:1000; Santa Cruz Biotechnology, Mississauga, ON, Canada) conjugated with horseradish peroxidase. In the specific case of CYP4F proteins, the membrane was washed, stripped in SDS/β-mercaptoethanol solution at 55 °C for 15 min to enhance the signal strength [28], and then incubated with the secondary antibody conjugated with horseradish peroxidase. Chemiluminescent immunodetection was performed by using the Luminata™ Crescendo Western HRP Substrate (EMD Millipore, Billerica, MA, USA) and the ChemiDoc™ imaging system from Bio-Rad. Expression of the proteins of interest was normalized against total lane density of loaded proteins based on Amido black staining (CYP4F) or stain-free gel technology (CYP4A and CYP2C). The linear dynamic range of sample was evaluated for each antibody to make sure that an appropriate sample loading was used.

2.3. Western Blots of Cardiac Protein

Samples of frozen ventricles were homogenized in an ice-cold lysis buffer (in mmol/L): Tris-HCl (pH 7.4) 15, NaCl 150, sodium vanadate 0.2, EGTA 1, $MgCl_2$ 1, β-mercaptoethanol 10, Triton 1%, sodium deoxycholate 0.5%, and a protease inhibitor cocktail 0.1% from Sigma-Aldrich. Total protein content was evaluated with the DC protein assay kit (Bio-Rad). Western blot analysis of 25 μg of proteins was used to assess the level of CYP2J protein in the ventricles. The membrane was incubated overnight at 4 °C with anti-CYP2J2 (Ab76176) polyclonal antibody (1:1000; Abcam). The membrane was washed and then incubated with a goat anti-rabbit IgG HRP-linked secondary antibody (SC2004; 1:1000; Santa Cruz Biotechnology) conjugated with horseradish peroxidase. Chemiluminescent immunodetection was performed using the Luminata™ Crescendo Western HRP Substrate (EMD Millipore) and the ChemiDoc™ imaging system from Bio-Rad. Expression of the proteins of interest was normalized against total protein loaded based on Amido black staining of whole lanes. Again, the linear dynamic range of the method was evaluated.

2.4. Data Analysis

Student's *t*-test followed by a Mann-Whitney rank sum test (when the test for normality failed) were used to evaluate the differences between groups (SigmaPlot 12.5, Jandel Scientific Software, San Rafael, CA, USA). All the results are expressed as mean ± SEM. Statistical significance was set at $p < 0.05$.

3. Results

Table 1 shows body weight and biochemical blood parameters of mice at sacrifice (week 12). Many clinical features of human Type II diabetes were shown to be present in the *db/db* mice (T2D) at sacrifice: severe obesity, hyperglycemia, hyperinsulinemia, hypertriglyceridemia, and hypercholesterolemia; thus confirming the validity of this T2D animal model.

Table 1. Body weight and biochemical blood parameters at sacrifice (week 12). (** $p < 0.01$, *** $p < 0.001$ vs. control).

Measures at Sacrifice (Week 12)	Control Mice (n = 17)	BKS.Cg-m +/+ Lepr^{db}/J Mice (*db/db*: T2D) (n = 20)
Weight (g)	23.5 ± 0.5	41.3 ± 0.9 ***
Glycemia (mM)	8.2 ± 0.7	31.3 ± 0.6 ***
Insulinemia (ng/mL)	0.67 ± 0.06	3.90 ± 0.50 ***
HDL-C (mM)	2.10 ± 0.05	3.18 ± 0.13 ***
Triglyceridemia (mM)	1.67 ± 0.07	2.33 ± 0.22 **
Cholesterolemia (mM)	2.32 ± 0.17	3.77 ± 0.11 ***

As shown in Figure 1 (lower panel), a significant reduction in relative expression of CYP2J proteins was observed in the cardiac ventricles of T2D mice, when compared to the control animals (0.80 ± 0.03 vs. 1.05 ± 0.06; $p < 0.001$). Upper panel shows the representative blot images of cardiac CYP2J and the total proteins loaded for both the control and T2D groups. Figure 2 (lower panel) also shows a significant reduction in relative expression of CYP2C proteins that was observed in the liver of T2D mice when compared to the control animals (1.56 ± 0.17 vs. 2.21 ± 0.19; $p < 0.01$). Upper panel shows the representative blot images of hepatic CYP2C and the total proteins loaded for both the control and T2D groups. In contrast, Figure 3 (lower panel) shows a significant increase in relative expression of CYP4A proteins that was observed in the liver of T2D mice when compared to the control animals (1.06 ± 0.09 vs. 0.18 ± 0.01; $p < 0.001$).

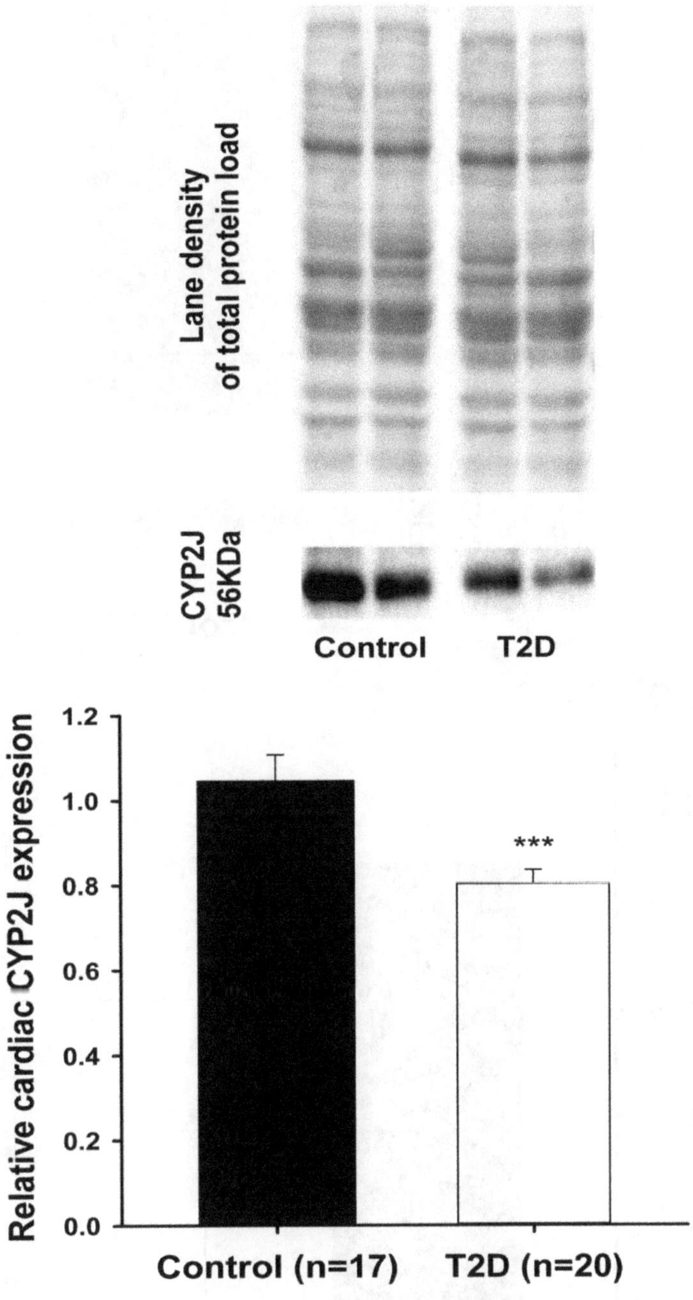

Figure 1. A significant decrease (*** $p < 0.001$) was observed in the relative protein expression of cardiac CYP2J in Type II diabetes (T2D) mice (0.80 ± 0.03) compared to controls (1.05 ± 0.06).

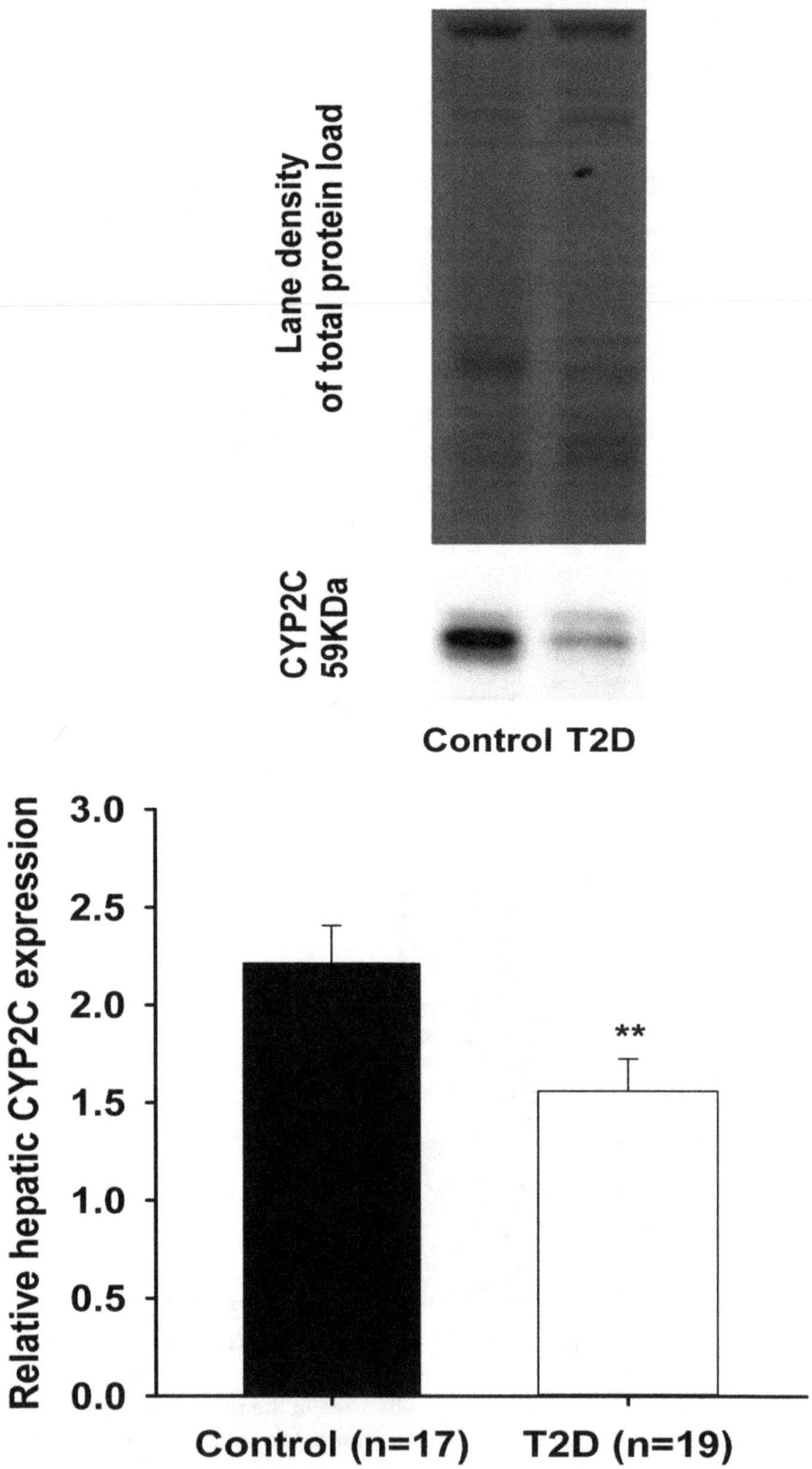

Figure 2. A significant decrease (** $p < 0.01$) was observed in the relative protein expression of hepatic CYP2C in T2D mice (1.56 ± 0.17) compared to controls (2.21 ± 0.19).

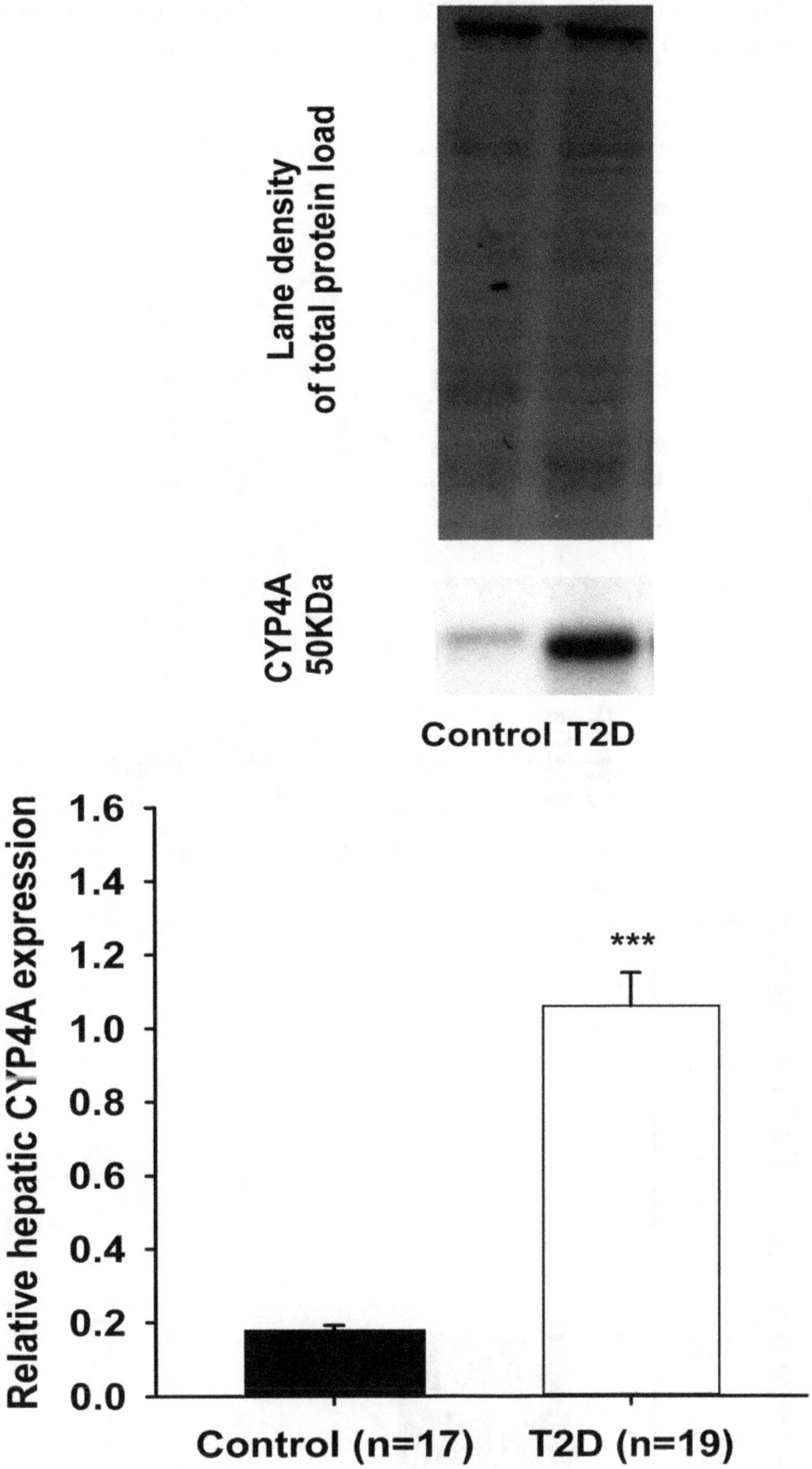

Figure 3. A significant increase (*** $p < 0.001$) was observed in the protein expression of hepatic CYP4A in T2D mice (1.06 ± 0.09) compared to controls (0.18 ± 0.01).

Upper panel shows the representative blot images of hepatic CYP4A and the total proteins loaded for both the control and T2D groups. Moreover, as seen with CYP4A, Figure 4 (lower panel) shows a significant increase in relative expression of CYP4F proteins that was observed in the liver of T2D mice when compared to the control animals (2.53 ± 0.22 vs. 1.10 ± 0.07; $p < 0.001$). Upper panel shows the representative blot images of hepatic CYP4F and the total proteins loaded for both the control and T2D groups.

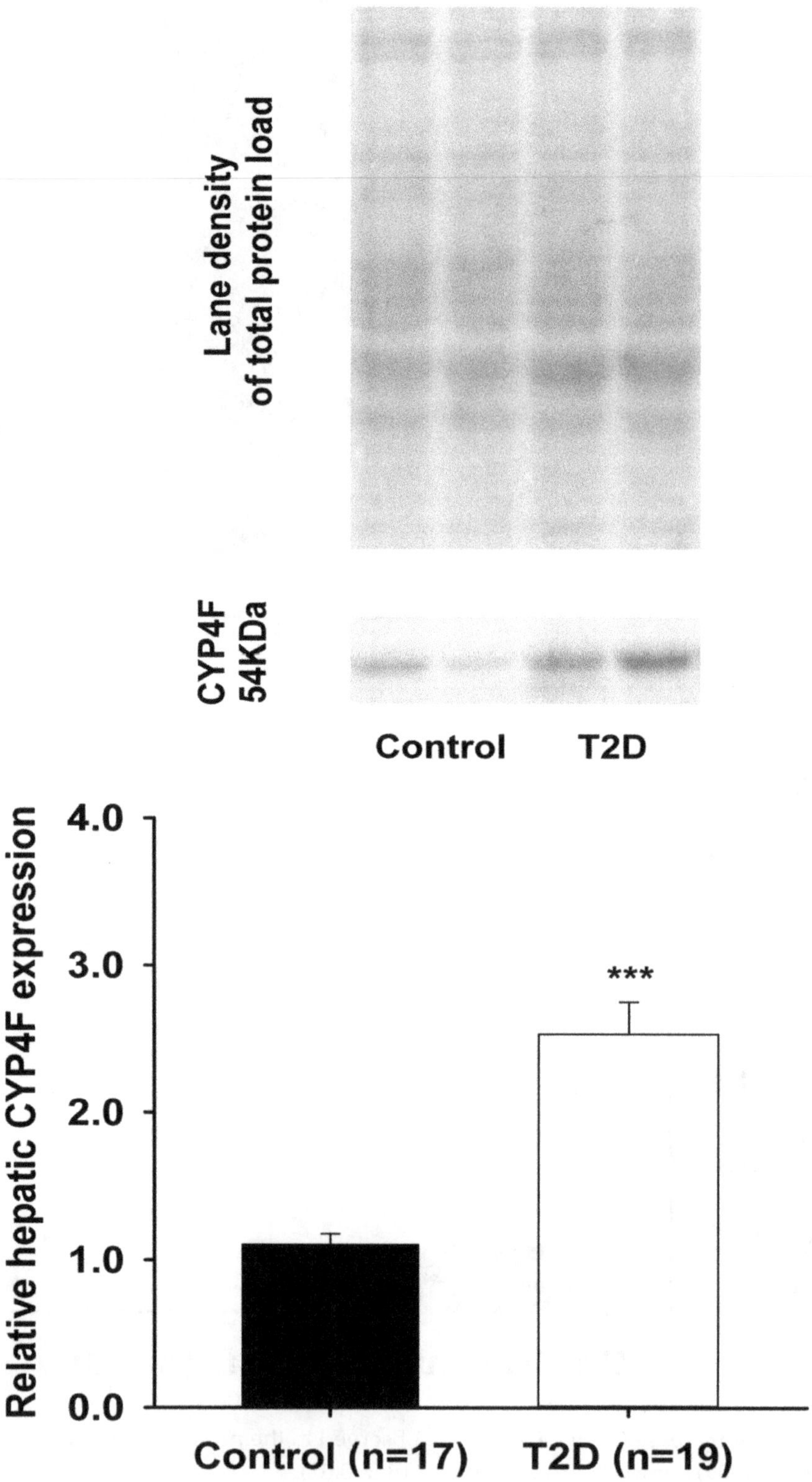

Figure 4. A significant increase (*** $p < 0.001$) was observed in the protein expression of hepatic CYP4F in T2D mice (2.53 ± 0.22) compared to controls (1.10 ± 0.07).

4. Discussion

The pathophysiology of CVD is highly complex, and a constellation of risk factors contribute to its development and progression. Consequence of the current worldwide obesity epidemic, one major risk factor of CVD that is becoming epidemic as well is Type II diabetes. Interestingly, we have already shown that CYPs expression and metabolic activity are altered in a number of conditions such as metabolic syndrome and renal insufficiency in different animal models [29,30]. Besides, Imig et al. demonstrated a decrease in renal expression of CYP2C epoxygenase enzymes in diabetic obese Zucker rats and in high fat diet-fed insulin resistant rats [31]. They concluded that eicosanoids metabolites are altered in Type II diabetes and contribute to the progression of renal injury. Moreover, Shimojo et al. reported an induction of hepatic and renal CYP4A subfamily enzymes in diabetic rats [32]. Yousif et al. demonstrated that CYP4 family expression is twice as high in the hearts of diabetic rats when compared to normal animals [33]. Enriquez et al. showed that expression of murine CYP4A10 and 4A14 in the obese mice, and 4A2 in the male fatty Zucker rat, were greatly increased [34]. Zhao et al. [35] studied the mesenteric artery protein expression in lean and obese Zucker rats. They concluded that mesenteric arterial CYP2C11 and CYP2J proteins were decreased by 38% and 43%, respectively, in obese Zucker rats. In contrast, sEH mRNA and protein expressions were significantly increased in obese Zucker rat mesenteric arteries [35]. A previous study has shown that the synthesis of renal CYP450 (CYP)-derived eicosanoids is downregulated in genetic or high-fat diet-induced obese rats [36]. These results demonstrated that the PPAR-alpha agonist fenofibrate increased renal CYP-derived eicosanoids and restored endothelial dilator function in obese Zucker rats [36]. A study from Theken et al. [37] evaluated CYP epoxygenase (EET+DHET) and ω-hydroxylase (20-HETE) metabolic activity in liver and kidney in wild-type mice fed with a high fat diet, which promoted weight gain and significantly increased insulinemia. Hepatic CYP epoxygenase metabolic activity was significantly suppressed, while renal CYP ω-hydroxylase metabolic activity was significantly induced in high fat diet-fed mice. A significantly higher 20-HETE:EET+DHET formation rate ratio was observed in both tissues [37]. They concluded that the observed changes in CYP epoxygenase and hydroxylase metabolic activity were driven by high fat diet rather than by genotype.

Interestingly, there are recent clinical studies that begin to bridge the gap between animal models of CYP-mediated arachidonic acid metabolism and cardiovascular disease in humans. Indeed, Akasaka et al. [38] examined CYP2C19 genotypes in 81 patients with microvascular angina (MVA) caused by coronary microvascular dysfunction. They found that CYP2C19 poor metabolizers had declined levels of EETs, suggesting insufficient defensive mechanism against chronic inflammation, a risk factor for MVA. Moreover, Theken et al. [39] evaluated the role of CYP-derived eicosanoids in humans with stable atherosclerotic cardiovascular disease (CVD, $n = 82$) versus healthy volunteers ($n = 36$). Among other things, they noted that obesity was significantly associated with low plasma EET levels and 14,15-EET:14,15 DHET ratios. Collectively, their findings suggest that CYP-mediated eicosanoid metabolism is dysregulated in certain subsets of CVD patients and demonstrate that biomarkers of CYP epoxygenase are altered in stable CVD patients relative to healthy individuals. Later on, the same group came up with a study [24] of 106 patients with stable coronary artery disease (CAD) in which relationships between biomarkers of CYP-mediated eicosanoid metabolism and vascular function phenotypes were evaluated. Collectively, their findings demonstrated that enhanced CYP ω-hydroxylases (generating HETEs) and sEH (degradating EETs) metabolic functions are associated with more advanced endothelial dysfunction and vascular inflammation, respectively, in patients with established atherosclerotic CVD.

In the present study, we show that Type II diabetes, a major CVD-associated pathological condition, significantly decreases the cardiac protein expression of cytochrome P450 CYP2J and of hepatic CYP2C in *db/db* mice. As CYP2J and CYP2C are the major AA epoxygenases in the cardiovascular and hepatic systems [2], where they are widely expressed respectively [40], down regulation of these two CYP epoxygenases could compromise the formation of EETs, which play many crucial roles in cardiovascular homeostasis. In fact, in addition to their potent vasodilating effect, EETs have potent anti-inflammatory properties, inhibit platelet aggregation, promote fibrinolysis, and reduce vascular smooth muscle cell proliferation [41]. In addition, our results also show increased hepatic protein expression of both cytochrome P450 CYP4A and CYP4F in *db/db* mice. CYP4F2 is known to be the key AA ω-hydroxylase in human liver and kidney with a more superior substrate specificity for AA than the already established AA ω-hydroxylase CYP4A11 [42]. The massive formation of 20-HETE, along with its potent detrimental pro-inflammatory effects during ischemia-reperfusion and vasoconstrictor effect in the coronary arteries [2], suggests that it could also serve as an intracellular second messenger underlying the regulation of vascular tone [43].

5. Conclusions

Taken together, Type II diabetes-induced combined alterations of cardiac CYP2J, and hepatic CYP2C, CYP4A, and CYP4F protein expression are likely to play a significant role in CVD. As these four CYP isoforms were shown to generate the most vasoactive eicosanoid metabolites, Type II diabetes likely generates deleterious in situ alterations in the endogenous disposition of AA. Their net effect is thought to further promote CVD by disrupting the fine equilibrium between cardioprotective (CYP2C/CYP2J-generated) and cardiotoxic (CYP4A/CYP4F-generated) AA metabolites, adding weight on the cardiotoxic side of the balance.

6. Limitation

CVD-associated pathophysiological features of the diabetic mice such as (coronary disease, vasoconstriction, endothelial dysfunction, atherosclerosis, etc.) were not compared to those of the control animals. Such further studies, beyond the scope of this article, would help to elucidate how and how much the altered CYPs in Type II diabetes may influence the onset and progression of cardiovascular disease.

Acknowledgments: This study received support from the Fondation de l'Institut universitaire de cardiologie et de pneumologie de Québec and from Diabète Québec (grants to Benoit Drolet and Chantale Simard). Carolanne Gélinas and Audrey Blais-Boilard were recipients of summer studentship awards from the Fonds d'Enseignement et de Recherche (FER) de la Faculté de pharmacie de l'Université Laval. Jessica Virgili was the recipient of a doctoral studentship award from the FER. Benoit Drolet and Chantale Simard were scholars of the Fonds de recherche du Québec-Santé (FRQ-S). The funding sponsors had no role in the design of the study; in the collection, analyses, or interpretation of data; in the writing of the manuscript; or in the decision to publish the results.

Author Contributions: Sylvie Pilote, Carolanne Gélinas, Alida-Douce Kamaliza, Audrey Blais-Boilard, Jessica Virgili, and Dany Patoine performed the experiments. Jessica Virgili, Sylvie Pilote, and Dany Patoine analysed the data. Benoit Drolet and Chantale Simard contributed reagents/materials/analysis tools. Benoit Drolet and Chantale Simard wrote the paper.

References

1. Kaspera, R.; Totah, R.A. Epoxyeicosatrienoic acids: Formation, metabolism and potential role in tissue physiology and pathophysiology. *Expert Opin. Drug Metab. Toxicol.* **2009**, *5*, 757–771. [CrossRef] [PubMed]
2. Seubert, J.M.; Zeldin, D.C.; Nithipatikom, K.; Gross, G.J. Role of epoxyeicosatrienoic acids in protecting the myocardium following ischemia/reperfusion injury. *Prostaglandins Other Lipid Mediat.* **2007**, *82*, 50–59. [CrossRef] [PubMed]
3. Jenkins, C.M.; Cedars, A.; Gross, R.W. Eicosanoid signalling pathways in the heart. *Cardiovasc. Res.* **2009**, *82*, 240–249. [CrossRef] [PubMed]
4. Kuhn, H.; Banthiya, S.; van Leyen, K. Mammalian lipoxygenases and their biological relevance. *Biochim. Biophys. Acta* **2015**, *1851*, 308–330. [CrossRef] [PubMed]
5. Luo, W.; Liu, B.; Zhou, Y. The endothelial cyclooxygenase pathway: Insights from mouse arteries. *Eur. J. Pharmacol.* **2016**, *780*, 148–158. [CrossRef] [PubMed]
6. Fleming, I. Epoxyeicosatrienoic acids, cell signaling and angiogenesis. *Prostaglandins Other Lipid Mediat.* **2007**, *82*, 60–67. [CrossRef] [PubMed]
7. Jamieson, K.L.; Endo, T.; Darwesh, A.M.; Samokhvalov, V.; Seubert, J.M. Cytochrome P450-derived eicosanoids and heart function. *Pharmacol Ther.* **2017**. [CrossRef] [PubMed]

8. Huwiler, A.; Pfeilschifter, J. Lipids as targets for novel anti-inflammatory therapies. *Pharmacol. Ther.* **2009**, *124*, 96–112. [CrossRef] [PubMed]
9. Ayajiki, K.; Okamura, T.; Fujioka, H.; Imaoka, S.; Funae, Y.; Toda, N. Involvement of CYP3A-derived arachidonic acid metabolite(s) in responses to endothelium-derived K+ channel opening substance in monkey lingual artery. *Br. J. Pharmacol.* **1999**, *128*, 802–808. [CrossRef] [PubMed]
10. Delozier, T.C.; Kissling, G.E.; Coulter, S.J.; Dai, D.; Foley, J.F.; Bradbury, J.A.; Murphy, E.; Steenbergen, C.; Zeldin, D.C.; Goldstein, J.A. Detection of human CYP2C8, CYP2C9, and CYP2J2 in cardiovascular tissues. *Drug Metab. Dispos.* **2007**, *35*, 682–688. [CrossRef] [PubMed]
11. Klose, T.S.; Blaisdell, J.A.; Goldstein, J.A. Gene structure of CYP2C8 and extrahepatic distribution of the human CYP2Cs. *J. Biochem. Mol. Toxicol.* **1999**, *13*, 289–295. [CrossRef]
12. Lee, C.A.; Neul, D.; Clouser-Roche, A.; Dalvie, D.; Wester, M.R.; Jiang, Y.; Jones, J.P.; Friewald, S.; Zientek, M.; Totah, R.A. Identification of novel substrates for human cytochrome P450 2J2. *Drug Metab. Dispos.* **2010**, *38*, 347–356. [CrossRef] [PubMed]
13. Wu, S.; Moomaw, C.R.; Tomer, K.B.; Falck, J.R.; Zeldin, D.C. Molecular cloning and expression of CYP2J2, a human cytochrome P450 arachidonic acid epoxygenase highly expressed in heart. *J. Biol. Chem.* **1996**, *271*, 3460–3468. [CrossRef] [PubMed]
14. Zeldin, D.C.; Foley, J.; Goldsworthy, S.M.; Cook, M.E.; Boyle, J.E.; Ma, J.; Moomaw, C.R.; Tomer, K.B.; Steenbergen, C.; Wu, S. CYP2J subfamily cytochrome P450s in the gastrointestinal tract: Expression, localization, and potential functional significance. *Mol. Pharmacol.* **1997**, *51*, 931–943. [CrossRef] [PubMed]
15. Zeldin, D.C.; Foley, J.; Ma, J.; Boyle, J.E.; Pascual, J.M.; Moomaw, C.R.; Tomer, K.B.; Steenbergen, C.; Wu, S. CYP2J subfamily P450s in the lung: Expression, localization, and potential functional significance. *Mol. Pharmacol.* **1996**, *50*, 1111–1117. [PubMed]
16. Zeldin, D.C.; Foley, J.; Boyle, J.E.; Moomaw, C.R.; Tomer, K.B.; Parker, C.; Steenbergen, C.; Wu, S. Predominant expression of an arachidonate epoxygenase in islets of Langerhans cells in human and rat pancreas. *Endocrinology* **1997**, *138*, 1338–1346. [CrossRef] [PubMed]
17. Borlak, J.; Walles, M.; Levsen, K.; Thum, T. Verapamil: metabolism in cultures of primary human coronary arterial endothelial cells. *Drug Metab. Dispos.* **2003**, *31*, 888–891. [CrossRef] [PubMed]
18. Graham, R.A.; Goodwin, B.; Merrihew, R.V.; Krol, W.L.; Lecluyse, E.L. Cloning, tissue expression, and regulation of beagle dog CYP4A genes. *Toxicol. Sci.* **2006**, *92*, 356–367. [CrossRef] [PubMed]
19. Zhang, D.; Xie, X.; Chen, Y.; Hammock, B.D.; Kong, W.; Zhu, Y. Homocysteine upregulates soluble epoxide hydrolase in vascular endothelium in vitro and in vivo. *Circ Res.* **2012**, *110*, 808–817. [CrossRef] [PubMed]
20. Davis, B.B.; Thompson, D.A.; Howard, L.L.; Morisseau, C.; Hammock, B.D.; Weiss, R.H. Inhibitors of soluble epoxide hydrolase attenuate vascular smooth muscle cell proliferation. *Proc. Natl. Acad. Sci. USA* **2002**, *99*, 2222–2227. [CrossRef] [PubMed]
21. Elbekai, R.H.; El-Kadi, A.O. Cytochrome P450 enzymes: Central players in cardiovascular health and disease. *Pharmacol. Ther.* **2006**, *112*, 564–587. [CrossRef] [PubMed]
22. Roman, R.J.; Maier, K.G.; Sun, C.W.; Harder, D.R.; Alonso-Galicia, M. Renal and cardiovascular actions of 20-hydroxyeicosatetraenoic acid and epoxyeicosatrienoic acids. *Clin. Exp. Pharmacol. Physiol.* **2000**, *27*, 855–865. [CrossRef] [PubMed]
23. Abdul-Ghani, M.; DeFronzo, R.A.; Del Prato, S.; Chilton, R.; Singh, R.; Ryder, R.E.J. Cardiovascular Disease and Type 2 Diabetes: Has the Dawn of a New Era Arrived? *Diabetes Care* **2017**, *40*, 813–820. [CrossRef] [PubMed]
24. Schuck, R.N.; Theken, K.N.; Edin, M.L.; Caughey, M.; Bass, A.; Ellis, K.; Tran, B.; Steele, S.; Simmons, B.P.; Lih, F.B.; et al. Cytochrome P450-derived eicosanoids and vascular dysfunction in coronary artery disease patients. *Atherosclerosis* **2013**, *227*, 442–448. [CrossRef] [PubMed]
25. Guo, Z.; Su, W.; Allen, S.; Pang, H.; Daugherty, A.; Smart, E.; Gong, M.C. COX-2 Up-regulation and vascular smooth muscle contractile hyperreactivity in spontaneous diabetic *db/db* mice. *Cardiovasc. Res.* **2005**, *67*, 723–735. [CrossRef] [PubMed]
26. Hatley, M.E.; Srinivasan, S.; Reilly, K.B.; Bolick, D.T. Increased Production of 12/15 Lipoxygenase Eicosanoids Accelerates Monocyte/Endothelial Interactions in Diabetic *db/db* Mice. *J. Biol. Chem.* **2003**, *278*, 25369–25375. [CrossRef] [PubMed]

27. Patoine, D.; Levac, X.; Pilote, S.; Drolet, B.; Simard, C. Decreased CYP3A expression and activity in guinea pig models of diet-induced metabolic syndrome: Is fatty liver infiltration involved? *Drug Metab. Dispos.* **2013**, *41*, 952–957. [CrossRef] [PubMed]
28. Pilote, S.; Virgili, J.; Patoine, D.; Drolet, B.; Simard, C. Altered hepatic protein expression of CYP4F in mouse models of Type I and Type II diabetes. In Proceedings of the 5th ICCR Congress on Chronic Societal Cardiometabolic Diseases, Quebec City, QC, Canada, 8–12 July 2015; Volume 7, p. 28.
29. Patoine, D.; Petit, M.; Pilote, S.; Picard, F.; Drolet, B.; Simard, C. Modulation of CYP3a expression and activity in mice models of Type 1 and Type 2 diabetes. *Pharmacol. Res. Perspect.* **2014**, *2*, e00082:1–8. [CrossRef] [PubMed]
30. Kingma, J.; Simard, D.; Patoine, D.; Pilote, S.; Drolet, B.; Rouleau, J.; Simard, C. Chronic kidney disease augments cardiovascular risk: Modulation of myocardial blood flow regulation and CYP450 arachidonic acid metabolites. International Academy of Cardiology Annual Scientific Sessions 2014. In Proceedings of the 19th World Congress on Heart Disease, Boston, MA, USA, 25–28 July 2014. *Cardiology* **2014**, *128* (Suppl. 1), 115.
31. Imig, J.D. Eicosanoids and renal damage in cardiometabolic syndrome. *Exp. Opin. Drug Metab. Toxicol.* **2008**, *4*, 165–174. [CrossRef] [PubMed]
32. Shimojo, N.; Ishizaki, T.; Imaoka, S.; Funae, Y.; Fujii, S.; Okuda, K. Changes in amounts of cytochrome P450 isozymes and levels of catalytic activities in hepatic and renal microsomes of rats with streptozocin-induced diabetes. *Biochem. Pharmacol.* **1993**, *46*, 621–627. [CrossRef]
33. Yousif, M.H.; Benter, I.F.; Roman, R.J. Cytochrome P450 metabolites of arachidonic acid play a role in the enhanced cardiac dysfunction in diabetic rats following ischaemic reperfusion injury. *Auton. Autacoid. Pharmacol.* **2009**, *29*, 33–41. [CrossRef] [PubMed]
34. Enriquez, A.; Leclercq, I.; Farrell, G.C.; Robertson, G. Altered expression of hepatic CYP2E1 and CYP4A in obese, diabetic ob/ob mice, and fa/fa Zucker rats. *Biochem. Biophys. Res. Commun.* **1999**, *255*, 300–306. [CrossRef] [PubMed]
35. Zhao, X.; Dey, A.; Romanko, O.P.; Stepp, D.W.; Wang, M.H.; Zhou, Y.; Jin, L.; Pollock, J.S.; Clinton Webb, R.; Imig, J.D. Decreased epoxygenase and increased epoxide hydrolase expression in the mesenteric artery of obese Zucker rats. *Am. J. Physiol. Regul. Integr. Comp. Physiol.* **2005**, *288*, R188–R196. [CrossRef] [PubMed]
36. Zhao, X.; Quigley, J.E.; Yuan, J.; Wang, M.H.; Zhou, Y.; Imig, J.D. PPAR-alpha activator fenofibrate increases renal CYP-derived eicosanoid synthesis and improves endothelial dilator function in obese Zucker rats. *Am. J. Physiol. Heart Circ. Physiol.* **2006**, *290*, H2187–H2195. [CrossRef] [PubMed]
37. Theken, K.N.; Deng, Y.; Schuck, R.N.; Oni-Orisan, A.; Miller, T.M.; Kannon, M.A.; Poloyac, S.M.; Lee, C.R. Enalapril reverses high-fat diet-induced alterations in cytochrome P450-mediated eicosanoid metabolism. *Am. J. Physiol. Endocrinol. Metab.* **2012**, *302*, E500–E509. [CrossRef] [PubMed]
38. Akasaka, T.; Sueta, D.; Arima, Y.; Tabata, N.; Takashio, S.; Izumiya, Y.; Yamamoto, E.; Tsujita, K.; Kojima, S.; Kaikita, K.; et al. CYP2C19 variants and epoxyeicosatrienoic acids in patients with microvascular angina. *IJC Heart Vasc.* **2017**, *15*, 15–20. [CrossRef] [PubMed]
39. Theken, K.N.; Schuck, R.N.; Edin, M.L.; Tran, B.; Ellis, K.; Bass, A.; Lih, F.B.; Tomer, K.B.; Poloyac, S.M.; Wu, M.C.; et al. Evaluation of cytochrome P450-derived eicosanoids in humans with stable atherosclerotic cardiovascular disease. *Atherosclerosis* **2012**, *222*, 530–536. [CrossRef] [PubMed]
40. Alsaad, A.M.; Zordoky, B.N.; Tse, M.M.; El-Kadi, A.O. Role of cytochrome P450-mediated arachidonic acid metabolites in the pathogenesis of cardiac hypertrophy. *Drug Metab. Rev.* **2013**, *45*, 173–195. [CrossRef] [PubMed]
41. Tacconelli, S.; Patrignani, P. Inside epoxyeicosatrienoic acids and cardiovascular disease. *Front Pharmacol.* **2014**, *5*, 239. [CrossRef] [PubMed]
42. Powell, P.K.; Wolf, I.; Jin, R.; Lasker, J.M. Metabolism of arachidonic acid to 20-hydroxy-5,8,11, 14-eicosatetraenoic acid by P450 enzymes in human liver: Involvement of CYP4F2 and CYP4A11. *J. Pharmacol. Exp. Ther.* **1998**, *285*, 1327–1336. [PubMed]
43. Roman, R.J. P-450 metabolites of arachidonic acid in the control of cardiovascular function. *Physiol. Rev.* **2002**, *82*, 131–185. [CrossRef] [PubMed]

6

Imbalance of Drug Transporter-CYP450s Interplay by Diabetes and its Clinical Significance

Yiting Yang and Xiaodong Liu *

Center of Drug Metabolism and Pharmacokinetics, China Pharmaceutical University, Nanjing 210009, China; 1821010209@stu.cpu.edu.cn

* Correspondence: xdliu@cpu.edu.cn

Abstract: The pharmacokinetics of a drug is dependent upon the coordinate work of influx transporters, enzymes and efflux transporters (i.e., transporter-enzyme interplay). The transporter–enzyme interplay may occur in liver, kidney and intestine. The influx transporters involving drug transport are organic anion transporting polypeptides (OATPs), peptide transporters (PepTs), organic anion transporters (OATs), monocarboxylate transporters (MCTs) and organic cation transporters (OCTs). The efflux transporters are P-glycoprotein (P-gp), multidrug/toxin extrusions (MATEs), multidrug resistance-associated proteins (MRPs) and breast cancer resistance protein (BCRP). The enzymes related to drug metabolism are mainly cytochrome P450 enzymes (CYP450s) and UDP-glucuronosyltransferases (UGTs). Accumulating evidence has demonstrated that diabetes alters the expression and functions of CYP450s and transporters in a different manner, disordering the transporter–enzyme interplay, in turn affecting the pharmacokinetics of some drugs. We aimed to focus on (1) the imbalance of transporter-CYP450 interplay in the liver, intestine and kidney due to altered expressions of influx transporters (OATPs, OCTs, OATs, PepTs and MCT6), efflux transporters (P-gp, BCRP and MRP2) and CYP450s (CYP3As, CYP1A2, CYP2E1 and CYP2Cs) under diabetic status; (2) the net contributions of these alterations in the expression and functions of transporters and CYP450s to drug disposition, therapeutic efficacy and drug toxicity; (3) application of a physiologically-based pharmacokinetic model in transporter–enzyme interplay.

Keywords: diabetes; transporter-enzyme interplay; influx transporter; efflux transporter; physiologically based pharmacokinetic model, pharmacokinetics, cytochrome P450 enzymes

1. Introduction

The pharmacokinetics of a drug is determined by absorption, distribution, excretion and metabolism. Drug absorption, distribution and excretion are mainly controlled by drug transporters, while drug metabolism is mediated by metabolic enzymes. These drug transporters are classified into the ATP binding cassette (ABC) family and the solute carrier (SLC) family. The main SLC transporters involved in drug transport are multidrug/toxin extrusions (MATEs), organic anion transporting polypeptides (OATPs), monocarboxylate transporters (MCTs), organic anion transporters (OATs), peptide transporters (PepTs), and organic cation transporters (OCTs). Most SLC transporters belong to influx transporters, except for MATEs. The identified ABC transporters related to drug efflux include P-glycoprotein (P-gp), multidrug resistance-associated proteins (MRPs) and breast cancer resistance protein (BCRP). These transporters are widely expressed in the intestine, liver and kidney. They affect drug therapeutic effects/toxicity via regulating drug uptake or secretion. Enzymes involved in drug metabolism mainly include cytochrome P450 enzymes (CYP450s) and UDP-glucuronosyltransferases (UGTs). These enzymes are also widely distributed in the liver, intestine and kidney. Drug disposition in tissues is highly dependent on the coordinate work of these influx transporters, enzymes and efflux transporters, termed as the "interplay of transporters and enzymes" [1–3]. Moreover, multiple SLC transporters, ABC transporters and enzymes often participate in the disposition of drugs. A typical example is atorvastatin. Atorvastatin is a substrate of P-gp, MRP2, BCRP, OATP1B1, OATP1B2, OATP2A1, CYP3A4/5 [4] and UGTs [5,6]. Sodium taurocholate co-transporting polypeptide (NTCP) also mediates hepatic uptake of atorvastatin [7]. In the liver, atorvastatin enters hepatocytes from portal blood mainly via influx transporters at the basolateral surface of hepatocytes. In hepatocytes, atorvastatin is metabolized via CYP3As or UGTs. Atorvastatin and its metabolites are excreted into bile via efflux transporters (MRP2, BCRP and P-gp) or returned to the blood via MRP3 [8]. The transporter–enzyme interplay also occurs in the intestine and kidney. Accumulating studies [9–12] have demonstrated that diabetes remarkably alters the expression and functions of drug transporters and CYP450s, disordering transporter-CYP450 interplay and in turning affecting the disposition of corresponding drugs, their therapeutic efficacy or drug toxicity. Here, we aimed to focus on (1) the imbalance of transporter-CYP450 interplay in the liver, intestine and kidney due to alterations in the expression of influx transporters, efflux transporters and CYP450s under diabetic status; (2) the net contributions of the altered expressions and functions of transporters and CYP450s to drug disposition, therapeutic efficacy and drug toxicity; (3) application of a physiologically based pharmacokinetic model (PBPK) in the imbalance of transporter–enzyme interplay under diabetic conditions.

2. Liver

Drugs are eliminated in the liver mainly via metabolism and biliary excretion. The liver highly expresses various drug transporters (such as P-gp, BCRP, MRPs, OATPs, OCTs, OATs and MATEs) (Figure 1A) and drug metabolic enzymes (such as CYP450s and UGTs). They work in series to control the disposition of drugs in the liver (Figure 1B).

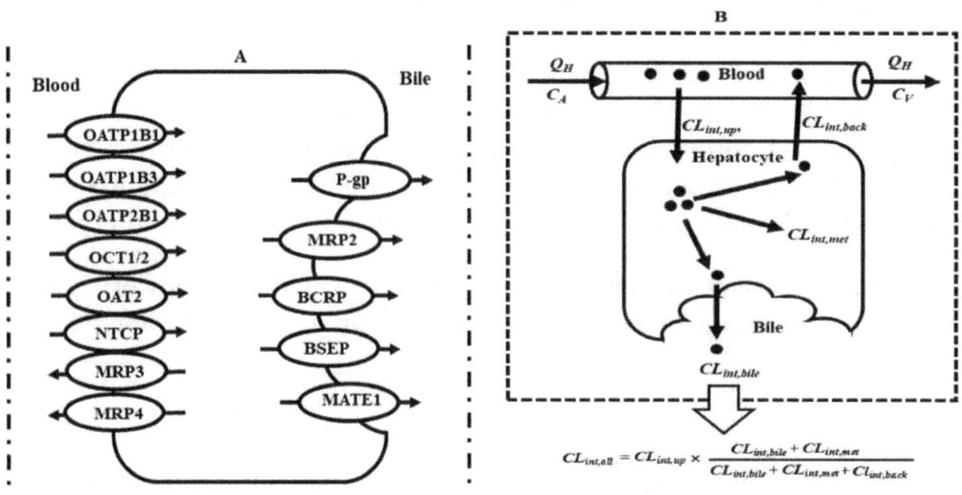

Figure 1. (**A**) Possible location of main transporters in liver. (**B**) Transporter–enzyme interplay in the elimination of drugs in the liver. Symbol: BCRP, breast cancer resistance protein; BSEP, bile salt export pump; C_A, concentrations of drug in arterial blood; $CL_{int,all}$, overall hepatic intrinsic clearance; $CL_{int,up}$, intrinsic uptake clearance; $CL_{int,back}$, intrinsic clearance of backflux to blood; $CL_{int,met}$, intrinsic metabolism clearances; $CL_{int,bile}$, biliary clearance of unbound drug; C_V, concentrations of drug in venous blood; MATEs, multidrug/toxin extrusion; MRPs, multidrug resistance-associated proteins; NTCP, sodium taurocholate co-transporting polypeptide; OATs, organic anion transporters; OATPs, organic anion transporting polypeptides; OCTs, organic cation transporters; Q_H, hepatic blood flow; P-gp, P-glycoprotein.

2.1. OATPs

OATPs, expressed at the basolateral membrane of hepatocytes, mediates hepatocyte uptake of many anions from the blood, which becomes a rate-limited process of hepatic clearances for some drugs [3]. It was found that in diabetic rats (type 2 diabetes) induced by a streptozocin (STZ) and high-fat diet (HFD) combination (termed as STZ/HFD), hepatic OATP1B2 (rodent orthologue of human OATP1B1 and OATP1B3) is remarkably induced, leading to increased hepatic uptake of repaglinide [9,10], atorvastatin [9,11] and simvastatin [12] as well as hepatic clearances [9,11]. In line with this, the diabetic rats showed lower plasma concentrations of atorvastatin [9,11], simvastatin [12] and pravastatin [13] compared with control rats. Clinical trials also showed that tuberculosis patients with diabetes showed significantly lower concentrations of rifampicin than non-diabetic patients [14,15], which may be attributed to the induction of hepatic OATPs by diabetes and rifampicin.

2.2. *P-gp*

P-gp, expressed at the canalicular membrane of hepatocytes, mediates biliary excretion of its substrates. Diabetes was reported to upregulate the expression of hepatic Mdr1b (ABCB1b) mRNA and P-gp protein in 8-day diabetic Wistar rats (type 1 diabetes) induced by STZ, which was associated with the activation of protein kinase C alpha (PKCα) and nuclear factor kappa-B (NF-κB) [16]. A similar increase in the expression of hepatic Mdr1b mRNA was found in STZ-induced diabetic rats [17]. The induction of hepatic P-gp protein expression was also observed in STZ/HFD-induced diabetic rats [11]. However, a report showed that in STZ-induced diabetic Sprague-Dawley rats, 5-week diabetes significantly increased Mdr1a (ABCB1a) and decreased Mdr1b mRNA expression, but significantly decreased expressions of both Mdr1a and Mdr1b mRNA were found in 8-week diabetic rats. Immunoblotting demonstrated that 5-week diabetes significantly reduced the expression of P-gp protein in rats, but the decreases were not found in 8-week diabetic rats, indicating that the regulation of P-gp protein occurred at post-transcriptional level under diabetic status [18].

2.3. *BCRP*

BCRP, expressed at the canalicular membrane of hepatocytes, is also involved in the biliary excretion of its substrates. Altered expressions of hepatic BCRP under diabetic status are dependent on the type of diabetes, and diabetic progression. For example, expressions of hepatic BCRP mRNA in 5-week and 8-week diabetic rats induced by STZ were significantly downregulated, but expression of BCRP protein only showed a trend to decrease [19]. Similarly, He et al. reported that hepatic BCRP mRNA level was decreased in STZ-induced diabetic rats, whereas in type 2 diabetic patients and Goto-Kakizaki (GK) rats BCRP mRNA expression was significantly increased, although BCRP protein was unaltered [20]. Decreased expression of hepatic BCRP protein was observed in 10-day (but not 22-day) diabetic rats induced by STZ/HFD [11]. Interestingly, pregnancy also affected the expression of hepatic BCRP under diabetic status. For example, STZ treatment upregulated the expression of BCRP mRNA and protein in non-pregnant mice, but not in pregnant mice [21].

2.4. *MRP2*

MRP2 is co-expressed with P-gp and BCRP at the canalicular membrane of hepatocytes. Alterations in the expression of MRP2 by diabetes are also dependent on species. STZ-induced diabetic Donryu rats showed significantly lower expression of hepatic MRP2 mRNA, which was in line with lower biliary excretion of pravastatin [13]. A similar decrease in the protein (not mRNA) of hepatic MRP2 was found in STZ-induced diabetic male Wistar rats [22]. However, STZ-induced diabetic Sprague-Dawley rats showed higher expression of hepatic MRP2 protein, which was in line with higher biliary excretion of sulfobromophthalein compared with control rats [23]. Moreover, STZ treatment upregulated the expression of MRP2 in non-pregnant mice but not in pregnant mice [21]. The induction of hepatic MRP2 may partly explain the increased biliary excretions of cefoperazone and some anions (such as bengal, indocyanine green and bromcresol green) under diabetic status [24,25].

2.5. CYP450s

Growing evidence has demonstrated that diabetes increases the expression of some CYP450s (such as CYP2A1, CYP1A2, CYP2B1/2, CYP2C6, CYP2C7, CYP3A1/2 and CYP2E1) in rats [9,11,12,26–30], although opposite reports have also been shown [31,32]. The induction of CYP3A1/2 led to lower plasma exposure of simvastatin [12], atorvastatin [9,11], verapamil [27,29] and lidocaine [30] following intravenous dose to diabetic rats. The formation of 1,3-dimethyluric acid from theophylline is mainly mediated via CYP1A2 and CYP2E1. Both alloxan-induced diabetes and STZ-induced diabetes were reported to increase expressions of hepatic CYP2E1 and CYP3A2 by three-fold, leading to a lower area under the curve (AUC) of theophylline and a higher AUC of 1,3-dimethyluric acid following oral and intravenous administration to rats [28]. The induction of CYP1A2 (and CYP3A1/2) may contribute to a lower AUC of oltipraz [33], higher non-renal clearances of omeprazole [34] and systemic clearance of antipyrine [35] in diabetic rats. Diazinon is metabolized to toxic metabolite diethylphosphate via CYP3A2 and CYP1A2. The increases in diazinon toxicity and urinary recovery of its metabolite diethylphosphate in diabetic rats may be attributed to the enhancement of hepatic CYP1A2 (and CYP3A2)-mediated metabolism of diazinon [35]. A report showed that protein expression and activity of hepatic CYP2E1 in STZ-induced diabetic rats were increased by three- and 2.5-fold in comparison to control rats, respectively. The increases were in line with the increased oxidative stress, demonstrating crucial roles of CYP2E1 in stress-induced pathological processes under diabetic status [31,32,36].

Hyperketonemia (such as acetone) is considered as a reason for diabetes inducing CYP2E1. Data from primary cultured rat hepatocytes demonstrated that insulin decreased the expression of CYP2E1 and CYP2B protein and mRNA, inferring that a deficiency of insulin is also a reason that diabetes induces the expression of CYP2El and CYP2B [37]. Furthermore, data from both Fa2N-4 cells and HepG2 cells demonstrated that fatty acids (palmitic acid, oleic acid, stearic acid and linoleic acid), but not insulin, upregulated the activity and expression of CYP3A4 mRNA and protein, indicating that increased levels of fatty acids may be one of the reasons that diabetes elevated the function and expression of CYP3A4 [38]. Recent studies showed that diabetes reduced the expression of hepatic peroxisome proliferator activated receptor γ (PPARγ) protein [39,40] and PPARα protein [41]. The decreased expression of hepatic PPARα was attributed to the increased palmitic acid [41]. A report showed that PPARα agonist gemfibrozil in PPARα-null mice showed more induction of the mRNA, protein and activity of CYP3a, CYP2b and CYP2c than in wild-type mice, indicating that the induction of gemfibrozil on CYP450s was suppressed by PPARα activation [42]. The downregulation of PPARα protein expression by diabetes [41] might attenuate the inhibition of PPARα on the expression of CYP450s, leading to the induction of hepatic CYP450s, which needs further investigation. Moreover, diabetes was reported to increase the expression of hepatic glucocorticoid receptor and increase the circulating level of corticosterone [43,44]. The increased level of corticosterone might induce expressions of CYP2B [45] and CYP2C [46] via activating glucocorticoid receptor. All these results demonstrate that alterations in the expressions of hepatic CYP450s were involved in various mechanisms. In contrast to CYP2C6 induction, diabetes significantly lowered the expression of CYP2C11 [26,47–50], impairing the metabolism of diclofenac [49], glibenclamide [48] and nateglinide [47]. The increase in CYP2C6 expression and decrease in CYP2C11 expression may partly explain why the AUC values of both phenytoin and 4′-hydroxylphenytoin in diabetic rats were comparable to control rats [51].

Some contradictory results have also been reported. In Goto-Kakizaki rats, it was found that expressions of hepatic CYP reductase and CYP3A2 were significantly upregulated, accompanied by increases in the activities of midazolam 4-hydroxylase and CYP reductase. In contrast, hepatic expressions of CYP1A2 and CYP3A1 were downregulated, and the activities of 7-methoxyresorufin-*O*-demethylase and 7-ethoxyresorufin-O-deethylase were decreased. Expressions of other CYP450s, such as CYP1B1, CYP2B1, CYP2C11 and CYP2E1, were unaltered, inferring that diabetes regulates the expression of hepatic CYP450s in an isoform-specific manner [30,52]. Similarly, in 20-week-old male db/db mice, testosterone-6β-hydroxylation but not midazolam-1-

hydroxylation was significantly decreased, the intrinsic clearance (CL_{int}) value of testosterone-6β-hydroxylation (CYP3A11) was less than 46% of control mice. Other metabolic reactions such as dextromethorphan-*O*-demethylation (CYP2D), phenacetin-*O*-deethylation (CYP1A2), coumarin-7-hydroxylation (CYP2A4/5), tolbutamide-4-hydroxylation (CYP2C), bupropion-hydroxylation (CYP2B10) and omeprazole-5-hydroxylation (CYP2C29), chlorzoxazone-6-hydroxylation (CYP2E1) were unaltered [53]. Expressions and functions of hepatic CYP450s are dependent on diabetic progression. It was reported that 25-week-old db/db mice showed substantial decreases in mRNA expressions and functions of CYP2B10 and CYP2C29 compared with those of the 10-week-old db/db mice. But mRNA expressions of CYP3A11 and CYP2E1 in the 25-week-old db/db mice were comparable to those of the 10-week-old db/db mice [54]. In Zucker diabetic fatty (ZDF) rats, CYP1A1/2, and CYP3A1 levels were similar among the livers of 5 and 11-week-old ZDF rats and control rats, although 11-week-old ZDF rats possessed the higher serum glucose and glycated hemoglobin levels, but not 5-week-old ZDF rats. Moreover, 5-week-old ZDF rats, but not 11-week-old ZDF rats, showed lower levels of cytochrome b5, CYP2B1, CYP2C11, CYP2E1 and CYP3A2. Consistently, pentoxyresorufin O-depentylation, testosterone 2α- and 16α-hydroxylation, chlorzoxazone 6-hydroxylation, and midazolam 1′- and 4-hydroxylation were decreased only in 5-week-old ZDF rats [55]. Expressions (mRNA and proteins) of CYP3A11/13 and their activities were significantly increased in STZ-induced diabetic C57BLKS/J mice and db/db mice [56]. In contrast, Wang et al. reported that the levels of hepatic CYP3A11 mRNA in C57BL/6 mice diabetic mice induced by HFD/STZ were less than 30% of control mice [31]. All these results indicate that alterations in the expressions of hepatic CYP450s are highly dependent on the type of diabetes, diabetic progression and animal species.

Expressions of hepatic CYP450s in diabetes patients have been widely investigated, although some results are often in contrast to findings in diabetic mice. Gravel et al. [57] assessed the activities of seven major CYP450s (CYP1A2, CYP2B6, CYP2C9, CYP2C19, CYP2D6, CYP2E1, and CYP3A4/5) in 38 type 2 diabetic patients and 35 non-diabetic subjects following the oral administration of a cocktail of probes (caffeine, bupropion, tolbutamide, omeprazole, dextromethorphan, chlorzoxazone and midazolam). They found that the activities of CYP2C19, CYP2B6, and CYP3A in diabetic patients were decreased by about 46%, 45%, and 38%, respectively. CYP1A2 and CYP2C9 activities showed a trend to slightly increase in subjects with diabetes, but activities of CYP2D6 and CYP2E1 were unaltered [57]. Meanwhile, obese children showed higher oral clearance of chlorzoxazone and lower AUC of chlorzoxazone. The AUC was only 46% of nonobese peers, inferring the increased CYP2E1 activity [58].

In vitro data demonstrated that protein expressions and activities of CYP3A4 in hepatic microsomes of diabetic livers were significantly lower than those in non-diabetic donors, although a great variability (8.2-fold) in CYP3A4 protein levels was observed. However, the expression and activity of CYP2E1 were significantly increased [59]. The disposition of nisoldipine in humans was investigated. The results show that the disposition of nisoldipine is enantioselective and nisoldipine is preferentially metabolized. Compared with non-diabetes patients, AUC values of (+)-nisoldipine and (−)-nisoldipine in diabetes patients were increased by 94% and 143%, respectively. Similar increases were also found in their peak concentration (C_{max}). Lidocaine tests demonstrated a decrease in activity of CYP3A (and CYP1A2) [60]. Similarly, pregnant women with gestational diabetes showed significantly higher C_{max} and AUC of lidocaine following peridural anesthesia administration of lidocaine than non-diabetic patients [61]. However, oral plasma concentrations of nifedipine [62] and metoprolol [63] in pregnant women with gestational diabetes were comparable to those in non-diabetic pregnant women. Adith et al. [64] investigated phenytoin kinetics in 10 male type 1 and 10 type 2 diabetic patients. Age- and sex-matched epileptic patients receiving phenytoin alone served as control groups. They found that steady-state concentrations of phenytoin were significantly lower in both types of diabetic patients compared to the respective controls. In line with this, diabetes patients showed significantly increased V_{max}/K_m values of phenytoin. Similarly, the AUCs of cyclosporin A in kidney transplant recipients with diabetes mellitus were approximately 50%~60% that of non-diabetic patients [65,66], which was partly attributed to the delayed gastric emptying [66]. Moreover, no difference in cyclosporine A trough levels between renal transplant patients and renal transplant patients with diabetes was found [67]. Diabetes patients were also reported to show a trend to increase in the expression and activity of CYP3A4, although no statistical significance was observed. Importantly, significant decreases were found in diabetic patients with non-alcoholic fatty liver or non-alcoholic steatohepatitis. Furthermore, the decrease in activity and protein level of CYP3A4 continued with the severity of disease as it progressed from non-alcoholic fatty liver to non-alcoholic steatohepatitis [68]. Matzke et al. [69] also investigated the activities of CYP1A2 and CYP2D6 in type 1 diabetes and type 2 diabetes patients using the probes antipyrine, caffeine and dextromethorphan. The results show that compared with controls, oral clearance of antipyrine was increased 72% in type 1 diabetes patients. Formation clearances of 4-hydroxyantipyrine and 3-hydroxymethylantipyrine were increased by 74% and 137%, respectively. The caffeine metabolic index (paraxanthine/caffeine) was increased by 34%, but no statistical significance was obtained. These alterations did not occur in type 2 diabetes patients. Similarly, although plasma clearance of theophylline in diabetic patients was comparable to that in healthy subjects, there was a positive correlation between hemoglobin A1c values and formation clearances of both 1,3-dimethyluric acid and 1-methyluric acid [70], in line with inductions of CYP1A2 and CYP2E1.

Although antipyrine is widely used to assess the activity of CYP450s in diabetic patients, the results are often confusing [69,71–73]. Sotaniemi et al. [73] assessed the effects of diabetes on hepatic drug metabolism clearance in men using antipyrine in 298 diabetic patients, who were classified by type of the disease, age, gender, duration of therapy and liver involvement. They found that a 13-fold individual variation in antipyrine metabolism existed among all the diabetic patients. Antipyrine was eliminated faster in untreated type 1 patients, which was reversed by insulin treatment. Males aged 16–59 years, who responded insufficiently to insulin therapy, had a rapid antipyrine elimination, which could be normalized by the readjustment of insulin. The antipyrine elimination rate in women with insufficient glucose control on insulin therapy was comparable to controls. In type 2 diabetic patients, the clearance of antipyrine was unaltered in women, but men over 40 years of age showed a reduced antipyrine metabolism. Diet/drinking-habits also affect the expression of hepatic CYP450s. Urry et al. [74] investigated CYP1A2 activity in diabetic patients using coffee as a probe in 57 type 2 diabetes and 146 non-type 2 diabetes. They found that diabetes patients showed higher activity of CYP1A2 than control groups. Further studies showed that participants habitually consuming more caffeine showed higher CYP1A2 activity than participants with lower caffeine consumption. Several studies have demonstrated that CYP2D6 activity is unaltered by diabetes [43,69,75].

2.6. Interplay of Transporter-CYP450s in Liver

In the liver, drugs enter hepatocytes from portal blood through passive diffusion or transporter-mediated transport. In hepatocytes, drugs are metabolized by metabolic enzymes. Parent drugs and their metabolites are pumped out of hepatocytes to bile through efflux transporters (such as P-gp, BCRP or MRP2) and are exported to the blood through passive diffusion or efflux transporters (such as MRP3 and MRP4) (Figure 1B). Typical examples are statins. Most statins are substrates of CYP450s, MRPs, OATPs, BCRP and P-gp, characterizing transporter–enzyme interplay. The overall hepatic intrinsic clearance ($CL_{int,all}$) is a hybrid parameter which is composed of intrinsic influx clearances ($CL_{int,up}$) from portal blood, intrinsic metabolism clearance ($CL_{int,met}$), biliary excretion clearance ($CL_{int,bile}$) and intrinsic efflux clearance ($CL_{int,back}$) of unbound drugs from hepatocytes to the blood, i.e.,

$$CL_{intt,all} = CL_{int,up} \times \frac{CL_{int,bile} + CL_{int,met}}{CL_{int,bile} + CL_{int,met} + CL_{int,back}} \tag{1}$$

According to the relative values of $CL_{int,bile}$ and $CL_{int,met}$, to $CL_{int,back}$, the drugs are classified into three groups.

1. $CL_{int,back}$ is much smaller than the sum of $CL_{int,bile}$ and $CL_{int,met}$, thus, $CL_{int,all}$ is equal to $CL_{int,up}$; this is to say, $CL_{int,all}$ is only controlled by uptake clearance, which is mainly mediated by influx transporters. Typical drugs are statins.
2. Sum of $CL_{int,bile}$ and $CL_{int,met}$ is much less than $CL_{int,back}$. $CL_{int,all} = CL_{int,up} \times (CL_{int,bile} + CL_{int,met})/CL_{int,back}$, indicating that $CL_{int,all}$ is determined by the net effect of $CL_{int,up}$, $CL_{int,back}$, $CL_{int,bile}$ and $CL_{int,met}$.
3. Some drugs (such as midazolam) are not substrates of transporters. These drugs also rapidly penetrate the sinusoidal membrane, i.e., $CL_{int,up} = CL_{int,back}$, thus, $CL_{int,all} = CL_{int,bile} + CL_{int,met}$.

Diabetes significantly disorders transporter-CYP450 interplay via altering expressions and functions of transporters and CYP450s, finally affecting pharmacokinetics and activity/toxicity of drugs. For example, diabetes upregulated expressions and functions of hepatic CYP3A and OATP1B2, enhanced hepatic uptake and metabolism of simvastatin [12], atorvastatin [9,11], in turn, increasing hepatoxicity of atorvastatin [76]. Data from PBPK also showed that both hepatic OATP1B2 and CYP3A contribute to the clearance of atorvastatin, but the roles of hepatic OATP1B2 were much larger than that of CYP3A [11]. Another example is cyclosporin A. Cyclosporin A is also a substrate of CYP3A, MRP2, P-gp, OATP1B1 and BCRP. Significantly increased systemic clearance of cyclosporin A in diabetic rats [77] should be attributed to the net effect of alterations in these transporters and CYP3A. Methotrexate transport in the liver is mediated by various transporters such as OATP1B1, MRP2, BCRP and OAT2. Moreover, induction of CYP2E1 also enhanced methotrexate-induced hepatocytoxicity [78]. These results indicate that the regulation of hepatic OATPs and CYP2E1 expressions and functions may explain clinic findings that diabetic patients were particularly at increased risk of methotrexate hepatotoxicity [79].

3. Intestine

A series of transporters (such as P-gp, BCRP, OATPs, OCT1, PepTs, MRP2, MRP3 and MCTs) and enzymes (such as CYP450s and UGTs) have been expressed in enterocytes, implicating intestinal absorption of drugs and first-pass effects (Figure 2).

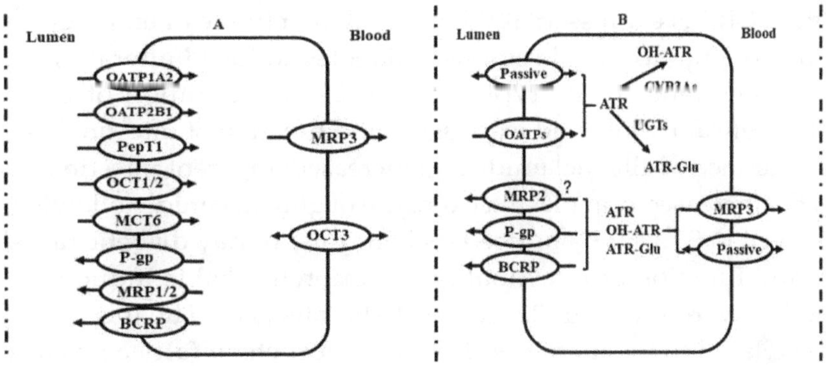

Figure 2. (**A**) Possible location of main transporters in human intestine and (**B**) roles of transporter-CYP3A interplay in disposition of atorvastatin in enterocytes. Symbol: ATR, atorvastatin; BCRP, breast cancer resistance protein; MCTs, monocarboxylate transporters; MRPs, multidrug resistance-associated proteins; OATPs, organic anion transporting polypeptides; OCTs, organic cation transporters; PepT1, peptide transporters; P-gp, P-glycoprotein; OH-ATR, hydroxyl atorvastatin; ATR-Glu, atorvastatin acyl glucuronide.

3.1. P-gp

P-gp is highly expressed at the apical membrane of the intestinal epithelium, pumping out of its substrates from enterocytes to the intestinal lumen. The expression of intestinal P-gp protein is region-dependent. P-gp protein progressively increases from proximal to distal regions. The highest expression of P-gp occurs at the ileum [80]. Several studies have demonstrated that diabetes impairs expression and function of intestinal P-gp, leading to the enhancement of intestinal absorption and increasing plasma exposure following oral administration of P-gp substrates such as arctigenin [81], protoberberine alkaloids [82], digoxin [83], grepafloxacin [84], paclitaxel [17] and morphine [85]. In line with the increased plasma levels of morphine, diabetic mice showed a stronger analgesic effect following an oral dose compared with control mice [85]. The decreased expression and function of intestinal P-gp under diabetes status may explain that clinic findings that diabetic patients also showed higher serum concentration of digoxin compared with non-diabetic patients following an oral dose of digoxin [86,87].

Downregulation of intestinal P-gp expression by diabetes was considered to be partly attributed to the acceleration of the ubiquitin-proteasome [88] via nitric oxide synthase (NOS) activation [89–91]. However, the role of NO in intestinal P-gp is time-dependent. In Caco-2 cells, it was reported that short-term exposure to sodium nitroprusside impaired P-gp function and expression, whereas long-term exposure stimulated P-gp function and expression [92]. Increased levels of short chain fatty acids (SCFAs) were also found in the intestinal content of diabetic rats [47]. A recent study showed that SCFAs downregulated the expression of intestinal P-gp via inhibiting histone deacetylase and NF-κB pathways [93].

3.2. MRP2

MRP2 (and MRP1) is co-located with phase II conjugating enzymes (such as UGTs and glutathione *S*-transferase) in the small intestine, pumping out of anions from enterocytes to the intestinal lumen. In contrast to P-gp, diabetes was reported to enhance the expression and function of intestinal MRP2 in rats [23]. Gliclazide is also a substrate of MRP2 [94]. C_{max} and AUC_{0-tn} of gliclazide following oral administration to diabetic rats were only 55% and 56% of those in control rats [94], respectively, which seemed to be attributed to the increased expression of intestinal MRP2. As expected, gliclazide administration significantly decreased glucose concentrations in healthy rats, but hypoglycemic effects of gliclazide were not observed in diabetic rats [95].

3.3. BCRP

Similarly to P-gp, BCRP is expressed at the luminal membrane of enterocytes. The BCRP protein gradually rises from proximal to distal regions. Diabetes-induced alterations in the expression of intestinal BCRP are dependent on the type of diabetes and duration of diabetes. STZ-induced diabetic rats showed significantly lowered expression and function of intestinal BCRP, accompanied by decreased intestinal clearance of glibenclamide and increased apparent intestinal effective permeability (P_{eff}) [48], leading to the increased oral plasma exposure of glibenclamide following oral administration to diabetic rats. However, in STZ/HFD-induced diabetic rats, 10-day diabetic rats showed significantly lowered expression and function of intestinal BCRP, but remarkable inductions of intestinal BCRP expression and function were found in 22-day diabetic rats [11]. The induction of intestinal BCRP was considered to be related to the increased levels of short chain fatty acids (SCFAs) via activating PPARγ [96].

3.4. PepT1

PepT1, located on the luminal membrane of enterocytes, is responsible for intestinal absorption of peptidomimetic drugs, dipeptides and tripeptides resulting from the dietary breakdown of proteins and bacterial peptidomimetics. Several investigations have demonstrated that diabetes downregulated the expression and function of intestinal PepT1 in experimental animals [47,97–99], decreasing oral plasma exposures of cephalexin and acyclovir following oral dose of cephalexin and valacyclovir [99]. Importantly, altered expression and function of intestinal PepT1 are also dependent on sex. For example, in Sprague-Dawley rats, it was reported that STZ-induced diabetes decreased the expression and function of intestinal PepT1 in male rats, but increased them in female rats [100]. Leptin and insulin deficiencies may contribute to the downregulation of intestinal PepT1 [101,102]. Dyshomeostasis of bile acid compositions was observed in intestinal content of diabetic rats. Bile acids downregulated the expression of intestinal PepT1 via activating farnesoid X receptor (FXR) [99].

3.5. MCT6

MCT6, located on the apical side of human intestinal villous epithelial cells, mediates intestinal absorption of nateglinide [103]. Loop diuretics such as furosemide, piretanide, azosemide, and torasemide may also be substrates of MCT6 [104]. Diabetes significantly decreased the expression of intestinal MCT6 and decreased plasma exposure of nateglinide following oral dose to rats. Further study demonstrated that SCFAs, especially butyrate, downregulated the expression of intestinal MCT6 via activating PPARγ [47]. The downregulation of intestinal MCT6 may also partly explain that diabetes significantly decreased plasma exposures of furosemide [105] and azosemide [106] following oral doses to rats.

3.6. CYP450s

Intestine also highly expresses CYP450s, especially CYP3As, which mediate drug metabolism, contributing to first-pass effects. In STZ-induced diabetes, it was found that diabetes significantly decreased CYP3A activity. In line with this, formations of norverapamil [27] and 6-β hydroxyltestosterone [107] were reduced to 21% and 50% that of control rats, respectively. Significant downregulation of intestinal CYP3A expression and function was also found in STZ/HFD-induced diabetic rats [11] and in Tsumura Suzuki obese diabetic (TSOD) mice [108]. Insulin treatment partly reversed the decreased CYP3A expression in STZ-induced diabetic rats [107], but not in TSOD mice [108]. However, the real mechanism leading to the decreased expression of intestinal CYP3A was unclear. In generally, expressions of CYP3A and P-gp were mainly controlled by pregnane X receptor (PXR). We recently reported upregulation of intestinal FXR [83]. A report showed that FXR agonist GW4064 remarkably induced expression of small heterodimer partner (SHP) [109], in turn, inhibiting the transcriptional activity of PXR [109,110]. Moreover, levels of bile acids, FXR agonist, were increased in intestinal contents of diabetic rats, which inhibited the expression of intestinal CYP3A and P-gp via the activation of FXR-SHP pathway.

3.7. Transporter-CYP450 Interplay in Intestine

Some drugs are often substrates of various transporters and CYP3As. Alterations in oral plasma exposure of drug should be attributed to common effects of the altered transporters and CYP3As. For example, atorvastatin is a substrate of intestinal P-gp, BCRP and OATPs, indicating that the P_{eff} of atorvastatin should be the integrated effects of passive diffusion, OATP1A5-mediated absorption, P-gp mediated efflux and BCRP-mediated efflux. Diabetes also downregulated the expression of intestinal OATP1A5 [11]. Thus, the P_{eff} of atorvastatin under diabetic status should be the net effects of these altered transporters. Downregulation of intestinal CYP3A expression by diabetes was also involved in the first-pass effect of atorvastatin. PBPK simulation demonstrated that contributions of intestinal transporters and CYP3A was intestinal BCRP > intestinal CYP3A > intestinal P-gp > intestinal OATP1A5 [11]. Cyclosporin A is also a substrate of BCRP, OATPs, CYP3A and P-gp, indicating that increased oral plasma exposure of cyclosporin A in diabetic rats [111] was also partly attributed to the common effects of the intestinal transporters and CYP3A. Verapamil is a substrate of P-gp and CYP3As. PBPK simulation also showed that the contribution of intestinal P-gp was much larger than that of intestinal CYP3A [93], indicating that increased oral plasma exposure of verapamil [27] was mainly attributed to downregulation of intestinal P-gp. Grepafloxacin [112] is also a substrate. Decreased expression of BCRP may partly explain why the decreased secretory transport of grepafloxacin was not in line with the decrease in expression of P-gp protein in diabetic rats [84]. Similarly, intestinal OATP1A5 also mediates intestinal absorption of glibenclamide [113], inferring that the increased P_{eff}

of glibenclamide by impairment of intestinal BCRP [48] may be partly weakened by the decreased expression of OATP1A5 protein.

4. Kidney

Drugs are eliminated in the kidney via urinary excretion. The process consists of glomerular filtration, secretion and reabsorption at the renal tubule. The secretion and reabsorption are mainly mediated by transporters. The identified renal transporters include OAT1/3, OCT1/2, PepT1/2, MATE1, MATE2/K, P-gp, BCRP, MCTs and urate transporter 1 (URAT1) (Figure 3A). Transporter interplay occurs at the kidney. For example, metformin, a substrate of OCTs and MATEs, is taken in renal epithelial cells via OCT1/2 at the basolateral membrane, then secreted into urine via MATEs at the brush-border membrane of renal tubular cells, mediating the renal excretion of metformin. The transporter interplay also participates in renal excretion of uric acid. URAT1, OAT1, OAT3, OAT4, OAT10, BCRP, sodium-dependent phosphate transport protein 1/4 (NPT1/4) and glucose transporter 9 (GLUT9) work together to regulate the excretion of uric acid via the kidney [114] (Figure 3B).

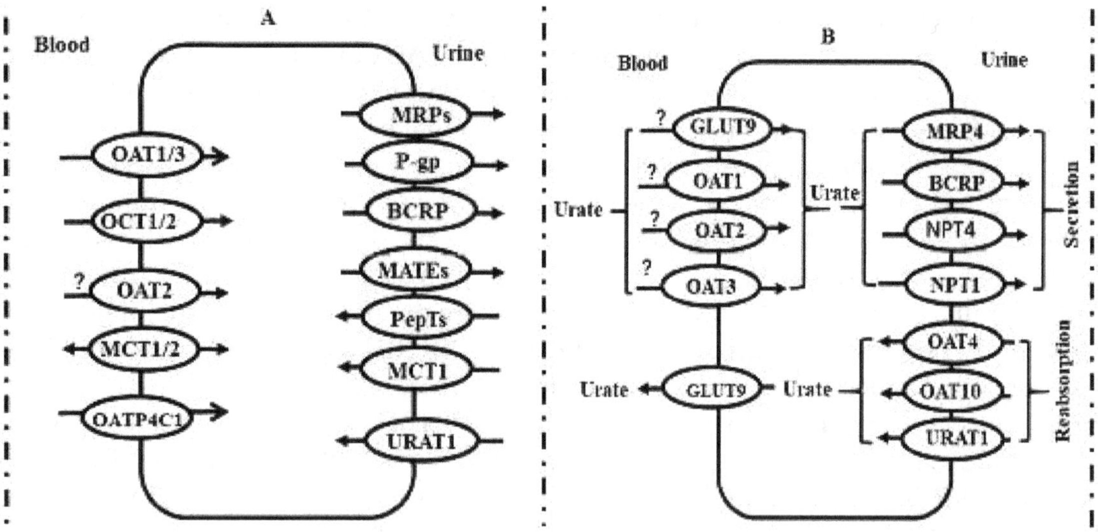

Figure 3. (**A**) Possible location of main transporters in human kidney and (**B**) roles of transporter interplay in renal excretion of uric acid. Symbol: OATPs, organic anion transporting polypeptides; OATs, organic anion transporters; OCTs, organic cation transporters; PepTs, peptide transporters; P-gp, P-glycoprotein; MRPs, multidrug resistance-associated proteins; BCRP, breast cancer resistance protein; MATEs, multidrug and toxin extrusion, NPTs, sodium-dependent phosphate transport proteins, GLUT9, glucose transporter 9, URAT1, urate transporter 1.

4.1. OAT1 and OAT3

The basolateral membrane of renal proximal tubule cells highly expresses OAT1 and OAT3, mediating the excretion of their substrates including ACE inhibitors, angiotensin II receptor blockers, diuretics, β-Lactam antibiotics, antiviral agents and endogenous compounds [3]. Several studies demonstrated that diabetes also impaired the function and expression of renal OATs. In STZ-induced diabetic rats, it was found that diabetes significantly decreased the membrane expression of renal OAT3, leading to lower uptake of [^{3}H] estrone sulfate in renal cortical slice. These decreases were in line with the activation of PKCα and NF-κB pathways, increased nuclear factor erythroid 2-related factor 2 (Nrf2) and oxidative stress [115,116]. Alteration in OATs by diabetes is dependent on sex. In lean and obese Zucker spontaneously hypertensive fatty (ZSF1) rats, it was found that the levels of renal OAT1 and OAT3 mRNA were higher in lean females than in lean males. Obesity remarkably reduced the expression of renal OAT1 and OAT3 in female ZSF1 rats but not in male ZSF1 rats [117]. Clinical trials showed that expressions of renal OAT1 and OAT3 in patients with diabetic kidney disease were less than 50% of the normal levels, which were in line with decreased urinary excretion of some organic acid metabolites and increased plasma levels of organic acid metabolites [118].

Diuretics show their diuretic effect via affecting proximal tubular epithelial cells. Some diuretics (such as torasemid and furosemide) are also substrates of OATs [3]. Several studies have showed that OAT1 or OAT3 deficiency damage the natriuretic effects of furosemide and bendroflumethiazide [119,120], inferring that the decreased expression of OATs by diabetes may impair the diuretic effect of diuretics. In line with the deduction, alloxan-induced diabetes significantly increased the plasma exposure of furosemide and decreased recovery from urine following intravenous dose to rats [105]. Importantly, diuretic efficiency, natriuretic efficiency, kaluretic efficiency and chloruretic efficiency of furosemide in diabetic rats showed a trend to decrease. Similarly, the diuretic efficiency, natriuretic efficiency, kaluretic efficiency and chloruretic efficiency of torasemide were significantly impaired both in alloxan-induced diabetic rats and STZ-induced diabetes, although its plasma exposure was unaltered [50]. These findings also may explain the clinical finding that diabetic patients need higher furosemide doses [121]. Moreover, sodium-glucose cotransporter (SGLT2) inhibitor empagliflozin is a substrate of OAT3. A report showed that OAT3 deficiency damaged the glucosuric effect of empagliflozin [122], indicating that the decreased expression of renal OAT3 by diabetes may attenuate the glucosuric effect of empagliflozin, which may also explain the clinic finding that compared with normal renal function and normal-to-mildly reduced renal function, diabetic patients with mild-to-moderately reduced renal function showed the lowest lowering glucose effect of luseogliflozin [123].

4.2. OCTs

Renal OCT1/2, mainly expressed at the basolateral membrane of tubule cells, transport a variety of organic cations, such as metformin, cisplatin, cephalexin and acyclovir. In STZ/HFD-induced diabetic rats, it was found that OCT2 protein expression was only 50% of control rats [124]. Similarly, in STZ-induced diabetic rats, the expressions of renal OCT1 and OCT2 were decreased by 50% and 70%, respectively [125]. The reduced mRNA and protein expressions of OCT1, OCT2 and OCT3 under diabetic status were also associated with a reduction in the clearance of N^1-methylnicotinamide [126,127]. The decreased mRNA and protein expressions of renal OCT2/3 were reported to be negatively correlated with the accumulation of renal and plasma advanced glycation end-products (AGEs) [127]. Insulin or AGE inhibitor aminoguanidine could reverse the decreased OCT2/3 by diabetes [125,127], inferring that the accumulation of AGEs may be involved in impaired expression of renal OCTs by diabetes [127]. Expressions of OCT1 and OCT2 are also be dependent on sex. In lean female ZSF1 rats, the mRNA expression level of OCT1 was significantly higher than that in their male counterparts. Obesity significantly reduced renal mRNA expressions of OCT1 and OCT2 in female ZSF1 rats, but not in male rats [117]. The decreased expression of renal OCTs by diabetes may affect pharmacokinetics of their substrates. For example, significantly higher AUC of metformin and lower renal clearance were observed in alloxan-induced diabetic rats than in normal rats following an intravenous dose [128]. A clinic trial [129] showed that renal clearance of metformin decreased along with diabetes progression. A report demonstrated the rank of the renal clearances of metformin in healthy subjects (525 ± 125 mL/min) > newly diagnosed maturity onset diabetic patients (322 ± 166 mL/min) > maturity onset diabetic patients (224 ± 38 mL/min). Interestingly, pregnancy seems to increase the functions of renal MATEs and OCTs [130]. Renal clearances of N^1-methylnicotinamide (endogenous probe for the renal OCTs and MATEs) in both mid (504 ± 293 mL/min) and late pregnancy (557 ± 305 mL/min) were reported to be higher than in postpartum (240 ± 106 mL/min). The renal secretion of N^1-methylnicotinamide was 3.5-fold higher in mid pregnancy and 4.5-fold higher in late pregnancy compared with postpartum [130]. In line, gestational diabetes mellitus pregnant women showed higher renal clearance and renal secretion [131], and lower plasma concentrations of metformin [131,132] compared with non-pregnant controls. Another example is cisplatin. Cisplatin is a substrate of OCTs. Its main toxicity is nephrotoxicity. Several studies have demonstrated that both insulin-dependent and insulin-independent diabetes show resistance against cisplatin-induced nephrotoxicity [133–135]. Animal experiments showed that diabetes prevented nephrotoxicity partly via decreasing the renal accumulation of cisplatin [136,137]. However, cisplatin treatment was not beneficial in diabetes due to its compromising its antitumor effect [136].

4.3. Other Transporters

Diabetes induced an approximately two-fold increase in renal PepT1 protein and slightly induced mRNA of PepT1 and PepT2 [138]. Reports on the expression of ABC transporters are often contradictory. For renal P-gp, it was reported that spontaneous type 1 and type 2 diabetic mice showed lower expressions of renal P-gp protein. The high glucose was considered to be a reason reducing the expression and function of P-gp [139]. However, the expression of P-gp protein was also reported to be unchanged [17,111,138], although level of Mdr1a mRNA was increased [17,138].

For MRP2, increased expression of renal MRP2 protein was found in STZ/HFD-diabetic rats [124] and in STZ-induced diabetic rats [23]. For BCRP, HFD/STZ-induced diabetes significantly increased the expression of BCRP protein in rats, but STZ-induced diabetes significantly decreased mRNA level of renal BCRP in rats [136]. These discrepancies may result from the duration of diabetes, sex and the type of diabetes. For example, in female rats, obesity decreased the expressions of MRP4 and Mdr1b mRNA, but the expression of MRP2 mRNA was unaltered. In male ZSF1 rats, expressions of MRP2, MRP4 and Mdr1b mRNA remained unchanged in obese rats compared to lean rats [117].

4.4. CYP450

The identified renal CYP450s include CYP2C, CYP2J, CYP2E1, CYP4As and CYP4Fs. They mainly mediate local biotransformation of endogenous compounds such as arachidonic acid. For example, arachidonic acid is metabolized by CYP4As and CYP4Fs to 20-hydroxyeicosatetraenoic acid (vasoconstrictor) and by CYP2C and CYP2J to epoxyeicosatrienoic acid (vasodilator), synergistically regulating renal vasoactivity. Several reports have shown that diabetes also affect the expressions of renal CYP450s. In mice, it was found that HFD feeding significantly decreased activities of CYP3A (1′-hydroxymidazolam), CYP2E1 (hydroxychlorzoxazone), CYP2J (ebastine hydroxylation) and CYP2B6 (hydroxybupropion) and CYP4A (12-hydroxydecanoic acid), but increased the activities of CYP2C (hydroxytolbutamide) and CYP2D (Hydroxybufuralol) [140]. Diabetes affects the expressions and activities of renal CYP450s in an isoform- and species-specific manner. In STZ-induced diabetic rats, formations of hydroxyandrostenedione and 2α-hydroxytestosterone were significantly increased by 250% and 300% compared to control rats, but formations of androstenedione and 6β-hydroxytestosterone were significantly decreased. The formations of 16α-hydroxytestosterone and 7α-hydroxytestosterone were unaltered [141]. Induction of CYP2E1, 4A2 and K-4 as well as increases in omega- and (omega-1) hydroxylation of lauric acid were also observed in kidney of STZ-induced rats [26]. Insulin treatment partly reversed these alterations by diabetes [26,141]. However, a recent report showed that expression of CYP4A protein in diabetic mice induced by HFD/STZ was downregulated by 29.16% of control mice [142]. The roles of altered renal CYP450s by diabetes in disposition of drugs needed further investigation.

4.5. Transporter Interplay in Kidney

Transporter interplay occurs in the kidney. For example, methotrexate is eliminated mainly via renal active excretion, which is involved in OAT1/3 at basolateral membrane of tubule and BCRP and MRP2 at brush-border membrane of tubule, these transporters in series work to regulate renal active excretion of methotrexate. Both higher plasma concentration of methotrexate and higher toxicity of methotrexate in STZ-diabetic rats [143] may partly be explained by the imbalance of expressions of renal OATs, BCRP and MRP2. Another example is β-lactam antibiotics. OATs mediate the uptake of β-lactam antibiotics into the tubule from the blood and PepT1/2 located in the brush-border membrane of the tubule, mediate reabsorption of antibiotics from the urine, and regulate urinary excretion of β-lactam antibiotics. Downregulation of renal OATs may partly contribute to a decrease in the renal clearance of DA-1131 (a carbapenem antibiotics) [144] and lower renal cortical cephaloridine accumulation in diabetic rats [145]. Creatinine is also substrate of OCT1/2, MATEs and OAT1/3, indicating that the decreased expressions of renal OATs and OCTs at least partly contribute to decreased clearance of creatinine under diabetic status.

5. Application of PBPK to Transporter-Enzyme Interplay

The above statements demonstrated that diabetes may simultaneously affect functions and expressions of transporters and enzymes in the intestine, liver and kidney. Their contributions to the disposition of drugs are often opposite. Moreover, some physiological parameters such as blood flow rates, intestinal transit and the free fraction of drug in plasma are often altered. Thus, the effects of diabetes on pharmacokinetics of drugs should be the integrated effects of these alterations, which may be accomplished using PBPK.

5.1. *Atorvastatin*

Atorvastatin is a substrate of P-gp, OATPs, BCRP and CYP3As. Diabetes reduced expressions of intestinal P-gp, CYP3A and OATP1A5, while induced expressions of liver OATP1B2 and CYP3A. Intestinal BCRP was highly dependent upon diabetes course, which was decreased at an early phase of diabetes (10-day) but induced at a late phase (22-day). A pharmacokinetic study showed that oral plasma exposure was increased in 10-day diabetic rats, but decreased in 22-day diabetic rats. PBPK simulation demonstrated that contributions of these targeted protein to altered oral plasma exposure of atorvastatin were intestinal BCRP > hepatic OATP1B2 > hepatic CYP3A > intestinal CYP3A > intestinal P-gp > intestinal OATP1A5. The increased oral plasma atorvastatin exposure in 10-day diabetic rats and the decreased oral plasma atorvastatin exposure in 22-day diabetic rats were attributed to the altered intestinal BCRP [11].

5.2. *Verapamil*

Verapamil is substrate of CYP3As and P-gp. Rat experiments showed that diabetes increased plasma exposure of verapamil following an oral dose but decreased plasma exposure of verapamil following an intravenous dose [29]. A semi-PBPK model (Figure 4) was successfully developed to simulate the pharmacokinetics of verapamil (Figure 5A,B) in rats using the parameters listed in Tables 1 and 2. Intestinal P-gp in diabetic rats was set to 60% of control rats [82]. The contributions of intestinal/hepatic CYP3A and intestinal P-gp to alterations in oral plasma concentration of verapamil in diabetic rats were investigated. The results demonstrate that increased oral plasma exposure of verapamil was mainly attributed to the impairment of intestinal P-gp (Figure 5E) and the role of intestinal CYP3As was minor (Figure 5D). Furthermore, the contribution of increased expression of hepatic CYP3As to the altered plasma concentration of verapamil following oral dose to rats was less than that of intestinal P-gp impairment, whose net effect was to increase oral plasma exposure of verapamil (Figure 5G).

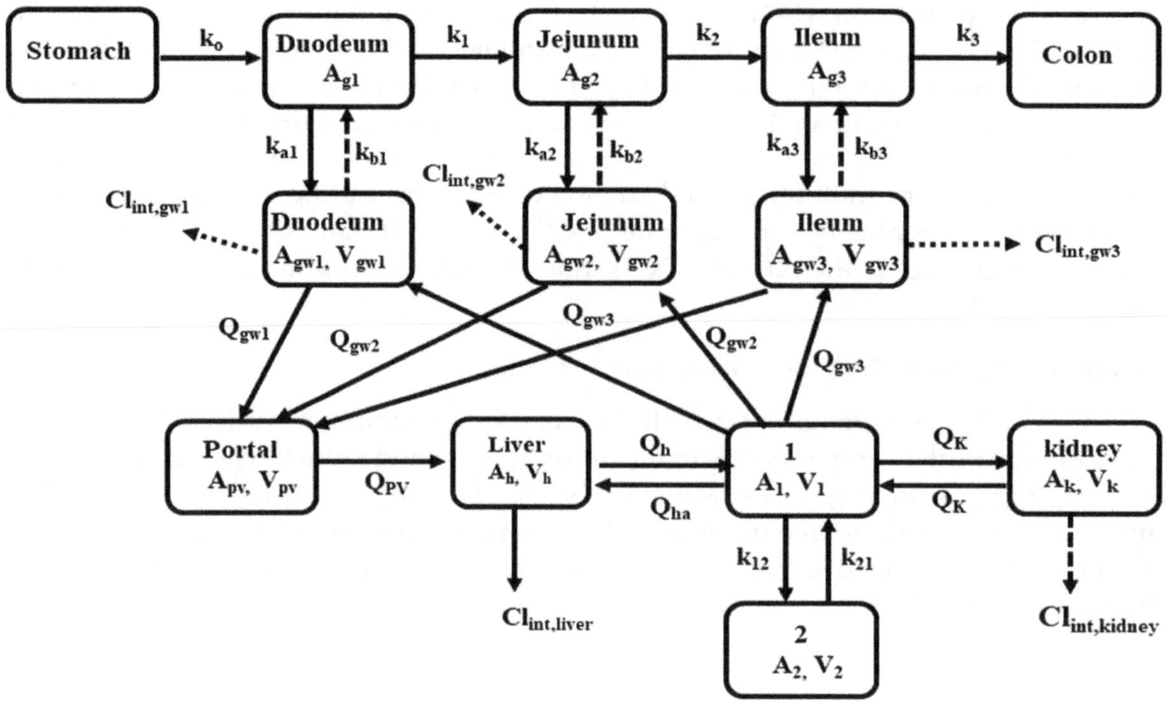

Figure 4. Schematic diagram of semi-physiologically based pharmacokinetic model (PBPK) model describing the pharmacokinetics of verapamil and furosemide in rats. A_i, Q_i and V_i indicate drug amount, blood flow and volume in corresponding compartment, respectively. k_i, $k_{a,i}$ and $k_{b,i}$ represent the transit rate constant, drug absorption rate constant and efflux rate constant from enterocytes to the gut lumen, respectively. $Cl_{int,gwi}$, $Cl_{int,liver}$ and $Cl_{int,kidney}$ mean the intrinsic clearance in enterocytes, hepatocytes and kidney, respectively.

Table 1. The physiological parameters of rats for the semi-PBPK model [11].

Parameters	Unit	Control Rats	Diabetic Rats
Gastric emptying rate	h^{-1}	20.8	20.8
Duodenum transit time	h^{-1}	28.74	28.74
Jejunum transit time	h^{-1}	4.2	4.2
Ileum transit time	h^{-1}	0.789	0.789
Intestinal radius	cm	0.2	0.2
Duodenum wall volume	mL	1.08	1.08
Jejunum wall volume	mL	9.94	9.94
Ileum wall volume	mL	0.32	0.32
Portal vein volume	mL	0.25	0.25
Liver volume	mL	10	10
Renal volume	mL	1.83 [146]	1.83
Duodenum wall blood flow	mL/min	0.972	2.223
Jejunum wall blood flow	mL/min	9.125	20.877
Ileum wall blood flow	mL/min	0.253	0.580
Portal vein blood flow	mL/min	16.043	23.68
Hepatic artery blood flow	mL/min	2.243	11.914
Liver blood flow	mL/min	18.286	35.594
Renal blood flow	ml/min	11.7 [146]	4.10 [a]
Hepatic microsomal protein	mg/g liver	44.8	44.8
Intestinal microsomal protein	mg/g intestine	25.9	25.9
Liver weight	g/kg body weight	40	36

[a] Renal blood flow was reduced by 65% of control rats [147].

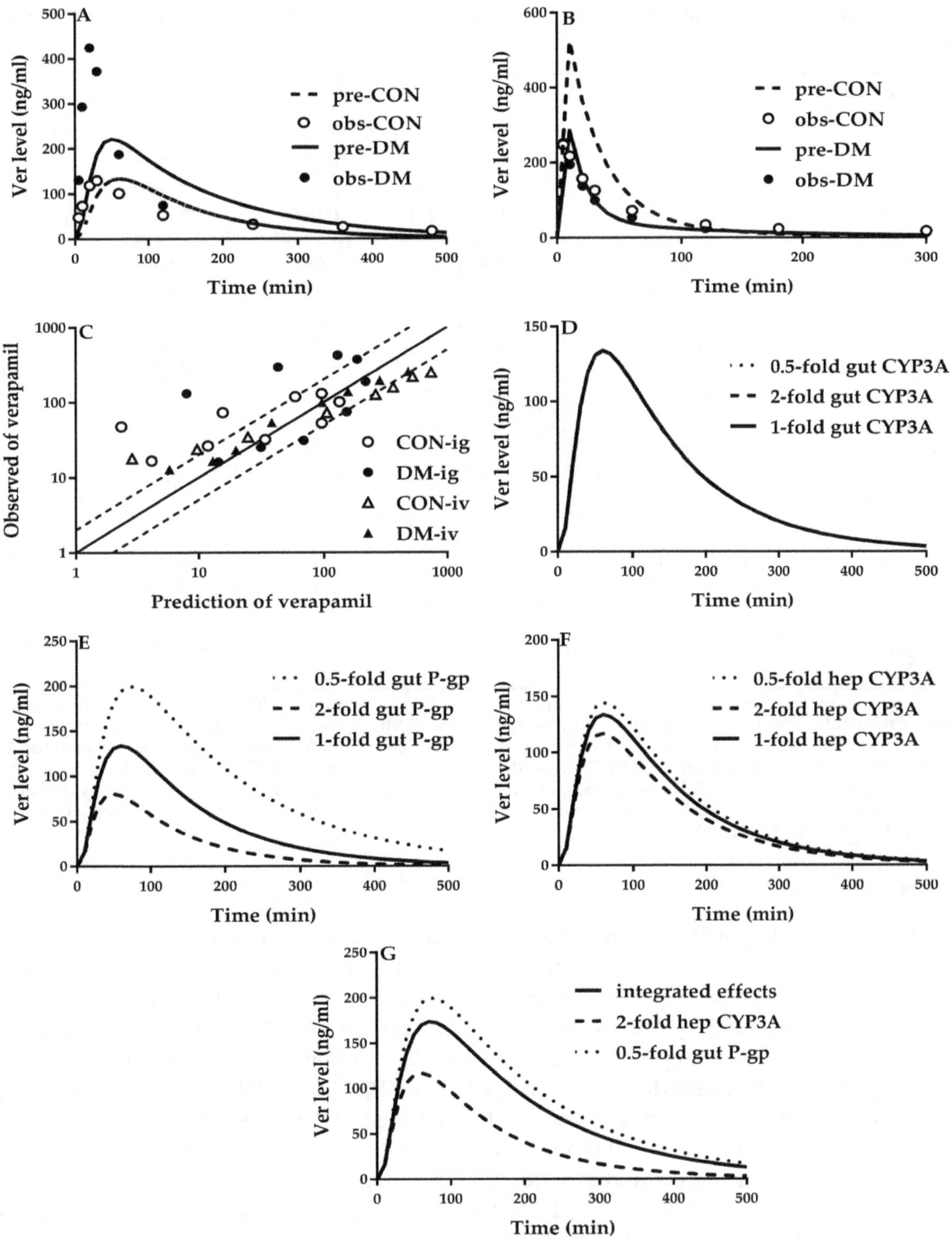

Figure 5. Observed (point) and predicted (line) plasma concentrations of verapamil (Ver) following (**A**) oral (10 mg/kg, ig) and (**B**) intravenous dose (1 mg/kg, iv) to diabetic rats (DM) and control rats (CON); (**C**) comparison of mean observed and predicted plasma concentrations of verapamil at each time point; (**D**) individual contributions of altered hepatic CYP3A, (**E**) intestinal CYP3A and (**F**) intestinal P-gp to oral plasma exposure of verapamil as well as (**G**) their integrated effects. The observations were obtained from the literature [27].

Table 2. Pharmacokinetic parameters of verapamil and furosemide for PBPK simulation in diabetic rats (DM) and control rats (CON).

Parameter	Unit	Furosemide		Verapamil	
		CON rats	DM rats	CON rats	DM rats
Vc	L/kg	0.127 [148]	0.127	0.505 [a]	0.505
k21	h^{-1}	0.835 [148]	0.835	11.880 [a]	11.88
k12	h^{-1}	0.989 [148]	0.989	10.740 [a]	10.74
fu	%	10.4 [105]	10.4 [89]	0.05 [93]	0.05
Kt:p	Liver	0.33 [148]	0.33	8.20 [b]	8.20
Kt:p	Intestine	0.517 [148]	0.517	319.39 [b]	319.39
Kt:p	Kidney	1.36 [148]	1.36	/	/
$P_{app,A\text{-}B}$ (caco-2)	cm/s × 10^{-6}	6.90 [149]	3.45 [c]	13.8	13.8
$P_{app,B\text{-}A}$ (caco-2)	cm/s × 10^{-6}	/	/	24.84	14.90 [d]
CL_{kidney}	mL/min/kg	4.33 [105]	/		
CL_{liver}	mL/min/kg	2.20 [105]	/		
Fu × $CL_{int,liver}$	mL/min/250 g	0.60 [e]	0.75 [f]	/	/
Fu × $CL_{int,kidney}$	mL/min/250 g	1.19 [e]	0.48 [g]	/	/
Microsomes					
Liver					
V_{max}	nmol/(min/mg prot)	/	/	1.60 [27]	2.38 [27]
K_m	μM	/	/	13.21 [27]	16.09 [27]
Intestine					
V_{max}	pmol/(min/mg prot)	/	/	49.04 [27]	22.70 [27]
K_m	μM	/	/	34.06 [27]	55.37 [27]

[a] Estimated using the reported data [150]; [b] estimated according to a method [151] reported by Ruark et al. and physicochemical properties of verapamil; [c] function of intestinal MCT6 was set to be 50% that of control rats [47]; [d] level of intestinal P-gp protein was 60% that of control rats [82]; [e] fu × Clint were estimated using equation fu*Clint = Q × CL/(Q − CL); [f] contribution of CYP2C11 was 61.5% of the total metabolism [152], rests (38.5%) were assumed to attributed to CYP2E1 and CYP3As. Diabetes increased the expression of CYP2E1 and CYP3As by 3-fold [28] and expression of CYP2C11 mRNA was decreased to 16% that of control rats [47]; [g] function of renal OATs was decreased to 40% that of control rats [115].

5.3. Furosemide

Rat experiments demonstrated that diabetes decreased plasma furosemide exposure following oral dose but increased plasma furosemide exposure following intravenous dose [105]. Intestinal absorption of furosemide may be involved in MCT6 [84]. It was assumed that intestinal absorption of furosemide was mediated by MCT6. Function of intestinal MCT6 under diabetic status was set to be 50% according previous report [47]. Furosemide is eliminated mainly via renal secretion due to OAT1/2 [3]. Part of furosemide is metabolized by CYP2C11, CYP3As and CYP2E1 [152]. The contribution of CYP2C11 was 61.5% of the total metabolism [152], rests (38.5%) were assumed to attributed to CYP2E1 and CYP3As. Hepatic clearance (CL_{liver}) of furosemide was reported to be 2.20 mL/min/kg [105] and the estimated value of fu × $CL_{int,liver}$ was 0.75 mL/min/250g. Diabetes increased the expression of CYP2E1 and CYP3As by 3-fold [28] and the expression of CYP2C11 mRNA was decreased to 16% that of control rats [47]. Thus, fu × $CL_{int,liver}$ and CL_{liver} were estimated to be 0.75 mL/min/250g and 2.20 mL/min/kg. The estimated CL_{liver} of furosemide was near to observed data (2.98) in diabetic rats [105]. Diabetes altered expression of these targeted proteins (CYP2C11, CYP3As, CYP2E1 and OATs), intestinal blood, liver blood flow and renal blood flow. It was assumed that intestinal absorption of furosemide was mediated by MCT6. All these contribute to the altered furosemide pharmacokinetics, whose integrated effects (Figure 6) were predicted using PBPK model. The results demonstrate that the contribution of increases in CYP3A and CYP2E1 to hepatic clearance of furosemide was partly attenuated by decreases in CYP2C11, which may explain why non-renal clearance of furosemide was only slightly increased under diabetic status [105]. PBPK simulation demonstrated that decreases in renal excretion of furosemide due to downregulation of renal OATs and renal blood flow rates mainly contributed the increased plasma exposure of furosemide following an intravenous dose. Decreased oral exposure of furosemide was mainly attributed to the impairment of intestinal absorption due to the suppression of intestinal MCT6. The contribution of decreased expression of renal OATs to the altered oral plasma exposure of furosemide was less than that of intestinal MCT6 impairment, whose net effect was to decrease oral plasma of furosemide (Figure 6G).

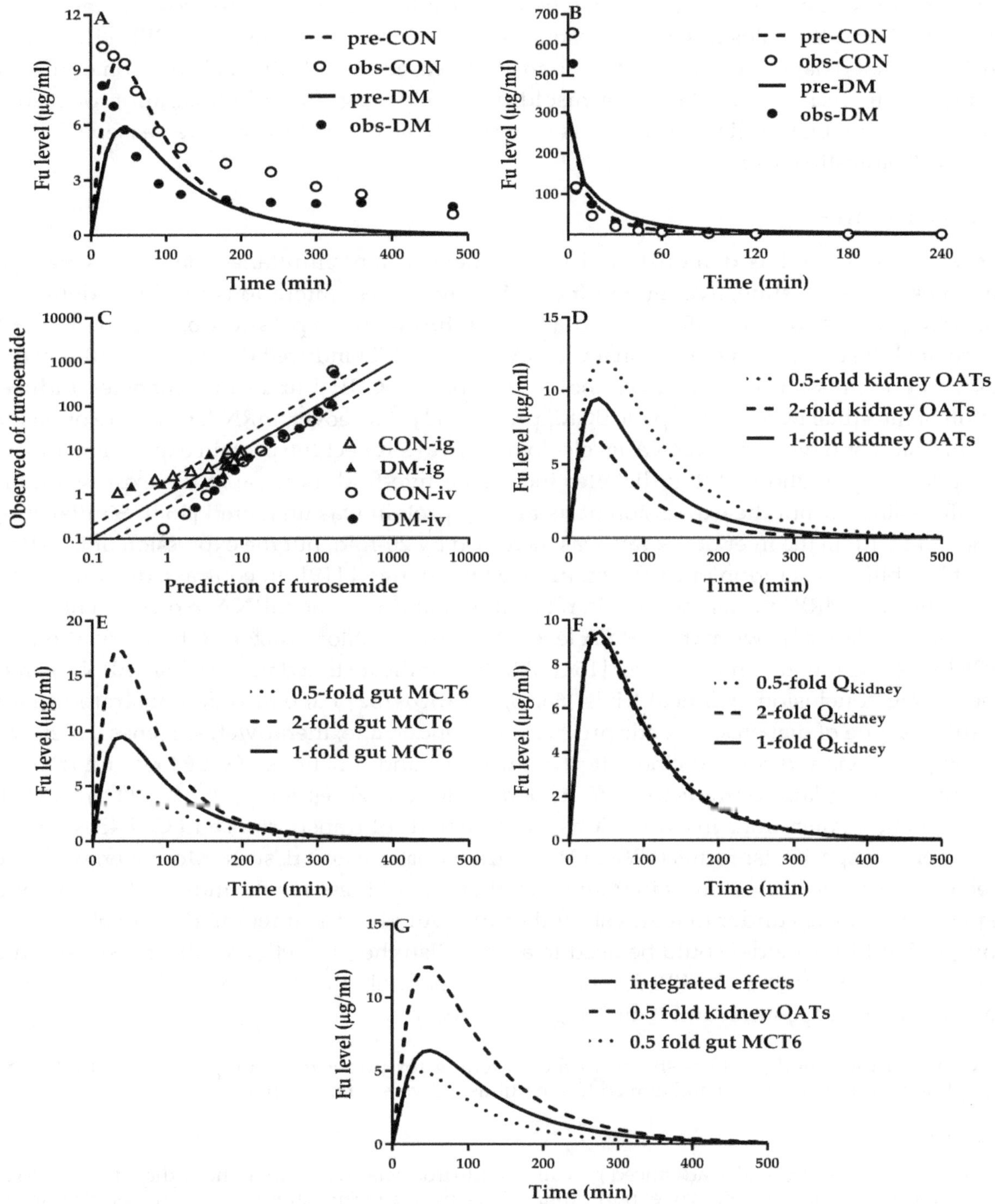

Figure 6. Observed (point) and predicted (line) plasma concentrations of furosemide (Fu) following (**A**) oral (6 mg/rat, ig) and (**B**) intravenous dose (6 mg/rat, iv) to diabetic rats (DM) and control rats (CON). Comparison of mean observed and predicted plasma concentrations of furosemide at each time point (**C**). Contributions of altered (**D**) renal OATs, (**E**) intestinal MCT6 and (**F**) renal blood flow (Q_{kidney}) to oral plasma exposure of furosemide as well as (**G**) integrated effects of intestinal MCT6 impairment and renal OATs impairment. The observations were obtained from the literature [89].

5.4. Metformin and Nisoldipine

A whole-body PBPK model was also used to predict the pharmacokinetics of metformin in diabetic patients [153]. The results show that increased plasma levels of metformin following oral dose mainly resulted from both the impairment of renal function and delaying gastrointestinal transit. The metabolism of nisoldipine is mediated by CYP3As. Decreased CYP3A activity may partly explain the increased oral plasma exposure. However, when nisoldipine, in controlled-release tablets, was given to diabetic patients, the roles of gastrointestinal transit were nonnegligible. PBPK simulation also demonstrated that delaying gastrointestinal transit increased the intestinal absorption of nisoldipine, indicating that increased oral plasma of nisoldipine following oral administration of nisoldipine controlled-release tablet in diabetes patients was mainly attributed to both decreased CYP3As and delaying gastrointestinal transit.

6. Future Perspective

Growing evidence has demonstrated that diabetes often simultaneously affects transporters and enzymes in the intestine, liver and kidney. Moreover, these alterations are dependent on tissue and diabetic progression. For example, diabetes induced the expression of hepatic CYP3A, but downregulated the expression of intestinal CYP3A. In STZ/HFD-induced diabetic rats, 10-day diabetes decreased the expression of both intestinal and hepatic BCRP, but 22-day diabetes induced the expression of intestinal BCRP not hepatic BCRP protein [11]. Moreover, mRNA levels are often indexed as the expression of targets, but mRNA levels do not always reflect the protein expression and activity. For example, a report showed that diabetes induced a five-fold increase in the expression of renal Mdr1a mRNA in rats, but the expression of renal P-gp protein was unaltered [138]. Similarly, mRNA expression of BCRP in the liver of GK rats was increased by 20-fold, but the expression of BCRP protein and function (biliary excretion of rosuvastatin) was unchanged [19]. In contrast, diabetes decreased the level of hepatic MRP2 protein by 80% in rats without affecting the mRNA expression of MRP2 [22]. Similarly, no correlation between the mRNA level and activity (chlorzoxazone 6-hydroxylation activity) of CYP2E1 was also found in human liver [154]. All these indicate that data based on mRNA sometimes give the wrong conclusion. Clinical trials [66,68,73,74,131,132] have also demonstrated that many factors such as type of diabetes, diabetic progression, gender, age, therapy/effectiveness, diet/drinking habits, complications and co-medicines affect expressions and functions of CYP450s and transporters, which may partly explain contradictory effects of diabetes on expressions of CYP450/transporters and pharmacokinetics. Alterations in expressions and functions of transporters and CYP450s by diabetes are dependent on specific isoforms (CYP450s and transporters) and tissues. Moreover, physiological parameters such as blood flow rates in tissues are altered. All these results indicate that alterations in the disposition of drugs under diabetes should be attributed to the integrated effect of these factors. We thought that PBPK model could be used to accomplish the prediction of drug disposition under diabetic status. Furthermore, the PBPK model could separately illustrate individual contributions of each factor to drug disposition and their integrated effects.

Author Contributions: Both authors shared in the searching for publication, preparation and editing of the manuscript. All authors have read and agreed to the published version of the manuscript.

Abbreviations

ABC, ATP binding cassette; AGEs, advanced glycation end-products; AUC, area under the curve; BCRP, breast cancer resistance protein; BSEP, bile salt export pump; C_{max}, peak concentration; CL_{int}, intrinsic clearance; CON, control rats; CYP450s cytochrome P450 enzymes; DM, diabetic rats; FXR, farnesoid X receptor; GLUT9, glucose transporter 9; HFD, high-fat diet; MATEs, multidrug/toxin extrusions; MCTs, monocarboxylate transporters; MRPs, multidrug resistance-associated proteins; NF-κB, nuclear factor kappa-B; NOS, nitric oxide synthase; NPT1/4, sodium-dependent phosphate transport protein 1/4; Nrf2, nuclear factor erythroid 2-related factor 2; NTCP, sodium taurocholate co-transporting polypeptide; OATPs, Organic anion transporting polypeptides; OATs, organic anion transporters; OCTs, organic cation transporters; PBPK, physiologically-based pharmacokinetic model; P_{eff}, apparent intestinal effective permeability; PepTs, peptide transporters; P-gp, P-glycoprotein; PKCα, protein kinase C alpha; PPAR, peroxisome proliferator activated receptor; PXR, pregnane X receptor; SCFAs, short chain fatty acids; SHP, small heterodimer partner; SGLT2, sodium-glucose cotransporter; SLC, solute carrier; STZ, streptozocin; TSOD, Tsumura, Suzuki, obese, diabetes; UGTs, UDP-glucuronosyltransferases; URAT1, urate transporter 1; ZSF1, Zucker spontaneously hypertensive fatty.

References

1. Lu, C.; Di, L. In vitro and in vivo methods to assess pharmacokinetic drug–drug interactions in drug discovery and development. *Biopharm. Drug Dispos.* **2020**, *41*, 3–31. [CrossRef]
2. Bteich, M.; Poulin, P.; Haddad, S. The potential protein-mediated hepatic uptake: Discussion on the molecular interactions between albumin and the hepatocyte cell surface and their implications for the in vitro-to-in vivo extrapolations of hepatic clearance of drugs. *Expert Opin. Drug Metab. Toxicol.* **2019**, *15*, 633–658. [CrossRef]
3. Liu, X. SLC Family Transporters. *Adv. Exp. Med. Biol.* **2019**, *1141*, 101–202. [CrossRef] [PubMed]
4. Park, J.E.; Kim, K.B.; Bae, S.K.; Moon, B.S.; Liu, K.H.; Shin, J.G. Contribution of cytochrome P450 3A4 and 3A5 to the metabolism of atorvastatin. *Xenobiotica* **2008**, *38*, 1240–1251. [CrossRef] [PubMed]
5. Goosen, T.C.; Bauman, J.N.; Davis, J.A.; Yu, C.; Hurst, S.I.; Williams, J.A.; Loi, C.M. Atorvastatin glucuronidation is minimally and nonselectively inhibited by the fibrates gemfibrozil, fenofibrate, and fenofibric acid. *Drug Metab. Dispos.* **2007**, *35*, 1315–1324. [CrossRef] [PubMed]
6. Li, J.; Volpe, D.A.; Wang, Y.; Zhang, W.; Bode, C.; Owen, A.; Hidalgo, I.J. Use of transporter knockdown Caco-2 cells to investigate the in vitro efflux of statin drugs. *Drug Metab. Dispos.* **2011**, *39*, 1196–1202. [CrossRef] [PubMed]
7. Choi, M.K.; Shin, H.J.; Choi, Y.L.; Deng, J.W.; Shin, J.G.; Song, I.S. Differential effect of genetic variants of Na^+-taurocholate co-transporting polypeptide (NTCP) and organic anion-transporting polypeptide 1B1 (OATP1B1) on the uptake of HMG-CoA reductase inhibitors. *Xenobiotica* **2011**, *41*, 24–34. [CrossRef]
8. Keppler, D.; Konig, J. Hepatic secretion of conjugated drugs and endogenous substances. *Semin. Liver Dis.* **2000**, *20*, 265–272. [CrossRef]
9. Shu, N.; Hu, M.; Liu, C.; Zhang, M.; Ling, Z.; Zhang, J.; Xu, P.; Zhong, Z.; Chen, Y.; Liu, L.; et al. Decreased exposure of atorvastatin in diabetic rats partly due to induction of hepatic Cyp3a and Oatp2. *Xenobiotica* **2016**, *46*, 875–881. [CrossRef]
10. Li, F.; Ling, Z.L.; Wang, Z.J.; Zhong, Z.Y.; Shu, N.; Zhang, M.; Liu, C.; Liu, L.; Liu, X.D. Differential effects of pravastatin on the pharmacokinetics of paroxetine in normal and diabetic rats. *Xenobiotica* **2017**, *47*, 20–30. [CrossRef]
11. Wang, Z.; Yang, H.; Xu, J.; Zhao, K.; Chen, Y.; Liang, L.; Li, P.; Chen, N.; Geng, D.; Zhang, X.; et al. Prediction of Atorvastatin Pharmacokinetics in High-Fat Diet and Low-Dose Streptozotocin Induced Diabetic Rats Using a Semiphysiologically Based Pharmacokinetic Model Involving Both Enzymes and Transporters. *Drug Metab. Dispos.* **2019**, *47*, 1066–1079. [CrossRef] [PubMed]
12. Xu, D.; Li, F.; Zhang, M.; Zhang, J.; Liu, C.; Hu, M.Y.; Zhong, Z.Y.; Jia, L.L.; Wang, D.W.; Wu, J.; et al. Decreased exposure of simvastatin and simvastatin acid in a rat model of type 2 diabetes. *Acta Pharm. Sin.* **2014**, *35*, 1215–1225. [CrossRef] [PubMed]
13. Hasegawa, Y.; Kishimoto, S.; Shibatani, N.; Inotsume, N.; Takeuchi, Y.; Fukushima, S. The disposition of pravastatin in a rat model of streptozotocin-induced diabetes and organic anion transporting polypeptide 2 and multidrug resistance-associated protein 2 expression in the liver. *Biol. Pharm. Bull.* **2010**, *33*, 153–156. [CrossRef] [PubMed]
14. Babalik, A.; Ulus, I.H.; Bakirci, N.; Kuyucu, T.; Arpag, H.; Dagyildizi, L.; Capaner, E. Plasma concentrations of isoniazid and rifampin are decreased in adult pulmonary tuberculosis patients with diabetes mellitus. *Antimicrob. Agents Chemother.* **2013**, *57*, 5740–5742. [CrossRef] [PubMed]
15. Nijland, H.M.; Ruslami, R.; Stalenhoef, J.E.; Nelwan, E.J.; Alisjahbana, B.; Nelwan, R.H.; van der Ven, A.J.; Danusantoso, H.; Aarnoutse, R.E.; van Crevel, R. Exposure to rifampicin is strongly reduced in patients with tuberculosis and type 2 diabetes. *Clin. Infect. Dis.* **2006**, *43*, 848–854. [CrossRef]
16. Kameyama, N.; Arisawa, S.; Ueyama, J.; Kagota, S.; Shinozuka, K.; Hattori, A.; Tatsumi, Y.; Hayashi, H.; Takagi, K.; Wakusawa, S. Increase in P-glycoprotein accompanied by activation of protein kinase Cα and NF- κB p65 in the livers of rats with streptozotocin-induced diabetes. *Biochim. Biophys. Acta* **2008**, *1782*, 355–360. [CrossRef]

17. Lee, J.H.; Lee, A.; Oh, J.H.; Lee, Y.J. Comparative pharmacokinetic study of paclitaxel and docetaxel in streptozotocin-induced diabetic rats. *Biopharm. Drug Dispos.* **2012**, *33*, 474–486. [CrossRef]
18. Zhang, L.L.; Lu, L.; Jin, S.; Jing, X.Y.; Yao, D.; Hu, N.; Liu, L.; Duan, R.; Liu, X.D.; Wang, G.J.; et al. Tissue-specific alterations in expression and function of P-glycoprotein in streptozotocin-induced diabetic rats. *Acta Pharm. Sin.* **2011**, *32*, 956–966. [CrossRef]
19. zhang, L.L.; Jin, S.; Li, J.; Duan, R.; Liu, X.D. Tissue species damage in expression and function of breast cancer resistance protein streptotozocin-induced diabetic rats. *J. China Pharmceut Unversit.* **2011**, *42*, 544–550.
20. He, L.; Yang, Y.; Guo, C.; Yao, D.; Liu, H.H.; Sheng, J.J.; Zhou, W.P.; Ren, J.; Liu, X.D.; Pan, G.Y. Opposite regulation of hepatic breast cancer resistance protein in type 1 and 2 diabetes mellitus. *Eur. J. Pharm.* **2014**, *724*, 185–192. [CrossRef]
21. Aleksunes, L.M.; Xu, J.; Lin, E.; Wen, X.; Goedken, M.J.; Slitt, A.L. Pregnancy represses induction of efflux transporters in livers of type I diabetic mice. *Pharm. Res.* **2013**, *30*, 2209–2220. [CrossRef] [PubMed]
22. van Waarde, W.M.; Verkade, H.J.; Wolters, H.; Havinga, R.; Baller, J.; Bloks, V.; Muller, M.; Sauer, P.J.; Kuipers, F. Differential effects of streptozotocin-induced diabetes on expression of hepatic ABC-transporters in rats. *Gastroenterology* **2002**, *122*, 1842–1852. [CrossRef] [PubMed]
23. Mei, D.; Li, J.; Liu, H.; Liu, L.; Wang, X.; Guo, H.; Liu, C.; Duan, R.; Liu, X. Induction of multidrug resistance-associated protein 2 in liver, intestine and kidney of streptozotocin-induced diabetic rats. *Xenobiotica* **2012**, *42*, 709–718. [CrossRef] [PubMed]
24. Nakashima, E.; Matsushita, R.; Takeda, M.; Nakanishi, T.; Ichimura, F. Comparative pharmacokinetics of cefoperazone and cephradine in untreated streptozotocin diabetic rats. *Drug Metab. Dispos.* **1992**, *20*, 730–735. [PubMed]
25. Watkins, J.B.; Noda, H. Biliary excretion of organic anions in diabetic rats. *J. Pharm. Exp. Ther.* **1986**, *239*, 467–473.
26. Shimojo, N.; Ishizaki, T.; Imaoka, S.; Funae, Y.; Fujii, S.; Okuda, K. Changes in amounts of cytochrome P450 isozymes and levels of catalytic activities in hepatic and renal microsomes of rats with streptozocin-induced diabetes. *Biochem. Pharm.* **1993**, *46*, 621–627. [CrossRef]
27. Hu, N.; Xie, S.; Liu, L.; Wang, X.; Pan, X.; Chen, G.; Zhang, L.; Liu, H.; Liu, X.; Liu, X.; et al. Opposite effect of diabetes mellitus induced by streptozotocin on oral and intravenous pharmacokinetics of verapamil in rats. *Drug Metab. Dispos.* **2011**, *39*, 419–425. [CrossRef]
28. Kim, Y.C.; Lee, A.K.; Lee, J.H.; Lee, I.; Lee, D.C.; Kim, S.H.; Kim, S.G.; Lee, M.G. Pharmacokinetics of theophylline in diabetes mellitus rats: Induction of CYP1A2 and CYP2E1 on 1,3-dimethyluric acid formation. *Eur. J. Pharm. Sci.* **2005**, *26*, 114–123. [CrossRef]
29. Chen, G.M.; Hu, N.; Liu, L.; Xie, S.S.; Wang, P.; Li, J.; Xie, L.; Wang, G.J.; Liu, X.D. Pharmacokinetics of verapamil in diabetic rats induced by combination of high-fat diet and streptozotocin injection. *Xenobiotica* **2011**, *41*, 494–500. [CrossRef]
30. Gawronska-Szklarz, B.; Musial, D.H.; Pawlik, A.; Paprota, B. Effect of experimental diabetes on pharmacokinetic parameters of lidocaine and MEGX in rats. *Pol. J. Pharm.* **2003**, *55*, 619–624.
31. Wang, X.; Wang, F.; Zhang, Y.; Xiong, H.; Zhang, Y.; Zhuang, P.; Zhang, Y. Diabetic cognitive dysfunction is associated with increased bile acids in liver and activation of bile acid signaling in intestine. *Toxicol. Lett.* **2018**, *287*, 10–22. [CrossRef] [PubMed]
32. Drolet, B.; Pilote, S.; Gelinas, C.; Kamaliza, A.D.; Blais-Boilard, A.; Virgili, J.; Patoine, D.; Simard, C. Altered Protein Expression of Cardiac CYP2J and Hepatic CYP2C, CYP4A, and CYP4F in a Mouse Model of Type II Diabetes-A Link in the Onset and Development of Cardiovascular Disease? *Pharmaceutics* **2017**, *9*, 44. [CrossRef] [PubMed]
33. Bae, S.K.; Kim, J.Y.; Yang, S.H.; Kim, J.W.; Kim, T.; Lee, M.G. Pharmacokinetics of oltipraz in rat models of diabetes mellitus induced by alloxan or streptozotocin. *Life Sci.* **2006**, *78*, 2287–2294. [CrossRef] [PubMed]
34. Lee, D.Y.; Lee, M.G.; Shin, H.S.; Lee, I. Changes in omeprazole pharmacokinetics in rats with diabetes induced by alloxan or streptozotocin: Faster clearance of omeprazole due to induction of hepatic CYP1A2 and 3A1. *J. Pharm. Pharm. Sci.* **2007**, *10*, 420–433. [CrossRef]
35. Ueyama, J.; Wang, D.; Kondo, T.; Saito, I.; Takagi, K.; Takagi, K.; Kamijima, M.; Nakajima, T.; Miyamoto, K.; Wakusawa, S.; et al. Toxicity of diazinon and its metabolites increases in diabetic rats. *Toxicol. Lett.* **2007**, *170*, 229–237. [CrossRef]

36. Maksymchuk, O.; Shysh, A.; Rosohatska, I.; Chashchyn, M. Quercetin prevents type 1 diabetic liver damage through inhibition of CYP2E1. *Pharm. Rep.* **2017**, *69*, 1386–1392. [CrossRef]
37. Woodcroft, K.J.; Novak, R.F. Insulin effects on CYP2E1, 2B, 3A, and 4A expression in primary cultured rat hepatocytes. *Chem. Biol. Interact.* **1997**, *107*, 75–91. [CrossRef]
38. Hu, N.; Hu, M.; Duan, R.; Liu, C.; Guo, H.; Zhang, M.; Yu, Y.; Wang, X.; Liu, L.; Liu, X. Increased levels of fatty acids contributed to induction of hepatic CYP3A4 activity induced by diabetes-in vitro evidence from HepG2 cell and Fa2N-4 cell lines. *J. Pharm. Sci.* **2014**, *124*, 433–444. [CrossRef]
39. Elaidy, S.M.; Hussain, M.A.; El-Kherbetawy, M.K. Time-dependent therapeutic roles of nitazoxanide on high-fat diet/streptozotocin-induced diabetes in rats: Effects on hepatic peroxisome proliferator-activated receptor-gamma receptors. *Can. J. Physiol. Pharm.* **2018**, *96*, 485–497. [CrossRef]
40. Zhang, C.; Deng, J.; Liu, D.; Tuo, X.; Xiao, L.; Lai, B.; Yao, Q.; Liu, J.; Yang, H.; Wang, N. Nuciferine ameliorates hepatic steatosis in high-fat diet/streptozocin-induced diabetic mice through a PPARα/PPARγ coactivator-1α pathway. *Br. J. Pharm.* **2018**, *175*, 4218–4228. [CrossRef]
41. Ahmad, A.; Ali, T.; Kim, M.W.; Khan, A.; Jo, M.H.; Rehman, S.U.; Khan, M.S.; Abid, N.B.; Khan, M.; Ullah, R.; et al. Adiponectin homolog novel osmotin protects obesity/diabetes-induced NAFLD by upregulating AdipoRs/PPARα signaling in ob/ob and db/db transgenic mouse models. *Metabolism* **2019**, *90*, 31–43. [CrossRef] [PubMed]
42. Shi, C.; Min, L.; Yang, J.; Dai, M.; Song, D.; Hua, H.; Xu, G.; Gonzalez, F.J.; Liu, A. Peroxisome Proliferator-Activated Receptor α Activation Suppresses Cytochrome P450 Induction Potential in Mice Treated with Gemfibrozil. *Basic Clin. Pharm. Toxicol.* **2017**, *121*, 169–174. [CrossRef] [PubMed]
43. Liu, Y.; Nakagawa, Y.; Wang, Y.; Sakurai, R.; Tripathi, P.V.; Lutfy, K.; Friedman, T.C. Increased glucocorticoid receptor and 11β-hydroxysteroid dehydrogenase type 1 expression in hepatocytes may contribute to the phenotype of type 2 diabetes in db/db mice. *Diabetes* **2005**, *54*, 32–40. [CrossRef] [PubMed]
44. Liu, Y.; Yan, C.; Wang, Y.; Nakagawa, Y.; Nerio, N.; Anghel, A.; Lutfy, K.; Friedman, T.C. Liver X receptor agonist T0901317 inhibition of glucocorticoid receptor expression in hepatocytes may contribute to the amelioration of diabetic syndrome in db/db mice. *Endocrinology* **2006**, *147*, 5061–5068. [CrossRef] [PubMed]
45. Schuetz, E.G.; Schmid, W.; Schutz, G.; Brimer, C.; Yasuda, K.; Kamataki, T.; Bornheim, L.; Myles, K.; Cole, T.J. The glucocorticoid receptor is essential for induction of cytochrome P-4502B by steroids but not for drug or steroid induction of CYP3A or P-450 reductase in mouse liver. *Drug Metab. Dispos.* **2000**, *28*, 268–278. [PubMed]
46. Gerbal-Chaloin, S.; Daujat, M.; Pascussi, J.M.; Pichard-Garcia, L.; Vilarem, M.J.; Maurel, P. Transcriptional regulation of CYP2C9 gene. Role of glucocorticoid receptor and constitutive androstane receptor. *J. Biol. Chem.* **2002**, *277*, 209–217. [CrossRef]
47. Xu, F.; Zhu, L.; Qian, C.; Zhou, J.; Geng, D.; Li, P.; Xuan, W.; Wu, F.; Zhao, K.; Kong, W.; et al. Impairment of Intestinal Monocarboxylate Transporter 6 Function and Expression in Diabetic Rats Induced by Combination of High-Fat Diet and Low Dose of Streptozocin: Involvement of Butyrate-Peroxisome Proliferator-Activated Receptor-γ Activation. *Drug Metab. Dispos.* **2019**, *47*, 556–566. [CrossRef]
48. Liu, H.; Liu, L.; Li, J.; Mei, D.; Duan, R.; Hu, N.; Guo, H.; Zhong, Z.; Liu, X. Combined contributions of impaired hepatic CYP2C11 and intestinal breast cancer resistance protein activities and expression to increased oral glibenclamide exposure in rats with streptozotocin-induced diabetes mellitus. *Drug Metab. Dispos.* **2012**, *40*, 1104–1112. [CrossRef]
49. Kim, Y.C.; Oh, E.Y.; Kim, S.H.; Lee, M.G. Pharmacokinetics of diclofenac in rat model of diabetes mellitus induced by alloxan or steptozotocin. *Biopharm. Drug Dispos.* **2006**, *27*, 85–92. [CrossRef]
50. Kim, Y.C.; Oh, E.Y.; Kim, S.H.; Lee, M.G. Pharmacokinetics and pharmacodynamics of intravenous torasemide in diabetic rats induced by alloxan or streptozotocin. *Biopharm. Drug Dispos.* **2005**, *26*, 371–378. [CrossRef]
51. Kim, Y.C.; Kang, H.E.; Lee, M.G. Pharmacokinetics of phenytoin and its metabolite, 4′-HPPH, after intravenous and oral administration of phenytoin to diabetic rats induced by alloxan or streptozotocin. *Biopharm. Drug Dispos.* **2008**, *29*, 51–61. [CrossRef] [PubMed]
52. Oh, S.J.; Choi, J.M.; Yun, K.U.; Oh, J.M.; Kwak, H.C.; Oh, J.G.; Lee, K.S.; Kim, B.H.; Heo, T.H.; Kim, S.K. Hepatic expression of cytochrome P450 in type 2 diabetic Goto-Kakizaki rats. *Chem. Biol. Interact.* **2012**, *195*, 173–179. [CrossRef] [PubMed]

53. Shi, R.; Wu, J.; Meng, C.; Ma, B.; Wang, T.; Li, Y.; Ma, Y. Cyp3a11-mediated testosterone-6beta-hydroxylation decreased, while UGT1a9-mediated propofol O-glucuronidation increased, in mice with diabetes mellitus. *Biopharm. Drug Dispos.* **2016**, *37*, 433–443. [CrossRef] [PubMed]
54. Lam, J.L.; Jiang, Y.; Zhang, T.; Zhang, E.Y.; Smith, B.J. Expression and functional analysis of hepatic cytochromes P450, nuclear receptors, and membrane transporters in 10-and 25-week-old db/db mice. *Drug Metab. Dispos.* **2010**, *38*, 2252–2258. [CrossRef]
55. Park, S.Y.; Kim, C.H.; Lee, J.Y.; Jeon, J.S.; Kim, M.J.; Chae, S.H.; Kim, H.C.; Oh, S.J.; Kim, S.K. Hepatic expression of cytochrome P450 in Zucker diabetic fatty rats. *Food Chem. Toxicol.* **2016**, *96*, 244–253. [CrossRef]
56. Patoine, D.; Petit, M.; Pilote, S.; Picard, F.; Drolet, B.; Simard, C. Modulation of CYP3a expression and activity in mice models of type 1 and type 2 diabetes. *Pharm. Res. Perspect.* **2014**, *2*, e00082. [CrossRef]
57. Gravel, S.; Chiasson, J.L.; Turgeon, J.; Grangeon, A.; Michaud, V. Modulation of CYP450 Activities in Patients With Type 2 Diabetes. *Clin. Pharm. Ther.* **2019**, *106*, 1280–1289. [CrossRef]
58. Gade, C.; Dalhoff, K.; Petersen, T.S.; Riis, T.; Schmeltz, C.; Chabanova, E.; Christensen, H.R.; Mikus, G.; Burhenne, J.; Holm, J.C.; et al. Higher chlorzoxazone clearance in obese children compared with nonobese peers. *Br. J. Clin. Pharm.* **2018**, *84*, 1738–1747. [CrossRef]
59. Dostalek, M.; Court, M.H.; Yan, B.; Akhlaghi, F. Significantly reduced cytochrome P450 3A4 expression and activity in liver from humans with diabetes mellitus. *Br. J. Pharm.* **2011**, *163*, 937–947. [CrossRef]
60. Marques, M.P.; Coelho, E.B.; Dos Santos, N.A.; Geleilete, T.J.; Lanchote, V.L. Dynamic and kinetic disposition of nisoldipine enantiomers in hypertensive patients presenting with type-2 diabetes mellitus. *Eur. J. Clin. Pharm.* **2002**, *58*, 607–614. [CrossRef]
61. Moises, E.C.; Duarte Lde, B.; Cavalli Rde, C.; Marques, M.P.; Lanchote, V.L.; Duarte, G.; da Cunha, S.P. Pharmacokinetics of lidocaine and its metabolite in peridural anesthesia administered to pregnant women with gestational diabetes mellitus. *Eur. J. Clin. Pharm.* **2008**, *64*, 1189–1196. [CrossRef] [PubMed]
62. Filgueira, G.C.O.; Filgueira, O.A.S.; Carvalho, D.M.; Marques, M.P.; Moises, E.C.D.; Duarte, G.; Lanchote, V.L.; Cavalli, R.C. Effect of type 2 diabetes mellitus on the pharmacokinetics and transplacental transfer of nifedipine in hypertensive pregnant women. *Br. J. Clin. Pharm.* **2017**, *83*, 1571–1579. [CrossRef] [PubMed]
63. Antunes Nde, J.; Cavalli, R.C.; Marques, M.P.; Moises, E.C.; Lanchote, V.L. Influence of gestational diabetes on the stereoselective pharmacokinetics and placental distribution of metoprolol and its metabolites in parturients. *Br. J. Clin. Pharm.* **2015**, *79*, 605–616. [CrossRef] [PubMed]
64. Adithan, C.; Srinivas, B.; Indhiresan, J.; Shashindran, C.H.; Bapna, J.S.; Thakur, L.C.; Swaminathan, R.P. Influence of type I and type II diabetes mellitus on phenytoin steady-state levels. *Int. J. Clin. Pharm. Ther. Toxicol.* **1991**, *29*, 310–313.
65. Akhlaghi, F.; Dostalek, M.; Falck, P.; Mendonza, A.E.; Amundsen, R.; Gohh, R.Y.; Asberg, A. The concentration of cyclosporine metabolites is significantly lower in kidney transplant recipients with diabetes mellitus. *Ther. Drug Monit.* **2012**, *34*, 38–45. [CrossRef]
66. Mendonza, A.E.; Gohh, R.Y.; Akhlaghi, F. Blood and plasma pharmacokinetics of ciclosporin in diabetic kidney transplant recipients. *Clin. Pharm.* **2008**, *47*, 733–742. [CrossRef]
67. Wadhawan, S.; Jauhari, H.; Singh, S. Cyclosporine trough levels in diabetic and nondiabetic renal transplant patients. *Transplant. Proc.* **2000**, *32*, 1683–1684. [CrossRef]
68. Jamwal, R.; de la Monte, S.M.; Ogasawara, K.; Adusumalli, S.; Barlock, B.B.; Akhlaghi, F. Nonalcoholic Fatty Liver Disease and Diabetes Are Associated with Decreased CYP3A4 Protein Expression and Activity in Human Liver. *Mol. Pharm.* **2018**, *15*, 2621–2632. [CrossRef]
69. Matzke, G.R.; Frye, R.F.; Early, J.J.; Straka, R.J.; Carson, S.W. Evaluation of the influence of diabetes mellitus on antipyrine metabolism and CYP1A2 and CYP2D6 activity. *Pharmacotherapy* **2000**, *20*, 182–190. [CrossRef]
70. Korrapati, M.R.; Vestal, R.E.; Loi, C.M. Theophylline metabolism in healthy nonsmokers and in patients with insulin-dependent diabetes mellitus. *Clin. Pharm. Ther.* **1995**, *57*, 413–418. [CrossRef]
71. Adithan, C.; Danda, D.; Shashindran, C.H.; Bapna, J.S.; Swaminathan, R.P.; Chandrasekar, S. Differential effect of type I and type II diabetes mellitus on antipyrine elimination. *Methods Find. Exp. Clin. Pharm.* **1989**, *11*, 755–758.
72. Zysset, T.; Wietholtz, H. Differential effect of type I and type II diabetes on antipyrine disposition in man. *Eur. J. Clin. Pharm.* **1988**, *34*, 369–375. [CrossRef] [PubMed]

73. Sotaniemi, E.A.; Pelkonen, O.; Arranto, A.J.; Tapanainen, P.; Rautio, A.; Pasanen, M. Diabetes and elimination of antipyrine in man: An analysis of 298 patients classified by type of diabetes, age, sex, duration of disease and liver involvement. *Pharm. Toxicol.* **2002**, *90*, 155–160. [CrossRef] [PubMed]
74. Urry, E.; Jetter, A.; Landolt, H.P. Assessment of CYP1A2 enzyme activity in relation to type-2 diabetes and habitual caffeine intake. *Nutr. Metab. (Lond.)* **2016**, *13*, 66. [CrossRef] [PubMed]
75. Porazka, J.; Szalek, E.; Polom, W.; Czajkowski, M.; Grabowski, T.; Matuszewski, M.; Grzeskowiak, E. Influence of Obesity and Type 2 Diabetes Mellitus on the Pharmacokinetics of Tramadol After Single Oral Dose Administration. *Eur. J. Drug Metab. Pharm.* **2019**, *44*, 579–584. [CrossRef] [PubMed]
76. Shu, N.; Hu, M.; Ling, Z.; Liu, P.; Wang, F.; Xu, P.; Zhong, Z.; Sun, B.; Zhang, M.; Li, F.; et al. The enhanced atorvastatin hepatotoxicity in diabetic rats was partly attributed to the upregulated hepatic Cyp3a and SLCO1B1. *Sci. Rep.* **2016**, *6*, 33072. [CrossRef]
77. Brunner, L.J.; Iyer, L.V.; Vadiei, K.; Weaver, W.V.; Luke, D.R. Cyclosporine pharmacokinetics and effect in the type I diabetic rat model. *Eur. J. Drug Metab. Pharm.* **1989**, *14*, 287–292. [CrossRef]
78. Neuman, M.G.; Cameron, R.G.; Haber, J.A.; Katz, G.G.; Malkiewicz, I.M.; Shear, N.H. Inducers of cytochrome P450 2E1 enhance methotrexate-induced hepatocytoxicity. *Clin. Biochem.* **1999**, *32*, 519–536. [CrossRef]
79. Malatjalian, D.A.; Ross, J.B.; Williams, C.N.; Colwell, S.J.; Eastwood, B.J. Methotrexate hepatotoxicity in psoriatics: Report of 104 patients from Nova Scotia, with analysis of risks from obesity, diabetes and alcohol consumption during long term follow-up. *Can. J. Gastroenterol. Hepatol.* **1996**, *10*, 369–375. [CrossRef]
80. Liu, X. ABC Family Transporters. *Adv. Exp. Med. Biol.* **2019**, *1141*, 13–100. [CrossRef]
81. Zeng, X.Y.; Dong, S.; He, N.N.; Jiang, C.J.; Dai, Y.; Xia, Y.F. Comparative pharmacokinetics of arctigenin in normal and type 2 diabetic rats after oral and intravenous administration. *Fitoterapia* **2015**, *105*, 119–126. [CrossRef] [PubMed]
82. Yu, S.; Yu, Y.; Liu, L.; Wang, X.; Lu, S.; Liang, Y.; Liu, X.; Xie, L.; Wang, G. Increased plasma exposures of five protoberberine alkaloids from Coptidis Rhizoma in streptozotocin-induced diabetic rats: Is P-GP involved? *Planta Med.* **2010**, *76*, 876–881. [CrossRef] [PubMed]
83. Novak, A.; Godoy, Y.C.; Martinez, S.A.; Ghanem, C.I.; Celuch, S.M. Fructose-induced metabolic syndrome decreases protein expression and activity of intestinal P-glycoprotein. *Nutrition* **2015**, *31*, 871–876. [CrossRef] [PubMed]
84. Watanabe, M.; Kobayashi, M.; Ogura, J.; Takahashi, N.; Yamaguchi, H.; Iseki, K. Alteration of pharmacokinetics of grepafloxacin in type 2 diabetic rats. *J. Pharm. Pharm. Sci.* **2014**, *17*, 25–33. [CrossRef] [PubMed]
85. Nawa, A.; Fujita-Hamabe, W.; Kishioka, S.; Tokuyama, S. Decreased expression of intestinal P-glycoprotein increases the analgesic effects of oral morphine in a streptozotocin-induced diabetic mouse model. *Drug Metab. Pharm.* **2011**, *26*, 584–591. [CrossRef]
86. Joshi, S.D.; Santani, D.D.; Sheth, J.J.; Mehta, H.C.; Dave, K.C.; Goyal, R.K. Investigation into the possible mechanisms involved in altered digoxin levels in diabetic patients. *Indian J. Physiol. Pharm.* **1996**, *40*, 65–69.
87. Gitanjali, B.; Adithan, C.; Raveendran, R.; Shashindran, C.H.; Chandrasekar, S. Pharmacokinetics of single dose oral digoxin in patients with uncomplicated type II diabetes mellitus. *Int. J. Clin. Pharm. Ther. Toxicol.* **1992**, *30*, 113–116.
88. Nawa, A.; Fujita-Hamabe, W.; Tokuyama, S. Involvement of ubiquitination in the decrease of intestinal P-glycoprotein in a streptozotocin-induced diabetic mouse model. *Drug Metab. Pharm.* **2012**, *27*, 548–552. [CrossRef]
89. Nawa, A.; Fujita-Hamabe, W.; Tokuyama, S. Regulatory action of nitric oxide synthase on ileal P-glycoprotein expression under streptozotocin-induced diabetic condition. *Biol. Pharm. Bull.* **2011**, *34*, 436–438. [CrossRef]
90. Nawa, A.; Fujita-Hamabe, W.; Tokuyama, S. Altered intestinal P-glycoprotein expression levels in a monosodium glutamate-induced obese mouse model. *Life Sci.* **2011**, *89*, 834–838. [CrossRef]
91. Nawa, A.; Fujita Hamabe, W.; Tokuyama, S. Inducible nitric oxide synthase-mediated decrease of intestinal P-glycoprotein expression under streptozotocin-induced diabetic conditions. *Life Sci.* **2010**, *86*, 402–409. [CrossRef] [PubMed]
92. Duan, R.; Hu, N.; Liu, H.Y.; Li, J.; Guo, H.F.; Liu, C.; Liu, L.; Liu, X.D. Biphasic regulation of P-glycoprotein function and expression by NO donors in Caco-2 cells. *Acta Pharm. Sin.* **2012**, *33*, 767–774. [CrossRef] [PubMed]

93. Zhang, J.; Xie, Q.; Kong, W.; Wang, Z.; Wang, S.; Zhao, K.; Chen, Y.; Liu, X.; Liu, L. Short-chain fatty acids oppositely altered expressions and functions of intestinal cytochrome P4503A and P-glycoprotein and affected pharmacokinetics of verapamil following oral administration to rats. *J. Pharm. Pharm.* **2020**, *72*, 448–460. [CrossRef] [PubMed]
94. Al-Salami, H.; Butt, G.; Tucker, I.; Skrbic, R.; Golocorbin-Kon, S.; Mikov, M. Probiotic Pre-treatment Reduces Gliclazide Permeation (ex vivo) in Healthy Rats but Increases It in Diabetic Rats to the Level Seen in Untreated Healthy Rats. *Arch. Drug Inf.* **2008**, *1*, 35–41. [CrossRef] [PubMed]
95. Mikov, M.; Al-Salami, H.; Golocorbin-Kon, S.; Skrbic, R.; Raskovic, A.; Fawcett, J.P. The influence of 3alpha,7alpha-dihydroxy-12-keto-5beta-cholanate on gliclazide pharmacokinetics and glucose levels in a rat model of diabetes. *Eur. J. Drug Metab. Pharm.* **2008**, *33*, 137–142. [CrossRef] [PubMed]
96. Xie, Q.S.; Zhang, J.X.; Liu, M.; Liu, P.H.; Wang, Z.J.; Zhu, L.; Liang, L.; Jin, M.M.; Liu, X.N.; Liu, L.; et al. Short-chain fatty acids down-regulate expression and function of p-glycoprotein but up-regulate expression and function of breast cancer resistance protein in intestine of rats. *Acta Pharm. Sin.* **2020**, in press.
97. Hindlet, P.; Bado, A.; Farinotti, R.; Buyse, M. Long-term effect of leptin on H^+-coupled peptide cotransporter 1 activity and expression in vivo: Evidence in leptin-deficient mice. *J. Pharm. Exp. Ther.* **2007**, *323*, 192–201. [CrossRef]
98. Bikhazi, A.B.; Skoury, M.M.; Zwainy, D.S.; Jurjus, A.R.; Kreydiyyeh, S.I.; Smith, D.E.; Audette, K.; Jacques, D. Effect of diabetes mellitus and insulin on the regulation of the PepT 1 symporter in rat jejunum. *Mol. Pharm.* **2004**, *1*, 300–308. [CrossRef]
99. Liang, L.M.; Zhou, J.J.; Xu, F.; Li, X.W.; Liu, P.H.; Qin, L.; Liu, L.; Liu, X.D. Diabetes downregulates peptide transporter 1 in rat jejunum: Possible involvement of cholate-induced FXR activation. *Acta Pharm. Sin.* **2020**, in press.
100. Der-Boghossian, A.H.; Saad, S.R.; Perreault, C.; Provost, C.; Jacques, D.; Kadi, L.N.; Issa, N.G.; Sibai, A.M.; El-Majzoub, N.W.; Bikhazi, A.B. Role of insulin on jejunal PepT1 expression and function regulation in diabetic male and female rats. *Can. J. Physiol. Pharm.* **2010**, *88*, 753–759. [CrossRef]
101. Watanabe, K.; Terada, K.; Jinriki, T.; Sato, J. Effect of insulin on cephalexin uptake and transepithelial transport in the human intestinal cell line Caco-2. *Eur. J. Pharm. Sci.* **2004**, *21*, 87–95. [CrossRef] [PubMed]
102. Thamotharan, M.; Bawani, S.Z.; Zhou, X.; Adibi, S.A. Hormonal regulation of oligopeptide transporter pept-1 in a human intestinal cell line. *Am. J. Physiol.* **1999**, *276*, C821–C826. [CrossRef] [PubMed]
103. Kohyama, N.; Shiokawa, H.; Ohbayashi, M.; Kobayashi, Y.; Yamamoto, T. Characterization of monocarboxylate transporter 6: Expression in human intestine and transport of the antidiabetic drug nateglinide. *Drug Metab. Dispos.* **2013**, *41*, 1883–1887. [CrossRef] [PubMed]
104. Murakami, Y.; Kohyama, N.; Kobayashi, Y.; Ohbayashi, M.; Ohtani, H.; Sawada, Y.; Yamamoto, T. Functional characterization of human monocarboxylate transporter 6 (SLC16A5). *Drug Metab. Dispos.* **2005**, *33*, 1845–1851. [CrossRef] [PubMed]
105. Park, J.H.; Lee, W.I.; Yoon, W.H.; Park, Y.D.; Lee, J.S.; Lee, M.G. Pharmacokinetic and pharmacodynamic changes of furosemide after intravenous and oral administration to rats with alloxan-induced diabetes mellitus. *Biopharm. Drug Dispos.* **1998**, *19*, 357–364. [CrossRef]
106. Park, K.J.; Yoon, W.H.; Shin, W.G.; Lee, M.G. Pharmacokinetics and pharmacodynamics of azosemide after intravenous and oral administration to rats with alloxan-induced diabetes mellitus. *J. Pharm. Pharm.* **1996**, *48*, 1093–1097. [CrossRef] [PubMed]
107. Borbas, T.; Benko, B.; Dalmadi, B.; Szabo, I.; Tihanyi, K. Insulin in flavin-containing monooxygenase regulation. Flavin-containing monooxygenase and cytochrome P450 activities in experimental diabetes. *Eur J. Pharm. Sci.* **2006**, *28*, 51–58. [CrossRef]
108. Kudo, T.; Toda, T.; Ushiki, T.; Ohi, K.; Ikarashi, N.; Ochiai, W.; Sugiyama, K. Differences in the pharmacokinetics of Cyp3a substrates in TSOD and streptozotocin-induced diabetic mice. *Xenobiotica* **2010**, *40*, 282–290. [CrossRef]
109. Zhang, S.; Pan, X.; Jeong, H. GW4064, an agonist of farnesoid X receptor, represses CYP3A4 expression in human hepatocytes by inducing small heterodimer partner expression. *Drug Metab. Dispos.* **2015**, *43*, 743–748. [CrossRef]
110. Ourlin, J.C.; Lasserre, F.; Pineau, T.; Fabre, J.M.; Sa-Cunha, A.; Maurel, P.; Vilarem, M.J.; Pascussi, J.M. The small heterodimer partner interacts with the pregnane X receptor and represses its transcriptional activity. *Mol. Endocrinol.* **2003**, *17*, 1693–1703. [CrossRef]

111. Ogata, M.; Iizuka, Y.; Murata, R.; Hikichi, N. Effect of streptozotocin-induced diabetes on cyclosporin A disposition in rats. *Biol. Pharm. Bull.* **1996**, *19*, 1586–1590. [CrossRef] [PubMed]
112. Ando, T.; Kusuhara, H.; Merino, G.; Alvarez, A.I.; Schinkel, A.H.; Sugiyama, Y. Involvement of breast cancer resistance protein (ABCG2) in the biliary excretion mechanism of fluoroquinolones. *Drug Metab. Dispos.* **2007**, *35*, 1873–1879. [CrossRef] [PubMed]
113. Jiang, S.; Zhao, W.; Chen, Y.; Zhong, Z.; Zhang, M.; Li, F.; Xu, P.; Zhao, K.; Li, Y.; Liu, L.; et al. Paroxetine decreased plasma exposure of glyburide partly via inhibiting intestinal absorption in rats. *Drug Metab. Pharm.* **2015**, *30*, 240–246. [CrossRef] [PubMed]
114. Liu, X. Overview: Role of Drug Transporters in Drug Disposition and Its Clinical Significance. *Adv. Exp. Med. Biol.* **2019**, *1141*, 1–12. [CrossRef]
115. Phatchawan, A.; Chutima, S.; Varanuj, C.; Anusorn, L. Decreased renal organic anion transporter 3 expression in type 1 diabetic rats. *Am. J. Med. Sci.* **2014**, *347*, 221–227. [CrossRef]
116. Thongnak, L.; Pongchaidecha, A.; Jaikumkao, K.; Chatsudthipong, V.; Chattipakorn, N.; Lungkaphin, A. The additive effects of atorvastatin and insulin on renal function and renal organic anion transporter 3 function in diabetic rats. *Sci. Rep.* **2017**, *7*, 13532. [CrossRef]
117. Babelova, A.; Burckhardt, B.C.; Wegner, W.; Burckhardt, G.; Henjakovic, M. Sex-differences in renal expression of selected transporters and transcription factors in lean and obese Zucker spontaneously hypertensive fatty rats. *J. Diabetes Res.* **2015**, *2015*, 483238. [CrossRef]
118. Sharma, K.; Karl, B.; Mathew, A.V.; Gangoiti, J.A.; Wassel, C.L.; Saito, R.; Pu, M.; Sharma, S.; You, Y.H.; Wang, L.; et al. Metabolomics reveals signature of mitochondrial dysfunction in diabetic kidney disease. *J. Am. Soc. Nephrol.* **2013**, *24*, 1901–1912. [CrossRef]
119. Vallon, V.; Rieg, T.; Ahn, S.Y.; Wu, W.; Eraly, S.A.; Nigam, S.K. Overlapping in vitro and in vivo specificities of the organic anion transporters OAT1 and OAT3 for loop and thiazide diuretics. *Am. J. Physiol. Renal. Physiol.* **2008**, *294*, F867–F873. [CrossRef]
120. Eraly, S.A.; Vallon, V.; Vaughn, D.A.; Gangoiti, J.A.; Richter, K.; Nagle, M.; Monte, J.C.; Rieg, T.; Truong, D.M.; Long, J.M.; et al. Decreased renal organic anion secretion and plasma accumulation of endogenous organic anions in OAT1 knock-out mice. *J. Biol. Chem.* **2006**, *281*, 5072–5083. [CrossRef]
121. Cunha, F.M.; Pereira, J.; Marques, P.; Ribeiro, A.; Bettencourt, P.; Lourenco, P. Diabetic patients need higher furosemide doses: A report on acute and chronic heart failure patients. *J. Cardiovasc. Med. (Hagerstown)* **2020**, *21*, 21–26. [CrossRef] [PubMed]
122. Fu, Y.; Breljak, D.; Onishi, A.; Batz, F.; Patel, R.; Huang, W.; Song, P.; Freeman, B.; Mayoux, E.; Koepsell, H.; et al. Organic anion transporter OAT3 enhances the glucosuric effect of the SGLT2 inhibitor empagliflozin. *Am. J. Physiol. Renal. Physiol.* **2018**, *315*, F386–F394. [CrossRef] [PubMed]
123. Jinnouchi, H.; Nozaki, K.; Watase, H.; Omiya, H.; Sakai, S.; Samukawa, Y. Impact of Reduced Renal Function on the Glucose-Lowering Effects of Luseogliflozin, a Selective SGLT2 Inhibitor, Assessed by Continuous Glucose Monitoring in Japanese Patients with Type 2 Diabetes Mellitus. *Adv. Ther.* **2016**, *33*, 460–479. [CrossRef] [PubMed]
124. Nowicki, M.T.; Aleksunes, L.M.; Sawant, S.P.; Dnyanmote, A.V.; Mehendale, H.M.; Manautou, J.E. Renal and hepatic transporter expression in type 2 diabetic rats. *Drug Metab. Lett.* **2008**, *2*, 11–17. [CrossRef] [PubMed]
125. Grover, B.; Buckley, D.; Buckley, A.R.; Cacini, W. Reduced expression of organic cation transporters rOCT1 and rOCT2 in experimental diabetes. *J. Pharm. Exp. Ther.* **2004**, *308*, 949–956. [CrossRef]
126. Thomas, M.C.; Tikellis, C.; Burns, W.C.; Thallas, V.; Forbes, J.M.; Cao, Z.; Osicka, T.M.; Russo, L.M.; Jerums, G.; Ghabrial, H.; et al. Reduced tubular cation transport in diabetes: Prevented by ACE inhibition. *Kidney Int.* **2003**, *63*, 2152–2161. [CrossRef]
127. Thomas, M.C.; Tikellis, C.; Kantharidis, P.; Burns, W.C.; Cooper, M.E.; Forbes, J.M. The role of advanced glycation in reduced organic cation transport associated with experimental diabetes. *J. Pharm. Exp. Ther.* **2004**, *311*, 456–466. [CrossRef]
128. Lee, M.G.; Choi, Y.H.; Lee, I. Effects of diabetes mellitus induced by alloxan on the pharmacokinetics of metformin in rats: Restoration of pharmacokinetic parameters to the control state by insulin treatment. *J. Pharm. Pharm. Sci.* **2008**, *11*, 88–103. [CrossRef] [PubMed]
129. Tucker, G.T.; Casey, C.; Phillips, P.J.; Connor, H.; Ward, J.D.; Woods, H.F. Metformin kinetics in healthy subjects and in patients with diabetes mellitus. *Br. J. Clin. Pharm.* **1981**, *12*, 235–246. [CrossRef]

130. Bergagnini-Kolev, M.C.; Hebert, M.F.; Easterling, T.R.; Lin, Y.S. Pregnancy Increases the Renal Secretion of N(1)-methylnicotinamide, an Endogenous Probe for Renal Cation Transporters, in Patients Prescribed Metformin. *Drug Metab. Dispos.* **2017**, *45*, 325–329. [CrossRef]
131. Liao, M.Z.; Flood Nichols, S.K.; Ahmed, M.; Clark, S.; Hankins, G.D.; Caritis, S.; Venkataramanan, R.; Haas, D.; Quinney, S.K.; Haneline, L.S.; et al. Effects of Pregnancy on the Pharmacokinetics of Metformin. *Drug Metab. Dispos.* **2020**. [CrossRef] [PubMed]
132. Hughes, R.C.; Gardiner, S.J.; Begg, E.J.; Zhang, M. Effect of pregnancy on the pharmacokinetics of metformin. *Diabet. Med.* **2006**, *23*, 323–326. [CrossRef] [PubMed]
133. Cacini, W.; Singh, Y. Renal metallothionein and platinum levels in diabetic and nondiabetic rats injected with cisplatin. *Proc. Soc. Exp. Biol. Med.* **1991**, *197*, 285–289. [CrossRef] [PubMed]
134. Cacini, W.; Harden, E.A.; Skau, K.A. Reduced renal accumulation and toxicity of cisplatin in experimental galactosemia. *Proc. Soc. Exp. Biol. Med.* **1993**, *203*, 348–353. [CrossRef]
135. Scott, L.A.; Madan, E.; Valentovic, M.A. Attenuation of cisplatin nephrotoxicity by streptozotocin-induced diabetes. *Toxicol. Sci.* **1989**, *12*, 530–539. [CrossRef]
136. da Silva Faria, M.C.; Santos, N.A.; Carvalho Rodrigues, M.A.; Rodrigues, J.L.; Barbosa Junior, F.; Santos, A.C. Effect of diabetes on biodistribution, nephrotoxicity and antitumor activity of cisplatin in mice. *Chem. Biol. Interact.* **2015**, *229*, 119–131. [CrossRef]
137. Valentovic, M.A.; Scott, L.A.; Madan, E.; Yokel, R.A. Renal accumulation and urinary excretion of cisplatin in diabetic rats. *Toxicology* **1991**, *70*, 151–162. [CrossRef]
138. Tramonti, G.; Xie, P.; Wallner, E.I.; Danesh, F.R.; Kanwar, Y.S. Expression and functional characteristics of tubular transporters: P-glycoprotein, PEPT1, and PEPT2 in renal mass reduction and diabetes. *Am. J. Physiol. Renal. Physiol.* **2006**, *291*, F972–F980. [CrossRef]
139. Yeh, S.Y.; Pan, H.J.; Lin, C.C.; Kao, Y.H.; Chen, Y.H.; Lin, C.J. Hyperglycemia induced down-regulation of renal P-glycoprotein expression. *Eur. J. Pharm.* **2012**, *690*, 42–50. [CrossRef]
140. Maximos, S.; Chamoun, M.; Gravel, S.; Turgeon, J.; Michaud, V. Tissue Specific Modulation of cyp2c and cyp3a mRNA Levels and Activities by Diet-Induced Obesity in Mice: The Impact of Type 2 Diabetes on Drug Metabolizing Enzymes in Liver and Extra-Hepatic Tissues. *Pharmaceutics* **2017**, *9*, 40. [CrossRef]
141. Del Villar, E.; Gaule, C.; Vega, P. Kidney drug metabolizing activities in streptozotocin diabetic rats. *Gen. Pharm.* **1995**, *26*, 137–141. [CrossRef]
142. Ding, S.; Huang, J.; Qiu, H.; Chen, R.; Zhang, J.; Huang, B.; Cheng, O.; Jiang, Q. Effects of PPARs/20-HETE on the renal impairment under diabetic conditions. *Exp. Cell Res.* **2019**, *382*, 111455. [CrossRef] [PubMed]
143. Park, J.M.; Moon, C.H.; Lee, M.G. Pharmacokinetic changes of methotrexate after intravenous administration to streptozotocin-induced diabetes mellitus rats. *Res. Commun. Mol. Pathol. Pharm.* **1996**, *93*, 343–352.
144. Kim, S.H.; Kim, W.B.; Lee, M.G. Pharmacokinetics of a new carbapenem, DA-1131, after intravenous administration to rats with alloxan-induced diabetes mellitus. *Biopharm. Drug Dispos.* **1998**, *19*, 303–308. [CrossRef]
145. Valentovic, M.A.; Ball, J.G.; Rogers, B.A. Comparison of cephaloridine renal accumulation and urinary excretion between normoglycemic and diabetic animals. *Toxicology* **1996**, *108*, 93–99. [CrossRef]
146. Kong, W.M.; Sun, B.B.; Wang, Z.J.; Zheng, X.K.; Zhao, K.J.; Chen, Y.; Zhang, J.X.; Liu, P.H.; Zhu, L.; Xu, R.J.; et al. Physiologically based pharmacokinetic-pharmacodynamic modeling for prediction of vonoprazan pharmacokinetics and its inhibition on gastric acid secretion following intravenous/oral administration to rats, dogs and humans. *Acta Pharm. Sin.* **2020**. [CrossRef]
147. Yusuksawad, M.; Chaiyabutr, N. Restoration of renal hemodynamics and functions during black cumin (Nigella sativa) administration in streptozotocin-induced diabetic rats. *J. Exp. Pharm.* **2012**, *4*, 1–7. [CrossRef]
148. Kitani, M.; Ozaki, Y.; Katayama, K.; Kakemi, M.; Koizumi, T. A kinetic study on drug distribution: furosemide in rats. *Chem. Pharm. Bull. (Tokyo)* **1988**, *36*, 1053–1062. [CrossRef]
149. Varma, M.V.; Sarkar, M.; Kapoor, N.; Panchagnula, R. PH-dependent functional activity of P-glycoprotein in limiting intestinal absorption of protic drugs 1. Simultaneous determination of quinidine and permeability markers in rat in situ perfusion samples. *J. Chromatogr. B Analyt. Technol. Biomed. Life Sci.* **2005**, *816*, 243–249. [CrossRef]
150. Choi, D.H.; Chang, K.S.; Hong, S.P.; Choi, J.S.; Han, H.K. Effect of atorvastatin on the intravenous and oral pharmacokinetics of verapamil in rats. *Biopharm. Drug Dispos.* **2008**, *29*, 45–50. [CrossRef]

151. Ruark, C.D.; Hack, C.E.; Robinson, P.J.; Mahle, D.A.; Gearhart, J.M. Predicting passive and active tissue:plasma partition coefficients: Interindividual and interspecies variability. *J. Pharm. Sci.* **2014**, *103*, 2189–2198. [CrossRef] [PubMed]
152. Yang, K.H.; Choi, Y.H.; Lee, U.; Lee, J.H.; Lee, M.G. Effects of cytochrome P450 inducers and inhibitors on the pharmacokinetics of intravenous furosemide in rats: Involvement of CYP2C11, 2E1, 3A1 and 3A2 in furosemide metabolism. *J. Pharm. Pharm.* **2009**, *61*, 47–54. [CrossRef]
153. Li, J.; Guo, H.F.; Liu, C.; Zhong, Z.; Liu, L.; Liu, X.D. Prediction of drug disposition in diabetic patients by means of a physiologically based pharmacokinetic model. *Clin. Pharm.* **2015**, *54*, 179–193. [CrossRef] [PubMed]
154. Sumida, A.; Kinoshita, K.; Fukuda, T.; Matsuda, H.; Yamamoto, I.; Inaba, T.; Azuma, J. Relationship between mRNA levels quantified by reverse transcription-competitive PCR and metabolic activity of CYP3A4 and CYP2E1 in human liver. *Biochem. Biophys. Res. Commun.* **1999**, *262*, 499–503. [CrossRef]

7

Augmented Renal Clearance in Critical Illness: An Important Consideration in Drug Dosing

Sherif Hanafy Mahmoud * and Chen Shen

Faculty of Pharmacy and Pharmaceutical Sciences, University of Alberta, Edmonton, AB T6G 1C9, Canada; cshen2@ualberta.ca
* Correspondence: smahmoud@ualberta.ca

Abstract: Augmented renal clearance (ARC) is a manifestation of enhanced renal function seen in critically ill patients. The use of regular unadjusted doses of renally eliminated drugs in patients with ARC might lead to therapy failure. The purpose of this scoping review was to provide and up-to-date summary of the available evidence pertaining to the phenomenon of ARC. A literature search of databases of available evidence in humans, with no language restriction, was conducted. Databases searched were MEDLINE (1946 to April 2017), EMBASE (1974 to April 2017) and the Cochrane Library (1999 to April 2017). A total of 57 records were included in the present review: 39 observational studies (25 prospective, 14 retrospective), 6 case reports/series and 12 conference abstracts. ARC has been reported to range from 14 to 80%. ARC is currently defined as an increased creatinine clearance of greater than 130 mL/min/1.73 m^2 best measured by 8–24 h urine collection. Patients exhibiting ARC tend to be younger (<50 years old), of male gender, had a recent history of trauma, and had lower critical illness severity scores. Numerous studies have reported antimicrobials treatment failures when using standard dosing regimens in patients with ARC. In conclusion, ARC is an important phenomenon that might have significant impact on outcome in critically ill patients. Identifying patients at risk, using higher doses of renally eliminated drugs or use of non-renally eliminated alternatives might need to be considered in ICU patients with ARC. More research is needed to solidify dosing recommendations of various drugs in patients with ARC.

Keywords: augmented renal clearance; enhanced renal function; critically ill

---

1. Introduction

Studying the influence of renal dysfunction on the pharmacokinetics of drugs is an important consideration in drug development. In addition, clinicians are vigilant in adjusting the doses of renally eliminated drugs in patients with various degrees of renal impairment to avoid potential toxicities. On the other hand, little attention is given if patients exhibit an augmented renal clearance (ARC). Augmented renal clearance (ARC) is a manifestation of enhanced renal function seen in critically ill patients [1,2]. It is currently defined as an increased creatinine clearance of greater than 130 mL/min/1.73 m^2. ARC is a clinical phenomenon rapidly gaining recognition in the world of critical care. Although ARC may have existed long before our current recognition, it wasn't until the early 2010's, that the research group led by Andrew Udy put forth the concept of ARC as an independently existing medical phenomenon [3]. The increased renal clearance of endogenous by-products, various chemicals, toxins, and most importantly medications during ARC manifestation may have a significant impact on patient outcome. The use of regular unadjusted doses of renally eliminated drugs in patients with ARC might lead to therapy failure and worse patient outcome. The purpose of this scoping review was to provide and up-to-date summary of the available evidence pertaining to the phenomenon of ARC including epidemiology, risk factors and pathophysiology of ARC, pharmacokinetic changes of drugs in patients with ARC and suggested assessment and management approach of patients exhibiting ARC.

2. Methods

A literature search of databases of available evidence pertaining to augmented renal clearance (ARC) in humans, with no language restriction, was conducted. Databases searched were MEDLINE (1946 to 12 April 2017), EMBASE (1974 to 12 April 2017) and the Cochrane Library (1999 to 12 April 2017). To ensure that we captured all studies involving augmented renal clearance, we used the following keywords: "augmented renal clearance", "enchanc * renal clear *", "increase * renal clearance", "augmented kidney clearance", "enhance * kidney function *", "ren * ultrafiltrat *", "enhance * creatinine clear *", "increase * kidney function *", and "increase * creatinine clear *". Title and abstract screening were then conducted to identify duplicate studies and studies that were clearly not pertaining to the topic for exclusion. If any doubt arose regarding whether a study was related to ARC, the study was included for full text review. Studies on renal dysfunction (e.g., acute kidney injury, chronic kidney disease, renal dysfunction, etc.) or other clinical phenomena that would alter drug elimination (e.g., cystic fibrosis) were excluded. Non-human studies, non-English studies that could not be easily translated into English using an online translator tool, commentaries, opinion articles, editorials and review articles were excluded. Both authors independently conducted the processes of screening. Then, the full texts of the selected articles were assessed for inclusion in our review. Lastly, a manual search for additional relevant studies was performed by analyzing the reference lists of the selected studies. In case of any discrepancies between the reviewers, further discussion was done to reach a consensus. Data extraction from studies was confirmed by both authors.

3. Results and Discussion

As depicted in Figure 1, databases search resulted in 562 records. After duplicate removal and addition of records from other sources, 322 records remained. After title, abstract and full text screening, a total of 57 records were included in the present review: 39 observational studies (25 prospective, 14 retrospective), 6 case reports/case series and 12 conference abstracts. Because the main body of evidence was derived from observational studies, caution should be exercised while interpreting the results of the included records especially case reports. Table 1 summarizes the studies included in this review.

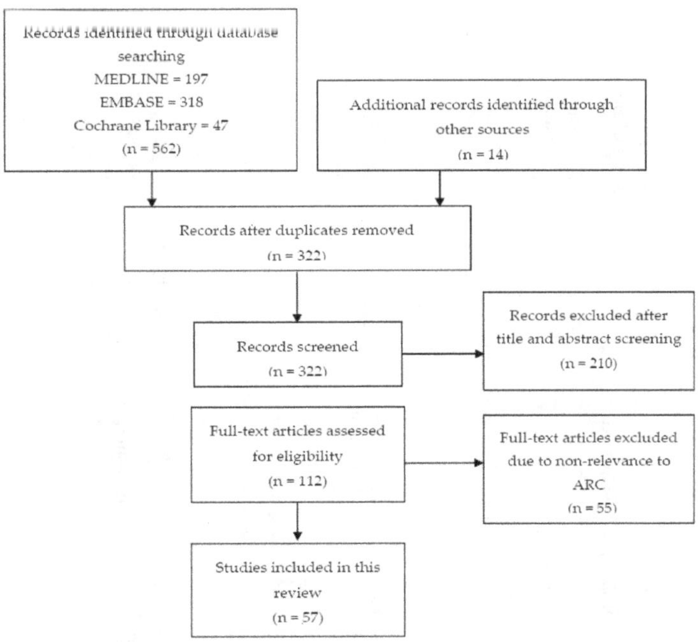

Figure 1. Flow diagram of the literature search for studies addressing augmented renal clearance (ARC).

Table 1. Summary of studies pertaining to ARC.

Author, Year	Study Type	Age (Years) Median (IQR)	Population	N	Sex (% Male)	Measured CrCl (mL/min)—Otherwise Specified	Intervention	Main Results
Barletta et al. [4], 2017	Retrospective observational	48 ± 19	ICU trauma patients where measured SCr available and SCr < 115 μmol/L	133	76	168 ± 65	ARCTIC (Augmented Renal Clearance in Trauma Intensive Care) Scoring system suggested	• 67% of patients identified to have ARC (CrCl > 130 mL/min) • ARC risk factors identified: from multivariate analysis were age < 56 years, age = 56–75 years, SCr < 62 μmol/L, male sex • ARCTIC score > 6 had sensitivity 84% and specificity 68%
Naeem et al. [5], 2017	Prospective observational	ARC: 37 ± 16 Non-ARC: 34 ± 14	ICU patients with SCr < 115 μmol/L	50	ARC: 70 Non-ARC: 60	ARC: 214 ± 46 Non-ARC: 112 ± 11	The effects of ARC on enoxaparin determined; Patients received enoxaparin 40 mg SC daily; Anti-Xa activity measured and compared among patients with and without ARC; measured 24 h CrCl	• 40% of patients identified to have ARC (CrCl > 130 mL/min) • Anti-Xa activity did not differ in both groups at baseline and 4 h after administration • ARC patients had significantly lower anti-Xa activity 12 and 24 h post enoxaparin administration; this implies short duration of action of enoxaparin in patients with ARC.
Udy et al. [6], 2017	Prospective observational (sub-study of BLING II RCT)	ARC: 52 (33–60) Non-ARC: 65 (55–73)	ICU patients with severe sepsis	254	ARC: 73 Non-ARC: 57	ARC: 165 (144–198) Non-ARC: 56 (27–83)	Conducted to determine the effect of ARC on patient outcome; patients randomized to receive beta lactam antibiotics (piperacillin/tazobactam, ticarcillin/clavulanic acid or meropenem) by intermittent or continuous infusion; measured 8 h CrCl	• 18% of patients identified to have ARC (CrCl > 130 mL/min); mainly younger, male and with less organ dysfunction • No outcome differences (ICU-free days or mortality) between ARC and non-ARC • No outcome differences were identified between continuous or intermittent infusion strategy
Udy et al. [7], 2017	Prospective observational	37 (24–49)	ICU (TBI patients with SCr < 120 μmol/L)	11	82	Median (day 1): 201 (76–239)	Measured 8-h CrCl, cardiac output and ANP were determined and correlated	• ARC complicates TBI patients (Measured CrCl generally > 150 mL/min); mainly males and with young age • CrCl was not significantly associated with changes in ANP or cardiac output

Table 1. *Cont.*

Author, Year	Study Type	Age (Years) Median (IQR)	Population	N	Sex (% Male)	Measured CrCl (mL/min)—Otherwise Specified	Intervention	Main Results
Barletta et al. [8], 2016	Retrospective observational	48 ± 18	ICU (trauma)	65	74	169 ± 70	Measured 12-h CrCl compared with CG method, CKD-EPI, and MDRD-4	• 69% of patients identified to have ARC (CrCl > 130 mL/min)—more common in younger patients and patients with SCr < 71 μmol/L • Measured CrCl was significantly higher ($p < 0.001$) than all estimates of CrCl • CG demonstrated lowest amount of bias (38 ± 56 mL/min) compared to CKD-EPI and MDRD-4
Chu et al. [9], 2016	Retrospective observational	Group A: 63 ± 15 Group B: 59 ± 14 Group C: 44 ± 16	Patients treated with vancomycin	148	66	Estimated by CG Group A: 54 ± 17 Group B: 106 ± 15 Group C: 188 ± 50	Vancomycin 1000 mg IV Q12H regimen given; vancomycin levels drawn pre 4th or 5th dose; levels compared across three groups: A (CrCl < 80), B (CrCl 80–129), C (CrCl ≥ 130; ARC)	• Patients with ARC (Group C) had higher percentage of subtherapeutic vancomycin • Vancomycin trough concentrations at steady state: Group A = 25 ± 10, Group B = 15 ± 8, Group C = 9 ± 5 mg/L • Vancomycin trough concentration below 10 mcg/mL: Group A = 0%, Group B = 28%, Group C = 63%
Declercq et al. [10], 2016	Prospective observational	Abdominal Surgery: 63 (51–71) Trauma Surgery: 62 (46–75)	Non-critically ill surgery patients	232	Abdo. Surgery: 74 Trauma Surgery: 58	Abdominal Surgery: 109 (82–135) Trauma Surgery: 109 (85–142)	Aim to assess the prevalence of ARC in non-critically ill surgical patients; Measured 8-h CrCl	• Abdominal surgery patients: 30% of patients identified to have ARC (CrCl > 130 mL/min) • Trauma surgery patients: 35% of patients identified to have ARC (CrCl > 130 mL/min) • The study identified presence of ARC in non-ICU surgery patients especially in younger male patients and undergoing trauma surgery
Hirai et al. [11], 2016	Retrospective observational	4.4 (range 1–15)	Pediatric ICU patients with normal renal function (Japan)	109	59	eGFR estimated by Schwartz formula 160 (range 90–323) mL/min/1.73 m^2	Vancomycin 40–60 mg/kg per day given in 2–4 divided doses; vancomycin clearance estimated	• ARC defined as eGFR ≥ 160 mL/min/1.73 m^2 • Febrile neutropenia is an independent risk factor for ARC • Age and eGFR significantly associated with vancomycin clearance ($p < 0.0001$)

Table 1. *Cont.*

Author. Year	Study Type	Age (Years) Median (IQR)	Population	N	Sex (% Male)	Measured CrCl (mL/min)—Otherwise Specified	Intervention	Main Results
Kawano et al. [12], 2016	Prospective observational	67 (53–77)	ICU (Japan)	111	56	Not reported	Measured 8-h CrCl	• 39% of patients identified to have ARC (CrCl > 130 mL/min/1.73 m^2) • Age < 63 years was identified as a risk factor for ARC
Roberts et al. [13], 2016	Prospective PK study	61 ± 17	Patients treated with levofloxacin	18	67	Estimated using CG 70 ± 67	Doses of levofloxacin 500 and 750 mg daily have been used; Monte-Carlo simulation conducted to determine PTA in ICU cohort compared to non ICU ones	• For CrCl > 130 and CrCl > 200, levofloxacin 1000 mg Q24H provided the highest target attainment for *S. pneumoniae*, *P. aeruginosa* and *S. aureus*. • For H. *influenza*, all levofloxacin doses/regimens analyzed were able to achieve >99% attainment
De Cock et al. [14], 2015	Prospective PK study	2.6 (range 0.08–15)	Pediatric ICU	50	60	Not reported	Population PK of amoxicillin/clavulanate in pediatric ICU population; Conventional dosing of 25–35 mg/kg every 6 h was tested.	• In ARC patients; the best dosing is 25 mg/kg over 1 h every 4 h; it produced the best median target attainment by Monte-Carlo Simulation
De Waele et al. [15], 2015	Retrospective observational	62 (50–72)	ICU	1081	63	ARC: 178 (140–243) Non-ARC: 54 (32–82)	Measured 24-h CrCl and ARC risk factors determined	• 56% of patients identified to have ARC (CrCl > 130 mL/min): mainly younger and less likely to be treated with vasopressors • Continuous ARC was present in 33% of patients • ARC incidence 37 per 100 ICU patient-days
Dias et al. [16], 2015	Retrospective observational	Mean 42 (range 20–66)	ICU (TBI patients)	18	89	CG method 199 (Range 62–471)	Cerebrovascular pressure reactivity index (PRx) correlated with CrCl	• A strong negative correlation between CG CrCl and PRX ($r = -0.82$, $p = 0.001$) have been reported • This correlation suggests that reduction in cerebral autoregulation (i.e., after TBI) is associated with an increase in creatinine clearance.

Table 1. *Cont.*

Author, Year	Study Type	Age (Years) Median (IQR)	Population	N	Sex (% Male)	Measured CrCl (mL/min)—Otherwise Specified	Intervention	Main Results
Huttner et al. [17], 2015	Prospective observational	ARC: 41 ± 12 Non-ARC: 51:10	ICU with CrCl ≥ 60 mL/min	100	75	Estimated with CG ARC: 166 (145–200) Non-ARC: 103 (87–113)	They determined the influence of ARC on patient outcome; Standard dose antibiotic regimens given (imipenem/cilastatin 500 mg IV QID; meropenem 2 g IV TID; piperacillin/tazobactam 4.5 g IV TID; cefepime 2 g IV BID)	• 64% of patients identified to have ARC (CrCl > 130 mL/min); mainly younger • ARC predicted undetectable antimicrobials concentrations but was not correlated with clinical failure
Morbitzer et al. [18], 2015	Retrospective observational	CN: 44 (29–52) TH/PI: 48 (40–62)	ICU (TBI)	27	63	Estimated using CG CN: 119 (91–166) TH/PI: 129 (100–156)	Vancomycin pharmacokinetics compared in patients with CN (T = 36–37 C), TH (T=33–34 C) or pentobarbital infusion	• Vancomycin clearance was higher in controlled normothermic patients compared to predicted values based on population parameters
Ruiz et al. [19], 2015	Prospective observational	ARC: 39 ± 16 No ARC: 55 ± 19	ICU (patients with normal SCr)	360	ARC: 75 No ARC: 65	ARC: 173 ± 44 No ARC: 79 ± 30	Measured 24-h CrCl compared with 4 formulas to estimate CrCl/GFR (CG, Robert, MDRD and CKD-EPI methods)	• 33% of patients identified to have ARC (CrCl > 130 mL/min/1.73 m^2): mainly trauma patients; younger • Different formulas tended to overestimate CrCl for low eGFR values and underestimate CrCl for normal and high eGFRs • Three factors suggested to identify ARC: Age ≤ 58 years, trauma and eGFR > 108.1 mL/min/1.73 m^2 as calculated by CKD-EPI
Spadaro et al. [20], 2015	Retrospective observational	Group A: 63 ± 11 Group B: 71 ± 10	ICU	348	Group A: 73 Group B: 69	Group A: 106 ± 41 Group B: 37 ± 16	Vancomycin administration protocol based on measured 24 h CrCl and vancomycin serum measurements; levels compared between two groups: A (CrCl > 50) and B (CrCl ≤ 50) Vancomycin serum trough target: 15–25 mg/L	• 66% of patients had subtherapeutic vancomycin on second determination ARC and increased to 80% on third determination • Patients who had a subtherapeutic vancomycin levels at the first determination had a significant correlation with in-hospital mortality (OR = 2, p = 0.003)

Table 1. *Cont.*

Author, Year	Study Type	Age (Years) Median (IQR)	Population	N	Sex (% Male)	Measured CrCl (mL/min)—Otherwise Specified	Intervention	Main Results
Steinke et al. [21], 2015	Prospective observational	66 (57–74)	ICU	100	61	73 (47–107)	Measured CrCl compared with estimated CrCl using serum cystatin C Hoek formula, CG, and CKD-EPI	• 16% of patients identified to have ARC (CrCl > 130 mL/min/1.73 m^2): mainly trauma patients; TBI or SAH • The Hoek formula's precision was higher than CG and CKD-EPI • Authors suggested more studies are needed to identify the rule of Hoek's formula in drug dosing.
Adnan et al. [22], 2014	Prospective observational	34 (24–47)	ICU patients with SCr < 120 μmol/L)	49	76	ARC: 173 (141–223) Non-ARC: 91 (64–112)	Measured 24-h CrCl compared with CG method	• 39% of patients identified to have ARC (CrCl > 130 mL/min) • CG method significantly underestimated CrCl in ARC patients
Akers et al. [23], 2014	Prospective observational	45 ± 19	ICU	13	62	Not reported	They determined the ability of the ARC score to predict piperacillin/tazobactam clearance; Piperacillin/tazobactam doses given were (3.375 g IV Q6H or 4.5 g Q6H)	• ARC score had sensitivity 100%, specificity 71% in detecting enhanced clearance of piperacillin/tazobactam
Baptista et al. [24], 2014	Prospective observational	ARC: 49 ± 15 No ARC: 60 ± 18	ICU patients with normal SCr	54	ARC: 64 No ARC: 36	ARC Patients: 161 ± 28 Non-ARC Patients: 105 ± 16	Measured 8-h CrCl compared with CG method, CKD-EPI, and MDRD	• 56% of patients identified to have ARC (CrCl > 130 mL/min) • All formulas underestimated 8h-CrCl for values >120 mL/min/1.73 m^2 and a overestimated for values <120 mL/min/1.73 m^2
Baptista et al. [25], 2014	Prospective observational (Group 1 data were retrospectively collected)	Group 1: 58 ± 16 Group 2: 60 ± 17	ICU	G 1: 79 G 2: 25	Group 1: 66 Group 2: 68	Group 1: 125 ± 67 mL/min/1.73 m^2 Group 2: 121 ± 54 mL/min/1.73 m^2	Continuous infusion Vancomycin dosing nomogram based on 8h measured CrCl was suggested Group 1: retrospective data Group 2: prospective assessment of the nomogram Target vancomycin level: 20–30 mg/L	• 36% and 40% of patients identified to have ARC in groups 1 and 2, respectively (CrCl > 130 mL/min/1.73 m^2) • Vancomycin clearance was significantly proportional to measured CrCl

Table 1. *Cont.*

Author, Year	Study Type	Age (Years) Median (IQR)	Population	N	Sex (% Male)	Measured CrCl (mL/min)—Otherwise Specified	Intervention	Main Results
Campassi et al. [26], 2014	Prospective observational	ARC: 48 ± 15 Non-ARC: 65 ± 17	ICU patients with SCr < 115 µmol/L	363	ARC: 48 Non-ARC: 47	ARC: 155 ± 33 Non-ARC: 78 ± 25	CrCl measured by 24 h urine collection; Vancomycin loading dose 15 mg/kg followed by continuous infusion 30 mg/kg/day was given Target trough 15–25 mg/L	• 28% of patients identified to have ARC (CrCl > 120 mL/min/1.73 m^2); generally younger; more trauma and obstetric admissions; lower APACHE II scores • 27% of patients who received vancomycin were identified to have ARC and had significantly lower vancomycin levels ($p < 0.05$) than non-ARC patients at 3 days; none of the ARC patients reached target trough despite being administered significantly higher vancomycin doses
Hites et al. [27], 2014	Prospective observational	61 (18–84)	Non-ICU obese (BMI ≥ 30 kg/m^2) patients treated with antibiotics	56	50	107 (6–389.0)	They assessed the adequacy of serum concentrations of antimicrobials when given to obese individuals; Standard doses of antibiotics given (Cefepime 2 g TID, Piperacillin/tazobactam 4 g QID, Meropenem 1 g TID); Measured 24-h CrCl determined	• Low levels of antimicrobials were detected following standard doses. • Elevated CrCl was the only predictor of those low concentrations underlining the role of ARC in under-dosing obese individuals.
Udy et al. [28], 2014	Prospective observational	Mean 37 (95% CI 29–44)	ICU patients with SCr < 120 µmol/L and age ≤ 60	20	60	Mean: 168 (95% CI 139–197)	Measured 24-h CrCl determined; various exogenous markers given to detect changes in nephron physiology	• ARC involves increased glomerular filtration, renal tubular secretion of anions and renal tubular reabsorption using various exogenous markers, suggesting that ARC affects many components of the nephron physiology
Udy et al. [29], 2014	Prospective observational	Mean 54 (95% CI 53–56)	ICU patients with SCr < 120 µmol/L	281	63.3	Mean: 108 (95% CI 102–115)	Measured 8-h CrCl determined daily	• 65% of patients identified to have ARC (CrCl > 120 mL/min/1.73 m^2); mainly younger, men, multi-trauma victims, and receiving mechanical ventilation • Presence of ICU admission day 1 ARC predicted sustained ARC during ICU stay

Table 1. *Cont.*

Author, Year	Study Type	Age (Years) Median (IQR)	Population	N	Sex (% Male)	Measured CrCl (mL/min)—Otherwise Specified	Intervention	Main Results
Carlier et al. [30], 2013	Prospective observational	56 (48–67)	ICU	61	85	125 (93–175)	Meropenem or piperacillin/tazobactam were given as extended IV infusions; antibiotics concentrations measured; measured 24 h CrCl determined; Meropenem dose: an IV loading of 1 g over 30 min then 1 g Q8H as extended infusion over 3 h; Piperacillin/tazobactam dose: an IV loading of 4.5 g over 30 min then 4.5 g Q6H extended infusion over 3 h.	• 80% of patients identified to have ARC (CrCl > 130 mL/min) • Elevated creatinine clearance is an independent predictor for not achieving meropenem and piperacillin/tazobactam target levels
Claus et al. [31], 2013	Prospective observational	ARC: 54 (44–61) Non-ARC: 66 (57–77)	ICU patients receiving antimicrobial therapies	128	ARC: 73 Non-ARC: 61	98 (57–164) mL/min/1.73 m^2	Measured 8 h-CrCl determined; measuring the effect of ARC on antimicrobial therapy failure	• 52% of patients identified to have ARC (CrCl > 130 mL/min/1.73 m^2); mainly younger and male • 27% of ARC patients had therapeutic failure (poor clinical response to antimicrobial therapy), more often than non-ARC patients (13%) ($p = 0.04$)
Minkute et al. [32], 2013	Retrospective observational	ARC: 46 (21–66) Non-ARC: 54 (22–86)	Patients treated with vancomycin	36	80	Estimated CG ARC: 151 (131–324) Non-ARC: 103 (90–127)	Vancomycin level comparison between ARC and non-ARC groups	• 50% of patients identified to have ARC (CrCl > 130 mL/min, using CG) • Vancomycin concentrations were lower in ARC group compared to Non-ARC • Vancomycin doses up to 44 mg/kg/day were needed in the ARC group to achieve target trough levels.
Roberts and Lipman [33], 2013	PK study (analysis of Phase III trial data)	58 ± 15	ICU patients with pneumonia	31	93	Estimated by CG 137 ± 71	Population PK of doripenem in critically ill.	• Doripenem clearance correlated with CrCl and was increased compared to non-ICU patients
Shimamoto et al. [34], 2013	Retrospective observational	Non-SIRS: 64 SIRS-2: 54 SIRS-3: 49 SIRS-4: 42	ICU (Septic patients on vancomycin)	105	66	Using CG No-SIRS: 121 ± 51 SIRS-2: 160 ± 65 SIRS-3: 195 ± 70 SIRS-4: 191 ± 77	Identified patients who had SIRS and categorized based on the number of SIRS criteria they had (non-SIRS, SIRS-2, 3 and 4); vancomycin CL and CrCL (CG) determined	• In patients age < 50: higher SIRS score predicted higher vancomycin clearance • In patients age > 50: higher SIRS does not reliably predict higher vancomycin clearance

Table 1. *Cont.*

Author, Year	Study Type	Age (Years) Median (IQR)	Population	N	Sex (% Male)	Measured CrCl (mL/min)—Otherwise Specified	Intervention	Main Results
Udy et al. [35], 2013	Prospective observational	42 ± 17	ICU (trauma, septic, SCr < 110 µmol/L)	71	63	Mean: 135 ± 52	They determined the prevalence and risk factors of ARC	• 58% of patients identified to have ARC; more in trauma patients; generally younger, males, with lower APACHE II , SOFA and higher cardiac index • Three risk factors suggested to predict ARC: age < 50 years, trauma, and SOFA score ≤ 4 (ARC score)
Udy et al. [36], 2013	Prospective observational	51 ± 17	ICU patients with SCr < 121 µmol/L	110	64	Mean: 125 ± 45 mL/min/1.73 m^2	Measured 8 h CrCl compared to estimated CrCl (CG and CKD-EPI)	• CKD-EPI and CG underestimated CrCl in patients with ARC • In patients with CKD-EPI eGFR = 60–119 mL/min/1.73 m^2, 42% had ARC
Baptista et al. [37], 2012	Prospective observational	Non-ARC: 70 (52–79) ARC: 41 (32–56)	ICU septic patients on vancomycin	93	Non-ARC: 71 ARC: 79	Non-ARC: 70 (58–104) ARC: 159 (141–194)	The effect of ARC on vancomycin PK: ARC patients compared to non-ARC patients; measured 24 h CrCl Vancomycin dosing: A loading dose of 1000 mg if wt. < 70 kg or 1500 mg if wt. > 70 kg then 30 mg/kg/day continuous infusion	• Serum vancomycin concentrations in ARC were significantly lower than control group for the 3 days of study
Grootaert et al. [38], 2012	Retrospective observational	59 (48–67)	ICU patients with measured CrCl > 120 mL/min (24-h method)	390	63	148 (132–172) mL/min/1.73 m^2	Measured 24-h CrCl compared with CG method (CrCl) and 4-variable MDRD method (eGFR)	• CG and MDRD underestimated measured CrCl in ARC patients
Udy et al. [39], 2012	Prospective observational	53 ± 21	ICU	48	71	134 ± 90	Measured 8 h CrCl; beta lactam antibiotic concentrations measured	• For patients with trough less than MIC and less than 4× MIC: 82 and 72% had CrCl > 130 mL/min/1.73 m^2, respectively • A 25 mL/min/1.73 m^2 increase in CrCl is associated with a 60% reduction in the probability of obtaining a trough concentration ≥ 4×MIC

Table 1. *Cont.*

Author, Year	Study Type	Age (Years) Median (IQR)	Population	N	Sex (% Male)	Measured CrCl (mL/min)—Otherwise Specified	Intervention	Main Results
Baptista et al. [40], 2011	Retrospective observational (post hoc analysis)	35 (25–51)	ICU patients with ARC	86	77	162 (145–190) mL/min/1.73 m^2	Measured 8-h (Australia) or 24 h (Portugal) CrCl compared with CG, modified CG, 4-variable MDRD and 6-variable MDRD	• All CrCl estimates underestimated measured CrCl • CG estimates had the greatest sensitivity→identified 62% of cohort with ARC; lower sensitivity observed with 4-variable MDRD (47%) and 6-variable MDRD (29%) formulae
Minville et al. [41], 2011	Retrospective observational	NPT: 58 ± 17 PT: 42 ± 18	ICU	284	NPT: 63 PT: 75	NPT: 85 ± 5 PT: 131 ± 5 mL/min/1.73 m^2	Measured 24-h CrCl; compared among patients with (NPT) and without polytrauma (PT)	• 37% of patients identified to have ARC (CrCl > 120 mL/min; significantly more trauma patients; younger; had lower SAPS II score; males • Age and trauma independently correlated to CrCl
Spencer et al. [42], 2011	Prospective PK study	54 ± 14	Neuro ICU	12	42	96 ± 32 (estimated, method not reported)	Patients received levetiracetam 500 mg iv every 12 h; levetiracetam levels measured	• Levetiracetam clearance was higher in neurocritical care population compared to healthy volunteers (drug clearance directly proportional to estimated CrCl $r^2 = 0.5$, $p = 0.01$); Higher doses of levetiracetam are recommended in neurocritical care population
Goboova et al. [43], 2015	Case Report	16	ICU (Polytrauma and sepsis)	1	100	Method not reported Day 29: 138 Days 41–51: 340 mL/min/1.73 m^2	Vancomycin initiated at doses of 1 g IV every 12 h then titrated up	• A trauma patient who developed ARC later during hospital stay • Vancomycin needed to be increased to up to 6 g per day to achieve therapeutic target trough level • Vancomycin increased to 2 g Q12H, which produced troughs of 15 mg/L and 10 mg/L • Increase in CrCl observed on day 46, vancomycin trough decreased to 5 mg/L, then dose increased to 2 g Q8H (67 mg/kg/day); trough: 19 mg/L

Table 1. *Cont.*

Author, Year	Study Type	Age (Years) Median (IQR)	Population	N	Sex (% Male)	Measured CrCl (mL/min)—Otherwise Specified	Intervention	Main Results
Abdul-Aziz et al. [44], 2014	Case Report	36	ICU (CNS infection)	1	100	234	Days 1–3: Flucloxacillin 2 g IV Q4H Days 4–16: Flucloxacillin 20 g/day via continuous infusion	• A case report of an ICU patient with CNS infection • Presence of ARC (Measured 8 h) lead to difficulty achieving therapeutic flucloxacillin concentration above MIC with conventional dosing (IV 2 g Q4H) • A continuous infusion of high dose flucloxaciilin (20 g/day) was required to achieve clinical cure
Cook et al. [45], 2013	Case Report	22	Neuro ICU (TBI)	1	0	Method not reported 153	They described a case of ARC leading to subtherapeutic vancomycin and levetiracetam levels	• A conventional vancomycin dose 750 mg IV Q12H (17.5 mg/kg/dose) yielded a trough level of 2.2 mg/L (subtherapeutic); dose had to be increased to 1.25 g iv Q8H (29 mg/kg/dose) to achieve a trough of 11 mg/L • Levetiracetam dose was increased from 1000 mg IV BID to 1000 mg Q8H to maintain a trough within reference range (usual dose 0.5–1 g iv Q12H)
Lonsdale et al. [46], 2013	Case Report	44	Neuro ICU (SAH with ventriculitis)	1	100	375 mL/min/1.73 m^2	They described a case of ARC leading to subtherapeutic vancomycin and meropenem levels	• The patient required dose escalation of vancomycin up to 6 g/day (Vancomycin 63 mg/kg/day) in order to achieve therapeutic trough levels (usual dose 45 mg/kg/d for CNS infections) • The patient required dose escalation of meropenem up to 2 g every 6 h in order to achieve therapeutic levels (usual dose 2 g iv Q8H for CNS infections)
Troger et al. [47], 2012	Case Reports	Pt 1: 37 Pt 2: 66	ICU patients with sepsis	2	100	Estimated with CG Pt 1: Initially: 138 Day 5: 276 Pt 2: Initially: 185 Later: 219	Described 2 cases of sepsis patients who required high doses of meropenem secondary to ARC Pt 1: meropenem 1 g IV Q8H then increased to meropenem 2 g IV Q4H Pt 2: meropenem 1 g Q8H then dose increased to1 g Q6H then to 2 g Q6H Meropenem trough target 4–10 mg/L	• Pt 1: meropenem dose was increased to 2 g IV Q4H × 1 week, trough was still <4 mg/L but procalcitonin decreased and clinical improvement was observed • Pt 2: meropenem dose was increased to 2 g Q6H, producing a trough concentration of 8.4 mg/L

Table 1. *Cont.*

Author, Year	Study Type	Age (Years) Median (IQR)	Population	N	Sex (% Male)	Measured CrCl (mL/min)—Otherwise Specified	Intervention	Main Results
Udy et al. [3], 2010	Case Series	Pt 1: 19 Pt 2: 41 Pt 3: 32	ICU Pt 1 TBI Pt 2 Surgery Pt 3 Burn	3	100	Pt 1: 224 Pt 2: 206 Pt 3: 151 Measured 8 h CrCl	Three case reports of patients with ARC Pt. 1: meropenem Pt 2: vancomycin + meropenem Pt 3: amikacin + ciprofloxacin	• Pt 1: meropenem 1 g Q8H, increased to 2 g Q8H due to undetectable trough serum concentration; pt. still did not have detectable concentration • Pt 2: vancomycin doses were increased up to 4 g (44 mg/kg) continuous infusion over 24-h for clinical cure; Meropenem increased to 1 g Q4H to reach target trough • Pt 3: Amikacin 1 g daily was increased up to 1.2 g Q12H due to undetectable trough levels
Caro et al. [48], 2016 Abstract	Phase I PK study	Range 29–50	ICU patients with ARC (CrCl ≥ 180 mL/min estimated by CG)	5	40	Estimated using CG 282 (207–417)	Determined the PK of ceftolozane/tazobactam in patients with ARC	• Study identified higher clearance of ceftolozane/tazobactam in ARC patients compared to non-ARC patients
Goboova et al. [49], 2016 Abstract	Retrospective observational	Mean 42 ± 14	Patients treated with gentamicin	204	78	Method not reported ARC Patients: 166 ± 28 mL/min/1.73 m^2	Identification of the influence of ARC on gentamicin dosing	• 14% of patients identified to have ARC (CrCl > 130 mL/min/1.73 m^2; • 93% of ARC patients were under-dosed (low peak levels) with standard gentamicin regimens
Morbitzer et al. [50], 2016 Abstract	Prospective observational	63 (56–71)	Neuro ICU (Hemorrhagic stroke)	17	27	131 (108–216) mL/min/1.73 m^2	Measured 8-h CrCl compared with CG method; vancomycin trough concentration determined	• CG method underestimated CrCl in ARC patients • Measured vancomycin trough was lower than predicted
Morimoto and Ishikura [51], 2016 Abstract	Prospective observational	Not reported	ICU (Japan)	33	Not reported	Not reported	CrCl measured (method not reported)	• 39% of patients identified to have ARC (CrCl > 130 mL/min/1.73 m^2); mainly younger, less males, had lower APACHE II score and not septic
Dunning and Roberts [52], 2015 Abstract	A survey	N/A	N/A	123	N/A	N/A	A survey of 123 ICU physicians about antibiotic prescribing and renal function assessment	• 15% responded that they would consider modifying the dosage regimen of beta-lactams and vancomycin antimicrobials in patients with ARC • This highlights the need for dosing guidance in patients with ARC.

Table 1. *Cont.*

Author, Year	Study Type	Age (Years) Median (IQR)	Population	N	Sex (% Male)	Measured CrCl (mL/min)—Otherwise Specified	Intervention	Main Results
Baptista et al. [53], 2014 Abstract	Retrospective observational	Not reported	ICU	477	Not reported	Not reported	CrCl measured by 8 h urine collection	• 33% of patients identified to have ARC (CrCl > 130 mL/min/1.73 m^2) • Urinary creatinine > 45 mg/mL and age < 65 are identified as best predictors of ARC (sensitivity 60%, specificity = 88%); specificity increased to 95% by adding BUN < 7 mmol/L
May et al. [54], 2014 Abstract	Prospective observational	Not reported	Neuro ICU (SAH)	20	Not reported	326 ± 135 mL/min/1.73 m^2	Measured 24-h CrCl determined; Monte-Carlo Simulation for levetiracetam doses to achieve trough levels ≥ 6 mg/L	• Estimated CrCl (method not reported) significantly underestimated CrCl • Monte Carlo Simulation suggested that levetiracetam dosing poorly achieved target attainment unless TID was used (as opposed to standard regimen)
Vermis et al. [55], 2014 Abstract	Retrospective observational	Not reported	Patients with hematological malignancies	96	Not reported	CrCl estimated using CG ARC pts: 147 Non-ARC pts: 79	Aimed to determine the prevalence of ARC in a hematological population; Vancomycin continuous infusion: loading 15 mg/kg, maintenance 30 mg/kg given and titrated based on levels Vancomycin trough target: 20 mg/L	• Therapeutic vancomycin trough targets were achieved with dose of 42 mg/kg/day in ARC patients (day 5 post initiation) and with 33 mg/kg/day in non-ARC (day 3 post initiation).
Weigel et al. [56], 2014 Abstract	Retrospective observational	55	ICU patients without renal replacement and receiving vancomycin infusion	287	69	ARC: MDRD eGFR > 130 Non ARC: MDRD eGFR < 130	A vancomycin loading dose of 20 mg/kg was given then adjusted by Therapeutic drug monitoring to target 20–25 mg/L; Vancomycin levels compared in patients with various degrees of eGFR using MDRD	• Subtherapeutic vancomycin levels were more frequent in patients with MDRD > 130 mL/min (55%) i.e., ARC vs. patients with MDRD < 130 mL/min (29%) $p < 0.001$ • Higher than conventional vancomycin dosing is recommended in patients with ARC
Neves et al. [57], 2013 Abstract	Prospective observational	55 ± 13	ICU	54	72	Mean: 138	Measured 8-h CrCl compared with CG method	• ARC identified in 50% of samples • Per subgroup analyses: CrCl > 120 mL/min/1.73 m^2, CG underestimated measured CrCl; CrCl < 120 mL/min/1.73 m^2, CG overestimated measured CrCl

Table 1. *Cont.*

Author, Year	Study Type	Age (Years) Median (IQR)	Population	N	Sex (% Male)	Measured CrCl (mL/min)—Otherwise Specified	Intervention	Main Results
Grootaert et al. [58], 2012 Abstract	Retrospective observational	66 (56–75)	ICU patients with measured CrCl available	1317	63	Not reported	Measured 24-h CrCl	• 16% of patients identified to have ARC (CrCl > 120 mL/min): mainly younger, taller, have lower BMI and had longer ICU stay • 30% patients had at least 1 episode of ARC Relative duration of ARC per patient was 5 days in all pts, and 7 days in antimicrobial group
Drust et al. [59], 2011 Abstract	Retrospective observational	Not reported	ICU patients with CrCl > 120 mL/min	15	Not reported	>120	Meropenem plasma concentrations measured	• 27% of patients had appropriate meropenem plasma levels • 67% of patients required higher doses of meropenem (up to 8 g/day) than recommended

ANP = atrial natriuretic peptide; APACHE II = Acute Physiology and Chronic Health Evaluation; ARC = Augmented Renal Clearance; CG = Cockcroft Gault equation; CKD-EPI = Chronic Kidney Disease Epidemiology; CN = controlled normothermia; CrCl = creatinine clearance; GFR = glomerular filtration rate; ICU = intensive care unit; IQR = interquartile range; MDRD = modification of diet in renal disease method; MIC = minimum inhibitory concentration; PK = pharmacokinetic; PT = patient; PTA = probability of target attainment; SAH = subarachnoid hemorrhage; SAPS II = Simplified Acute Physiology Score SCr = serum creatinine; SIRS = systemic inflammatory response syndrome; SOFA = sequential organ failure assessment score; TBI = traumatic brain injury; TH = therapeutic hypothermia. Age and CrCl reported in median (IQR) or mean ± SD.

3.1. ARC Definition and Prevalence

Augmented renal clearance (ARC), also reported as glomerular hyperfiltration or enhanced renal clearance, is an increase in kidney function that results in enhanced clearance of drugs with potential for therapy failure. ARC has been defined using creatinine clearance (CrCl). However, the definition of ARC in relation to CrCl cutoff has varied among studies, thus impeding accurate identification of ARC prevalence among intensive care unit (ICU) patients. Although, many research groups have defined ARC as patients with creatinine clearance > 130 mL/min/1.73 m^2 (Table 1), other creatinine clearance cutoffs have been suggested including ARC cutoff of CrCl > 120 mL/min/m^2 [26,38,41,55,58], and >160 mL/min/1.73 m^2 [11]. The definition of ARC was further complicated with the duration at which CrCl above the suggested cutoff. The majority of the studies have considered one occurrence of CrCl above cutoff is sufficient to acknowledge the presence of ARC. However, both Baptista et al. [24] and DeWaele et al. [15] elected to use the definition of ARC as CrCl > 130 mL/min/1.73 m^2 for more than half of the CrCl measures during a minimum of 72 h of ICU stay. This acknowledges the concern if the current definition of CrCl cutoff (without timeframe specification) truly captures the clinical implication (i.e., the point where changes must be made for renally cleared medications) to patient care. Furthermore, it is not clear if additional cutoffs beyond CrCl of 130 mL/min/1.73 m^2 are needed to stage ARC parallel the categories used to describe renal dysfunction i.e., mild, moderate and severe ARC. However, despite the various definitions observed, based on the large number of studies using the definition CrCl cutoffs of >130 mL/min/1.73 m^2, as well as associated clinical implications at this cut off point, we recommend a unified definition of ARC using CrCl > 130 mL/min/1.73 m^2 as the clinical cut-off in the adult population.

ARC has been reported to range from 14 to 80% (Table 1), suggesting that ARC is a commonly occurring clinical phenomenon. However, these studies may perhaps over- or under-estimate the true prevalence of ARC due to few reasons. First, the most common practice setting where ARC was identified is within the setting of the ICU. Since rigorous patient monitoring is a common practice within the ICU, including daily measures of renal function, it is much easier to identify ARC. In addition, critically ill are exposed to factors that may increase the likelihood of ARC occurrence, such as the use of intravenous fluids, vasopressors and inotropes [60,61]. Second, as discussed above, variations in ARC definitions might impede the true prevalence of ARC. Third, ARC prevalence needs to be interpreted in the context of the study patient selection criteria. For example, exclusion of patients with renal dysfunction will result in higher percentage of patients with ARC and vice versa.

The true onset and duration of ARC in critically ill is not known. In studies that assessed renal function more than one occasion throughout the ICU stay, it appears that the onset of ARC coincides with an acute insult to the body. In a prospective observational study of patients admitted to ICU, Udy et al. have reported that 65% of patients, identified to have ARC, had at least 1 occasion of measured ARC during the first 7 days of admission with 38% of those had ARC on the first day of ICU admission [29]. Occurrence of ARC on day 1 of ICU admission significantly predicted sustained CrCl elevation over the first seven days of the ICU stay (p = 0.019). Similarly, Huttner et al. have reported that 64% of patients had ARC at study enrollment [17]. Duration of ARC has varied among studies owing to difference in monitoring frequency and duration. While many studies have reported persistence of ARC for weeks [17,43,45,46,58], fewer patients exhibited transient ARC lasting for no more than 1 day [31]. Given the current unpredictability of ARC duration, continuous monitoring of patient's renal function is warranted as alteration in drug dosing might be required.

3.2. Pathophysiology

Our current understanding of the ARC pathophysiology remains limited. It has been reported that ARC is associated with increased glomerular filtration, renal tubular secretion of anions, and renal tubular reabsorption using various exogenous markers, suggesting that ARC affects many components of the nephron physiology [28]. It has been suggested that ARC is a hyperdynamic response to insults to the body. In the early study conducted by Ljungberg and Nilsson-Ehle, acute infection has been observed to be associated with enhanced renal clearance [62]. This has been attributed to changes in vascular permeability and increased renal blood flow secondary to elevated body temperature. Similarly, the effect of temperature changes on renal function has been reported in patients exposed to induced hypothermia. In a retrospective study comparing vancomycin pharmacokinetic in patients with controlled normothermia (median temperature = 37.2 °C) to patients with induced hypothermia (median temperature = 34 °C), Morbitzer et al. have demonstrated that vancomycin clearance was higher in controlled normothermic patients [18].

In addition to altered body temperature, insult to the brain could lead to ARC. Dias et al. have identified a possible link between the brain and the kidneys in their retrospective analysis of 18 severe traumatic brain injury (TBI) patients managed with intracranial pressure monitoring in the neurocritical care setting [16]. Analyzing cerebrovascular pressure reactivity index (PRx, a correlation index between intracranial pressure and arterial blood pressure that reflects the capability cerebral arteries to react to changes in blood pressure and is a key element of cerebral autoregulation) in ARC-manifesting patients showed a strong negative correlation ($r = -0.81$, $p < 0.001$) between PRx and creatinine clearance. This correlation suggests that reduction in cerebral autoregulation (i.e., after a TBI) is associated with an increase in creatinine clearance, adding an evidence to the theory that the central autoregulation plays a significant role in the manifestation of ARC. In another study of 11 TBI patients by Udy et al., atrial natriuretic peptide (ANP) levels have been found to be elevated in TBI patients suggesting that ANP following brain may play a role in enhancing glomerular filtration through increased natriuresis and diuresis [7]. The results of the correlation between ANP and CrCl, however, did not reach statistical significance.

Sime et al. have proposed a model of hyperdynamic state to bring forth a pathophysiology model to the occurrence of ARC [63]. It has been suggested that a number of factors consequential to critical illness combine to produce ARC. Systemic inflammatory response syndrome (SIRS) associated with critical illness results in the increase of inflammatory mediators. These mediators produce decrease in vascular resistance in the peripheries and increase in cardiac output. These two responses combine to produce a hyperdynamic state within the body system, resulting in increased renal blood flow, followed by glomerular hyperfiltration that manifest itself as ARC. Additionally, common to the ICU setting, critically ill patients are often subjected to fluid therapy and treatment with vasoactive drugs and inotropes thereby further increasing cardiac output that would more likely to contribute to the already-increased hyperdynamic state. Furthermore, critical illness also may have direct effect on the kidneys, further enhancing renal clearance in ARC. Although this model suggested by Sime et al. provides a logical explanation to the pathophysiology leading to ARC, the exact mechanism to which ARC, as a sequelae of physiological insult, remains uncertain.

3.3. ARC Risk Factors

Various studies (Table 1) have shown that patients exhibiting ARC tend to be younger (<50 years old), of male gender, had a recent history of trauma, and had lower critical illness severity scores such as sequential organ failure assessment score (SOFA) [35], Simplified Acute Physiology Score (SAPS) II [41] or Acute Physiology and Chronic Health Evaluation (APACHE II) [35,51]. Young age appears to be the only risk factor consistently recognized by various epidemiology studies to be able to reliably predict ARC (Table 1). In addition, Hirai et al. have identified febrile neutropenia to be an independent risk factor of ARC the pediatric cancer population [11].

Recognizing the need for a clinical prediction tool to identify patients at risk for manifesting ARC, Baptista et al. [53] have conducted a retrospective study in 447 patients admitted to an ICU at a tertiary hospital over a 1-year period, and assessed patient characteristics on its predictability of ARC occurrence. Urinary creatinine > 45 mg/mL and age < 65 years have been identified as best predictors of ARC (sensitivity 60%, specificity = 88%); specificity increased to 95% by adding BUN < 7 mmol/L. Furthermore, Udy et al. [35]. developed an ARC scoring system based on the risk of factors of age < 50 years old, presence of trauma, and SOFA score $\leq$ 4 (Table 2). This predictive tool was later validated by Akers et al., demonstrating a sensitivity of 100% and specificity of 71% for detecting patients with ARC, based on confirmation data from altered piperacillin/tazobactam pharmacokinetics in ICU patients [23]. Because of the impracticality need to complete a SOFA score in ARC scoring system, Barletta et al. have developed the augmented renal clearance in trauma intensive Care (ARCTIC) scoring system (Table 2) [4]. The ARCTIC scoring system employed the patient factors: serum creatinine, sex and age to identify those with high ARC risk (ARCTIC score > 6). The ARCTIC scoring system produced a sensitivity of 84% and specificity of 68%. Given the need for early recognition of ARC in the ICU setting, the use of the ARC or ARCTIC predictive tools allow for identification of at risk patients, and help direct clinicians to take appropriate interventions (e.g., obtain a measured creatinine clearance, employ more aggressive antibiotic dosing regimen/strategies, etc.).

Table 2. The ARC risk scoring systems.

	ARC Scoring System [23,35]	ARCTIC Scoring System [4]
Criteria	Age 50 or younger = 6 pts Trauma = 3 pts SOFA score ≤ 4 = 1 pt	SCr < 62 µmol/L = 3 pts Male sex = 2 pts Age <56 years = 4 pts Age: 56–75 years = 3 pts
Interpretation	0–6 points→low ARC risk 7–10 points→high ARC risk	>6 points→high ARC risk <6 points→low ARC risk
Sensitivity	100%	84%
Specificity	71%	68%

ARC = augmented renal clearance; ARCTIC = augmented renal clearance in trauma intensive Care (ARCTIC); SOFA = sequential organ failure assessment score; SCr = serum creatinine concentration; pt = point; pts = points.

3.4. Creatinine Clearance: Estimation Methods and ARC

Although risk factors and predictive models offer a method to screen for those at an increased risk for ARC, the actual identification of ARC requires accurate glomerular filtration rate (GFR) determination. While determination of inulin clearance is regarded as the gold standard for measuring GFR because CrCl might overestimate kidney function, affected by muscle mass and physical activity, urinary measurement of creatinine clearance (from 8 to 24 h of urine collection) is currently the most common measurement of renal function in the clinical setting [64]. That's because inulin clearance determination is labor intensive and requires administration of an exogenous substance. Because routine measurement of creatinine clearance is impractical, mathematical estimates of creatinine clearance based on population parameters are often employed to allow for prompt determination. Commonly used mathematical estimates of creatinine clearance/glomerular filtration rate (GFR) include the Cockcroft Gault equation (CG), the Modification of Diet in Renal Diseases (MDRD) formulae, and the Chronic Kidney Disease-Epidemiology (CKD-EPI) equation. These equations all have been validated in various populations, and their respective merits and deficiencies have been described elsewhere [65]. Measured creatinine clearance has been reported in 59% of the included studies. On the other hand creatinine clearance has been estimated only or not reported in 25 and 16% of the included studies, respectively (Table 1). In studies assessing the accuracy of mathematical estimates of creatinine clearance in the ARC population, all the mathematical estimations of creatinine clearance have been found to underestimate the actual measured creatinine clearance in patients with ARC [8,19,21,22,24,36,38,40,50,57].

Comparison of the various mathematical estimates suggest the Cockcroft Gault (CG) formula may be the best method of creatinine clearance estimation in the ARC population. To illustrate, Udy et al. have assessed the accuracy of the CKD-EPI estimation of creatinine clearance in comparison to 8-h measured creatinine clearance in 110 ICU patients [36]. Around 42% of the patients identified by the CKD-EPI equation to have creatinine clearance within the range of 60–119 mL/min/1.73 m^2 exhibited ARC (measured CrCl > 130). In a study conducted by Baptista et al., the CG and MDRD

(4- and 6-variable) estimations of creatinine clearance were compared to measured creatinine clearance using 8-h or 24-h urine sampling [40]. In patients exhibiting ARC, CG estimate was able to detect 62% of the cohort exhibiting ARC, while the MDRD estimations demonstrated lower sensitivity, with the 4-variable MDRD formula detecting 47% of the cohort while the 6-variable MDRD formula was only able to detect 27% of the cohort exhibiting ARC. Similarly, Barletta et al. have found that measured creatinine clearance were significantly higher ($p < 0.001$) than all estimates of creatinine clearance (CG, 4-variable MDRD, and CKD-EPI equation) with the CG method demonstrating the lowest bias [8]. However the CG method may only be used as a screening tool for ARC. Even if a CG estimate show an estimated creatinine clearance within the normal reference range, there is a still a high likelihood that ARC can be present in a patient. Therefore, in the setting of ICU, it would be prudent to assess a patient's measured creatinine clearance at least once, to determine whether a patient is truly experiencing ARC, and to also gauge the level of bias in the estimated creatinine clearance for that patient. Finally, we would like to mention that although serum creatinine used for determination of creatinine clearance is a reliable marker within the general population, consideration must be made when applying this measurement in patients with lower muscle mass, immobility, children or other conditions in which muscle mass are altered. Due to the reduced production of creatinine in these patients, falsely low measures of serum creatinine may inaccurately identify ARC in those populations.

3.5. Drug Therapy in ARC Population

3.5.1. Pharmacokinetic Changes in ARC

In the ICU setting, pharmacokinetic changes to drug therapy in the presence of ARC may have drastic implications on patient outcome. This is especially important to drugs that are renally cleared known to exhibit direct correlation between their renal clearance and creatinine clearance such as aminoglycoside antimicrobials, vancomycin and levetiracetam. Enhanced drug clearance will lead to shorter drug half-life ($t_{\frac{1}{2}}$), lower maximum drug concertation ($C_{\max}$) and lower area under the concentration curve (AUC) which could have direct implication on drugs' pharmacodynamic effects leading to therapy failure. This particularly important for antimicrobials that are time-dependent killers (efficacy depends on the duration of the drug concentration or AUC above the minimum inhibitory concentration (MIC) of the pathogen T > MIC) and concentration-dependent killers (efficacy depends on the Cmax of the drug relative to the MIC of the pathogen). Currently, antimicrobial monograms and various dosing guidelines have not acknowledged the need for alterations to drug dosing regimen in the ARC population. In a survey of ICU physicians in England clarifying their attitudes regarding antibiotic prescribing and assessment of renal function in septic patients, only 15% responded that they would consider modifying the dosage regimen of beta-lactams and vancomycin antimicrobials in patients with ARC [52]. This highlights the need for dosing guidance in patients with ARC.

3.5.2. Vancomycin

Vancomycin, a glycopeptide antibiotic, is one of the antimicrobials of choice for the treatment of serious, life-threatening infections by Gram-positive bacteria. It is a hydrophilic drug that is 80–90% excreted unchanged by the kidneys and its clearance is highly dependent on renal function. Previous pharmacokinetic and pharmacodynamic studies have established that steady state vancomycin trough level is a good surrogate of AUC:MIC which is in turn correlated with treatment success [66].

Currently, there is a growing body of evidence suggesting inadequate therapeutic vancomycin trough levels attained using conventional dosing in patients exhibiting ARC [9,25,26,32,43,45,50,55]. For example, Campassi et al. have reported that 100% of patients with ARC did not have vancomycin trough levels within the target 15–25 mg/L 3 days following vancomycin initiation despite getting high vancomycin doses [26]. Currently, studies on the clinical outcome of subtherapeutic serum concentration of vancomycin in ARC patients are scarce. However, it has been reported that in patients who did not reach therapeutic trough target 15–25 mg/L 48 h post treatment initiation, in-hospital mortality was significantly higher than those who have attained therapeutic target trough (OR = 2.1, $p = 0.003$) [20].

Various vancomycin dosing regimens have been suggested and tested in patients with ARC. In a study by Vermis et al., vancomycin therapeutic drug monitoring (TDM) has been implemented and vancomycin dose adjustment was based on vancomycin trough level 5 days post vancomycin initiation [55]. The average doses successful to achieve trough levels within target were 42 and 33 mg/kg/day in patients with ARC and without ARC, respectively. The authors proposed a loading dose of 25 mg/kg loading dose followed by 40 mg/kg/day for those with CrCl > 130 mL/min. Similarly, Minkute et al. have reported the need for vancomycin doses up to 44 mg/kg/day to achieve trough levels within target [32]. Baptista et al. [25] have suggested a vancomycin dosing strategy using 8 h measured creatinine clearance to achieve a target trough of 25 mg/L. The nomogram suggested has been validated in a second group of patients in the same study and has been found to produce 84% target attainment in patients with ARC.

3.5.3. Beta-Lactam Antimicrobials

Beta-lactams antibiotics are primarily renally eliminated thereby are affected by presence of ARC. Unlike vancomycin or aminoglycosides, therapeutic drug monitoring is not common for beta-lactam antibiotics. Clinicians generally prescribe guideline-recommended regimens without the need to conduct therapeutic drug monitoring. Although following the patients' clinical status after prescribing a beta-lactam is appropriate and acceptable in the general population, dismissal of beta-lactam concentration in the ARC population, where very little evidence exists and no dosing guidelines have been recommended, poses a substantial threat to treatment success and patient outcome. Numerous studies have reported beta-lactam treatment failures (based on sub-therapeutic serum level attainment) when using standard beta-lactam dosing regimens in patients with ARC (discussed below and in Table 1).

Carbapenems

Carbapenems (such as meropenem, imipenem, doripenem and ertapenem) are a family of broad spectrum beta-lactams used for the treatment of multi-drug resistant bacteria. They exhibit time-dependent antibacterial activity and their activity can be best illustrated by the T > MIC pharmacodynamic model [67]. Various studies have reported poor target achievement in ARC patients using conventional regimens. Binder et al. have reported that standard meropenem doses (500–1000 mg every 8 or 12 h) in ICU patients with estimated creatinine >60 mL/min result in lower meropenem AUC secondary to increased clearance suggesting the need for alternate regimen in this population [68]. Similarly, Drust et al. have reported that almost two-thirds of the ICU patents with CrCl > 120 mL/min required higher doses (up to 8 g/day) of meropenem than current recommended therapy to achieve effective plasma meropenem concentrations [59]. In addition, extended infusion have also been suggested for appropriate target T > MIC target attainment and treatment success. Carlier et al. have assessed the efficacy of whether meropenem extended infusion (1 g over 30 min, followed by a maintenance dose of meropenem 1 g infused over a period of 3 h every 8 h) would be a suitable alternative strategy for meropenem dosing in ARC patients [30]. Extended infusion did not improve meropenem plasma concentration by the end of the study, with lower percentage of ARC patients (61%) achieving T > MIC therapeutic target in comparison to non-ARC patients (94%, $p < 0.001$). In addition to meropenem, doripenem pharmacokinetics have been studied in critically ill patients with ARC [33]. Similarly, higher doses of doripenem have been suggested in patients with ARC.

Piperacillin/Tazobactam

Piperacillin/tazobactam is an extended spectrum beta-lactam antibiotic indicated for the treatment of severe multi-drug resistant infections. Like all beta-lactam antibiotics, piperacillin/tazobactam exhibits time-dependent bacterial eradication (T > MIC). Piperacillin/tazobactam is eliminated renally, and dose adjustment of piperacillin/tazobactam has been described for renally impaired population. There are many reports of subtherapeutic target attainment using conventional piperacillin/tazobactam dosing in ICU patients with ARC. Huttner et al. have assessed target attainment of various beta-lactams in the ICU population (ARC observed in 64% of the study cohort) [17]. Subtherapeutic serum concentrations have been reported with intravenous doses of piperacillin/tazobactam 4.5 g every eight hours in 61% of the treated patients. In addition, undetectable piperacillin/tazobactam concentrations were seen in 7% of the patients. To address the issue of subtherapeutic target attainment of piperacillin/tazobactam especially in ICU patients with ARC, various dosage regimens have been tested and suggested [6,23]. A Monte-Carlo simulation conducted by Akers et al. have suggested that doses above the FDA approved doses (up to 36 g per day) might be needed to achieve high probability of target achievement [23]. Unfortunately, the study by Akers et al. was not aimed to assess any of the dosing regimens modelled in their study and these proposed regimens still require validation.

Other Beta-Lactam Antimicrobials

Aside from few other studies [14,48], the evidence of the other members of the beta-lactams is scarce. However, as suggested by the body of evidence on meropenem and piperacillin/tazobactam, it is likely that all beta-lactams that are eliminated renally might be affected by the ARC phenomenon and require further research.

3.5.4. Other Medications

Aminoglycosides are mainly renally eliminated with predictable efficacy based on serum concentrations. Goboova et al. have conducted a retrospective analysis of 204 patients receiving gentamicin, in which 14% of the patients exhibited ARC [49]. The patients in the study were initially treated with conventional gentamicin regimen. Analysis of gentamicin peak concentration at steady state identified 93% of the ARC patients had subtherapeutic steady state concentrations which required dose escalation to attain target peak levels. This highlights the value of therapeutic drug monitoring in the setting of ARC.

Fluoroquinolones are another family of antibiotics affected by altering renal clearance. Due to predictability of current dosing in patients normal or impaired renal function, TDM is not necessary. However, TDM could be of value when using fluoroquinolones in patients with ARC and higher doses may be required. For example, using Monte Carlo simulation, levofloxacin doses of 1 g every 24 h have been suggested for infections caused by *S. pneumoniae*, *P. aeruginosa*, and *S. aureus* in patients with CrCl > 130 mL/min (conventional dosing 0.5–0.75 g every 24 h) [13].

In addition to antimicrobials, other agents have been tested such as levetiracetam and enoxaparin. Levetiracetam is a broad spectrum antiepileptic drug (AED) that has a more favorable side effect profile compared to older AEDs. It displays linear elimination kinetics; therefore dose changes produce relatively predictable changes in serum concentrations. However, it is renally eliminated and its clearance is directly proportional to CrCl and thus could be affected in patients with ARC. There are few reports discussing the enhanced elimination of levetiracetam in TBI and SAH patients with ARC [42,45,54]. Accordingly, Higher initial levetiracetam doses (1 g IV every 8 h) have been suggested in patients with high risk for ARC [42,54]. Enoxaparin, a low molecular weight heparin, also has been reported to be affected by presence of ARC suggested the need for more rigorous monitoring of anti-factor Xa activity in patients with ARC [5].

4. Conclusions

Augmented renal clearance (ARC) is a manifestation of enhanced renal function seen in critically ill patients. The current evidence presented in this review identified the significance of this phenomenon and the need for higher doses of renally eliminated drugs in patients with ARC. More research is needed to solidify dosing recommendations of various drugs in patients with ARC. However, based on the current evidence few recommendations could be put forward to guide clinicians in managing patients presenting with ARC (Figure 2).

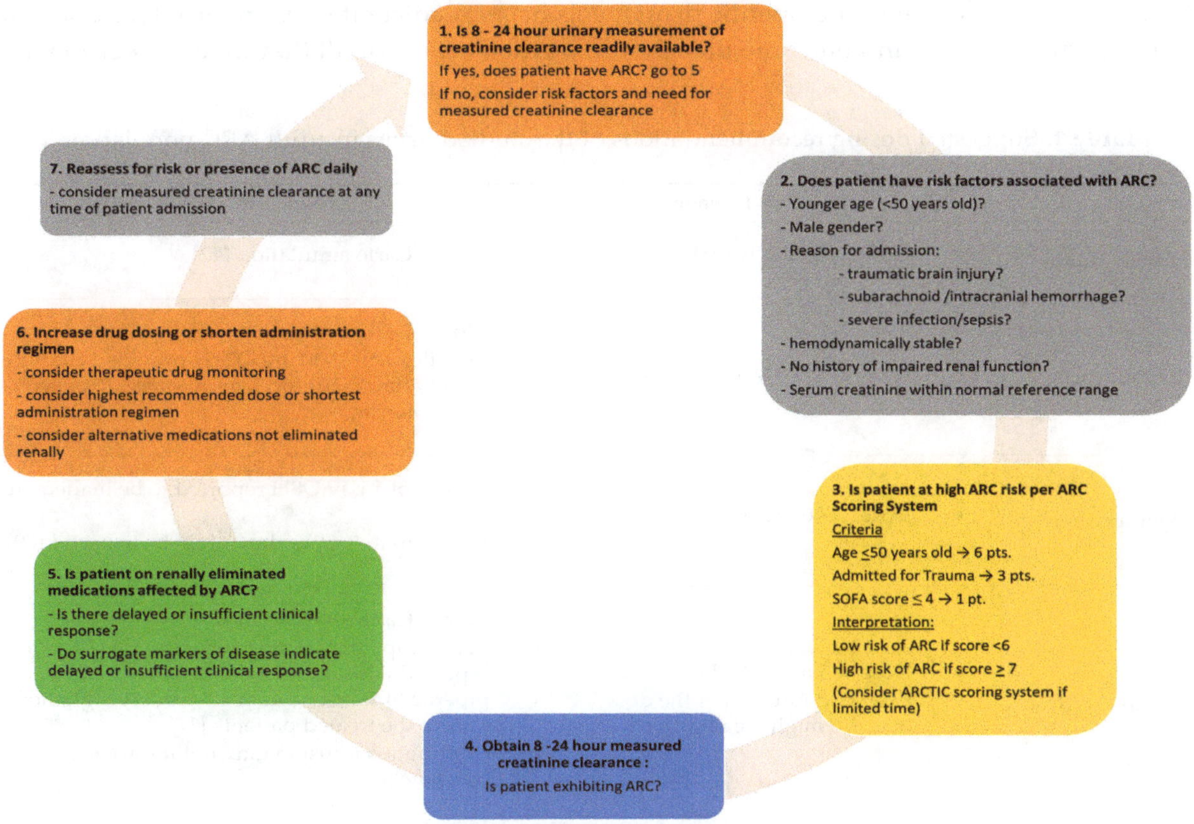

Figure 2. Assessment of ICU patients for augmented renal clearance (ARC).

The recognition of ARC risk factors allows clinicians to screen for at-risk patients. In the ICU setting, the ARC-scoring tool (Table 2) could be used to identify patients suitable for further investigation. If time does not permit the implementation of the ARC-scoring tool, the less time-consuming ARCTIC scoring system (Table 2) could still be considered. Other means of identifying at-risk patients include assessment of patient serum creatinine, estimated creatinine clearance, or delayed clinical response to medication interventions. Upon identification of at-risk patients, a measured 8–24 h creatinine clearance study should be undertaken. Evidence has shown that estimated creatinine clearance carry significant risk of underestimating the renal function of ARC patients in various settings. Therefore, at minimum, determination of a patient's creatinine clearance may be conducted by employing an 8-h urinary measurement, which will aid in the diagnosis of ARC and later-on be used for dosage adjustment of renally cleared medications. We also recommend continued daily monitoring of serum creatinine for those diagnosed with ARC. Due to the unpredictability of ARC manifestation (could be a transient 1-day occurrence or maintained for weeks), we can only determine the manifestation of ARC in an individual through continued measurement of renal function.

Despite many studies seem to suggest that ARC tends to manifest itself during initial ICU admission, any patients, including those with a recent history of acute kidney injury, could exhibit ARC at any time of their hospital admission. For those patients with confirmed ARC, considerations should be made for all renally cleared medications. Therapeutic drug monitoring and dose adjustment could be performed, when possible. Table 3 depicts suggested initial dosing of studied drugs in patients with ARC. For those medications where TDM is not routinely available and there is no sufficient evidence to guide dosage modification in ARC population, the use of the highest approved dose or most frequent administration regimen could be considered with close clinical monitoring. Furthermore, we suggest that consideration be made for alternative therapies that are not affected by altered renal function, such as those medications that are mainly metabolized rather than renally cleared (e.g., use of antiepileptic drugs that are eliminated via metabolism in place of levetiracetam). Finally, although attainment of therapeutic drug levels helps predict efficacy and safety, it is ultimately the patient's clinical status and outcome that should be the anchor for all therapeutic decision making.

Table 3. Suggested dosing recommendations of the studied drugs in adult ARC population.

Drug	Suggested Dosage	Suggestion Basis
Levetiracetam	• Dose: 1000 mg iv Q8H	• Monte-Carlo simulation [42]
Levofloxacin	• Dose: 750–1000 mg iv Q24H	• Monte-Carlo simulation [13] • Levofloxacin 1000 mg Q24H provided the highest target attainment for *S. pneumoniae*, *P. aeruginosa* and *S. aureus*.
Meropenem	• Dose: 2000 mg iv Q8H	• A dose of 1 g iv Q8H reported to be inadequate [27,30] • Doses up to 8 g per day might be required [59]
Piperacillin/Tazobactam	• Dose: 4.5 mg iv Q6H • Extended infusion of the dose over 4 h might be required	• Monte-Carlo simulation [23] • Subtherapeutic serum concentrations have been reported with intravenous doses of piperacillin/tazobactam 4.5 g every eight hours in 61% of the treated patients [17] • Continuous infusion may not improve treatment outcome [6]
Vancomycin	• Initial loading dose: 25–30 mg/kg followed by a maintenance dose of 45 mg/kg/day in divided doses Q8H or continuous infusion • Therapeutic drug monitoring is recommended (target 10–20 mg/L or 15–20 mg/L depending on the indication)	• Doses up to 44 mg/kg/day have been reported to be needed in patients with ARC [32] • Dosage regimens lower than the suggested dosage have resulted in subtherapeutic levels [9,20,37] • A dosing nomogram suggested by Baptista et al. allowed achievement of therapeutic vancomycin levels; average dose was ~47 mg/kg/day in patients with average weight 70 kg and measured CrCl 150 mL/min [25]

ARC = augmented renal clearance; CrCl = creatinine clearance; above recommended doses are based on observational studies and pharmacokinetics simulations. Above doses will need to be tested prospectively to assess its influence on patients' outcome; for antimicrobials, different doses might be needed based on the susceptibility pattern of the microorganisms.

Author Contributions: Sherif Hanafy Mahmoud and Chen Shen conducted literature review and wrote the paper.

References

1. Udy, A.A.; Putt, M.T.; Boots, R.J.; Lipman, J. ARC—Augmented renal clearance. *Curr. Pharm. Biotechnol.* **2011**, *12*, 2020–2029. [CrossRef] [PubMed]
2. Udy, A.A.; Roberts, J.A.; Boots, R.J.; Paterson, D.L.; Lipman, J. Augmented renal clearance: Implications for antibacterial dosing in the critically ill. *Clin. Pharmacokinet.* **2010**, *49*, 1–16. [CrossRef] [PubMed]

3. Udy, A.A.; Putt, M.T.; Shanmugathasan, S.; Roberts, J.A.; Lipman, J. Augmented renal clearance in the intensive care unit: An illustrative case series. *Int. J. Antimicrob. Agents* **2010**, *35*, 606–608. [CrossRef] [PubMed]
4. Barletta, J.F.; Mangram, A.J.; Byrne, M.; Sucher, J.F.; Hollingworth, A.K.; AliOsman, F.R.; Shirah, G.R.; Haley, M.; Dzandu, J.K. Identifying augmented renal clearance in trauma patients: Validation of the augmented renal clearance in trauma intensive care (arctic) scoring system. *J. Trauma Acute Care Surg.* **2017**, *82*, 665–671. [CrossRef] [PubMed]
5. Abdel El Naeem, H.E.M.; Abdelhamid, M.H.E.; Atteya, D.A.M. Impact of augmented renal clearance on enoxaparin therapy in critically ill patients. *Egypt. J. Anaesth.* **2017**, *33*, 113–117. [CrossRef]
6. Udy, A.A.; Dulhunty, J.M.; Roberts, J.A.; Davis, J.S.; Webb, S.A.R.; Bellomo, R.; Gomersall, C.; Shirwadkar, C.; Eastwood, G.M.; Myburgh, J.; et al. Association between augmented renal clearance and clinical outcomes in patients receiving β-lactam antibiotic therapy by continuous or intermittent infusion: A nested cohort study of the BLING-II randomised, placebo-controlled, clinical trial. *Int. J. Antimicrob. Agents* **2017**, *49*, 624–630. [CrossRef] [PubMed]
7. Udy, A.A.; Jarrett, P.; LassigSmith, M.; Stuart, J.; Starr, T.; Dunlop, R.; Deans, R.; Roberts, J.A.; Senthuran, S.; Boots, R.; et al. Augmented renal clearance in traumatic brain injury: A single-center observational study of atrial natriuretic peptide, cardiac output, and creatinine clearance. *J. Neurotrauma* **2017**, *34*, 137–144. [CrossRef] [PubMed]
8. Barletta, J.F.; Mangram, A.J.; Byrne, M.; Hollingworth, A.K.; Sucher, J.F.; AliOsman, F.R.; Shirah, G.R.; Dzandu, J.K. The importance of empiric antibiotic dosing in critically ill trauma patients: Are we under-dosing based on augmented renal clearance and inaccurate renal clearance estimates? *J. Trauma Acute Care Surg.* **2016**, *81*, 1115–1120. [CrossRef] [PubMed]
9. Chu, Y.; Luo, Y.; Qu, L.; Zhao, C.; Jiang, M. Application of vancomycin in patients with varying renal function, especially those with augmented renal clearance. *Pharm. Biol.* **2016**, *54*, 2802–2806. [CrossRef] [PubMed]
10. Declercq, P.; Nijs, S.; D'Hoore, A.; Van Wijngaerden, E.; Wolthuis, A.; De Buck Van Overstraeten, A.; Wauters, J.; Spriet, I. Augmented renal clearance in non-critically ill abdominal and trauma surgery patients is an underestimated phenomenon: A point prevalence study. *J. Trauma Acute Care Surg.* **2016**, *81*, 468–477. [CrossRef] [PubMed]
11. Hirai, K.; Ihara, S.; Kinae, A.; Ikegaya, K.; Suzuki, M.; Hirano, K.; Itoh, K. Augmented renal clearance in pediatric patients with febrile neutropenia associated with vancomycin clearance. *Ther. Drug Monit.* **2016**, *38*, 393–397. [CrossRef] [PubMed]
12. Kawano, Y.; Morimoto, S.; Izutani, Y.; Muranishi, K.; Kaneyama, H.; Hoshino, K.; Nishida, T.; Ishikura, H. Augmented renal clearance in Japanese intensive care unit patients: A prospective study. *J. Intensive Care* **2016**, *4*, 62. [CrossRef] [PubMed]
13. Roberts, J.A.; Cotta, M.O.; Cojutti, P.; Lugano, M.; Rocca, G.D.; Pea, F. Does critical illness change levofloxacin pharmacokinetics? *Antimicrob. Agents Chemother.* **2016**, *60*, 1459–1463. [CrossRef] [PubMed]
14. De Cock, P.A.J.G.; Standing, J.F.; Barker, C.I.S.; de Jaeger, A.; Dhont, E.; Carlier, M.; Verstraete, A.G.; Delanghe, J.R.; Robays, H.; De Paepe, P. Augmented renal clearance implies a need for increased amoxicillin-clavulanic acid dosing in critically ill children. *Antimicrob. Agents Chemother.* **2015**, *59*, 7027–7035. [CrossRef] [PubMed]
15. De Waele, J.J.; Dumoulin, A.; Janssen, A.; Hoste, E.A. Epidemiology of augmented renal clearance in mixed icu patients. *Minerva Anestesiol.* **2015**, *81*, 1079–1085. [PubMed]
16. Dias, C.; Gaio, A.R.; Monteiro, E.; Barbosa, S.; Cerejo, A.; Donnelly, J.; Felgueiras, O.; Smielewski, P.; Paiva, J.A.; Czosnyka, M. Kidney-brain link in traumatic brain injury patients? A preliminary report. *Neurocrit. Care* **2015**, *22*, 192–201. [CrossRef] [PubMed]
17. Huttner, A.; Von Dach, E.; Renzoni, A.; Huttner, B.D.; Affaticati, M.; Pagani, L.; Daali, Y.; Pugin, J.; Karmime, A.; Fathi, M.; et al. Augmented renal clearance, low beta-lactam concentrations and clinical outcomes in the critically ill: An observational prospective cohort study. *Int. J. Antimicrob. Agents* **2015**, *45*, 385–392. [CrossRef] [PubMed]
18. Morbitzer, K.A.; Jordan, J.D.; Rhoney, D.H. Vancomycin pharmacokinetic parameters in patients with acute brain injury undergoing controlled normothermia, therapeutic hypothermia, or pentobarbital infusion. *Neurocrit Care* **2015**, *22*, 258–264. [CrossRef] [PubMed]

19. Ruiz, S.; Minville, V.; Asehnoune, K.; Virtos, M.; Georges, B.; Fourcade, O.; Conil, J.M. Screening of patients with augmented renal clearance in ICU: Taking into account the ckd-epi equation, the age, and the cause of admission. *Ann. Intensiv. Care* **2015**, *5*, 49. [CrossRef] [PubMed]
20. Spadaro, S.; Berselli, A.; Fogagnolo, A.; Capuzzo, M.; Ragazzi, R.; Marangoni, E.; Bertacchini, S.; Volta, C.A. Evaluation of a protocol for vancomycin administration in critically patients with and without kidney dysfunction. *BMC Anesthesiol.* **2015**, *15*, 95. [CrossRef] [PubMed]
21. Steinke, T.; Moritz, S.; Beck, S.; Gnewuch, C.; Kees, M.G. Estimation of creatinine clearance using plasma creatinine or cystatin C: A secondary analysis of two pharmacokinetic studies in surgical ICU patients. *BMC Anesthesiol.* **2015**, *15*, 62. [CrossRef] [PubMed]
22. Adnan, S.; Ratnam, S.; Kumar, S.; Paterson, D.; Lipman, J.; Roberts, J.; Udy, A.A. Select critically ill patients at risk of augmented renal clearance: Experience in a malaysian intensive care unit. *Anaesth. Intensiv. Care* **2014**, *42*, 715–722.
23. Akers, K.S.; Niece, K.L.; Chung, K.K.; Cannon, J.W.; Cota, J.M.; Murray, C.K. Modified augmented renal clearance score predicts rapid piperacillin and tazobactam clearance in critically ill surgery and trauma patients. *J. Trauma Acute Care Surg.* **2014**, *77*, 163. [CrossRef] [PubMed]
24. Baptista, J.P.; Neves, M.; Rodrigues, L.; Teixeira, L.; Pinho, J.; Pimentel, J. Accuracy of the estimation of glomerular filtration rate within a population of critically ill patients. *J. Nephrol.* **2014**, *27*, 403–410. [CrossRef] [PubMed]
25. Baptista, J.P.; Roberts, J.A.; Sousa, E.; Freitas, R.; Deveza, N.; Pimentel, J. Decreasing the time to achieve therapeutic vancomycin concentrations in critically ill patients: Developing and testing of a dosing nomogram. *Crit. Care (Lond. Engl.)* **2014**, *18*, 654. [CrossRef] [PubMed]
26. Campassi, M.L.; Gonzalez, M.C.; Masevicius, F.D.; Vazquez, A.R.; Moseinco, M.; Navarro, N.C.; Previgliano, L.; Rubatto, N.P.; Benites, M.H.; Estenssoro, E.; et al. Augmented renal clearance in critically ill patients: Incidence, associated factors and effects on vancomycin treatment]. *Rev. Bras. Ter. Intensiv.* **2014**, *26*, 13–20. [CrossRef]
27. Hites, M.; Taccone, F.S.; Wolff, F.; Maillart, E.; Beumier, M.; Surin, R.; Cotton, F.; Jacobs, F. Broad-spectrum beta-lactams in obese non-critically ill patients. *Nutr. Diabetes* **2014**, *4*, e119. [CrossRef] [PubMed]
28. Udy, A.A.; Jarrett, P.; Stuart, J.; LassigSmith, M.; Starr, T.; Dunlop, R.; Wallis, S.C.; Roberts, J.A.; Lipman, J. Determining the mechanisms underlying augmented renal drug clearance in the critically ill: Use of exogenous marker compounds. *Crit. Care* **2014**, *18*, 657. [CrossRef] [PubMed]
29. Udy, A.A.; Baptista, J.P.; Lim, N.L.; Joynt, G.M.; Jarrett, P.; Wockner, L.; Boots, R.J.; Lipman, J. Augmented renal clearance in the ICU: Results of a multicenter observational study of renal function in critically ill patients with normal plasma creatinine concentrations. *Crit. Care Med.* **2014**, *42*, 520–527. [CrossRef] [PubMed]
30. Carlier, M.; Carrette, S.; Roberts, J.A.; Stove, V.; Verstraete, A.; Hoste, E.; Depuydt, P.; Decruyenaere, J.; Lipman, J.; Wallis, S.C.; et al. Meropenem and piperacillin/tazobactam prescribing in critically ill patients: Does augmented renal clearance affect pharmacokinetic/pharmacodynamic target attainment when extended infusions are used? *Crit. Care (Lond. Engl.)* **2013**, *17*, R84. [CrossRef] [PubMed]
31. Claus, B.O.M.; Hoste, E.A.; Colpaert, K.; Robays, H.; Decruyenaere, J.; De Waele, J.J. Augmented renal clearance is a common finding with worse clinical outcome in critically ill patients receiving antimicrobial therapy. *J. Crit. Care* **2013**, *28*, 695–700. [CrossRef] [PubMed]
32. Minkute, R.; Briedis, V.; Steponaviciute, R.; Vitkauskiene, A.; Maciulaitis, R. Augmented renal clearance—An evolving risk factor to consider during the treatment with vancomycin. *J. Clin. Pharm. Ther.* **2013**, *38*, 462–467. [CrossRef] [PubMed]
33. Roberts, J.A.; Lipman, J. Optimal doripenem dosing simulations in critically ill nosocomial pneumonia patients with obesity, augmented renal clearance, and decreased bacterial susceptibility. *Crit. Care Med.* **2013**, *41*, 489–495. [CrossRef] [PubMed]
34. Shimamoto, Y.; Fukuda, T.; Tanaka, K.; Komori, K.; Sadamitsu, D. Systemic inflammatory response syndrome criteria and vancomycin dose requirement in patients with sepsis. *Intensive Care Med.* **2013**, *39*, 1247–1252. [CrossRef] [PubMed]
35. Udy, A.A.; Roberts, J.A.; Shorr, A.F.; Boots, R.J.; Lipman, J. Augmented renal clearance in septic and traumatized patients with normal plasma creatinine concentrations: Identifying at-risk patients. *Crit. Care (Lond. Engl.)* **2013**, *17*, R35. [CrossRef] [PubMed]

36. Udy, A.A.; Morton, F.J.A.; NguyenPham, S.; Jarrett, P.; LassigSmith, M.; Stuart, J.; Dunlop, R.; Starr, T.; Boots, R.J.; Lipman, J. A comparison of CKD-EPI estimated glomerular filtration rate and measured creatinine clearance in recently admitted critically ill patients with normal plasma creatinine concentrations. *BMC Nephrol.* **2013**, *14*, 250. [CrossRef] [PubMed]
37. Baptista, J.P.; Sousa, E.; Martins, P.J.; Pimentel, J.M. Augmented renal clearance in septic patients and implications for vancomycin optimisation. *Int. J. Antimicrob. Agents* **2012**, *39*, 420–423. [CrossRef] [PubMed]
38. Grootaert, V.; Willems, L.; Debaveye, Y.; Meyfroidt, G.; Spriet, I. Augmented renal clearance in the critically ill: How to assess kidney function. *Ann. Pharmacother.* **2012**, *46*, 952–959. [CrossRef] [PubMed]
39. Udy, A.A.; Varghese, J.M.; Altukroni, M.; Briscoe, S.; McWhinney, B.C.; Ungerer, J.P.; Lipman, J.; Roberts, J.A. Subtherapeutic initial β-lactam concentrations in select critically ill patients: Association between augmented renal clearance and low trough drug concentrations. *Chest* **2012**, *142*, 30–39. [CrossRef] [PubMed]
40. Baptista, J.P.; Udy, A.A.; Sousa, E.; Pimentel, J.; Wang, L.; Roberts, J.A.; Lipman, J. A comparison of estimates of glomerular filtration in critically ill patients with augmented renal clearance. *Crit. Care (Lond. Engl.)* **2011**, *15*, R139. [CrossRef] [PubMed]
41. Minville, V.; Asehnoune, K.; Ruiz, S.; Breden, A.; Georges, B.; Seguin, T.; Tack, I.; Jaafar, A.; Saivin, S.; Fourcade, O.; et al. Increased creatinine clearance in polytrauma patients with normal serum creatinine: A retrospective observational study. *Crit. Care (Lond. Engl.)* **2011**, *15*, R49. [CrossRef] [PubMed]
42. Spencer, D.D.; Jacobi, J.; Juenke, J.M.; Fleck, J.D.; Kays, M.B. Steady-state pharmacokinetics of intravenous levetiracetam in neurocritical care patients. *Pharmacotherapy* **2011**, *31*, 934–941. [CrossRef] [PubMed]
43. Goboova, M.; Kuzelova, M.; Kissova, V.; Bodakova, D.; Martisova, E. An adjustment of vancomycin dosing regimen for a young patient with augmented renal clearance: A case report. *Acta Fac. Pharm. Univ. Comen.* **2015**, *62*, 1–4.
44. Abdul-Aziz, M.; McDonald, C.; McWhinney, B.; Ungerer, J.P.J.; Lipman, J.; Roberts, J.A. Low flucloxacillin concentrations in a patient with central nervous system infection: The need for plasma and cerebrospinal fluid drug monitoring in the ICU. *Ann. Pharmacother.* **2014**, *48*, 1380–1384. [CrossRef] [PubMed]
45. Cook, A.M.; Arora, S.; Davis, J.; Pittman, T. Augmented renal clearance of vancomycin and levetiracetam in a traumatic brain injury patient. *Neurocrit. Care* **2013**, *19*, 210–214. [CrossRef] [PubMed]
46. Lonsdale, D.O.; Udy, A.A.; Roberts, J.A.; Lipman, J. Antibacterial therapeutic drug monitoring in cerebrospinal fluid: Difficulty in achieving adequate drug concentrations. *J. Neurosurg.* **2013**, *118*, 297–301. [CrossRef] [PubMed]
47. Troger, U.; Drust, A.; Martens-Lobenhoffer, J.; Tanev, I.; Braun-Dullaeus, R.; Bode-Boger, S. Decreased meropenem levels in intensive care unit patients with augmented renal clearance: Benefit of therapeutic drug monitoring. *Int. J. Antimicrob. Agents* **2012**, *40*, 370–372. [CrossRef] [PubMed]
48. Caro, L.; Larson, K.; Nicolau, D.; DeWaele, J.; Kuti, J.; Gadzicki, E.; Yu, B.; Rhee, E. PK/PD and safety of 3 g ceftolozane/tazobactam in critically ill augmented renal clearance patients. In Proceedings of the 46th Critical Care Medicine Conference, Honolulu, HI, USA, 21–25 January 2017; p. 661.
49. Goboova, M.; Kuzelova, M.; Fazekas, T.; Kissova, V.; Kakosova, V.; Salkovska, L. The impact of therapeutic drug monitoring (TDM) in optimizing dosage regimens of gentamicin in patients with augmented renal clearance. *Int. J. Clin. Pharm.* **2016**, *38*, 596.
50. Morbitzer, K.; Jordan, D.; Sullivan, K.; Durr, E.; OlmShipman, C.; Rhoney, D. Enhanced renal clearance and impact on vancomycin trough concentration in patients with hemorrhagic stroke. In Proceedings of the Annual Meeting of the American College of Clinical Pharmacy (ACCP), Hollywood, FL, USA, 23–26 October 2016; Volume 36, p. e218.
51. Morimoto, S.; Ishikura, H. An observational prospective study on the onset of augmented renal clearance: The first report. *Crit. Care* **2016**, *20* (Suppl. 2), 182. [CrossRef]
52. Dunning, J.; Roberts, J. Assessment of renal function in dosing antibiotics in septic patients: A survey of current practice within critical care units in england. *Anaesthesia* **2015**, *70*, 21.
53. Baptista, J.P.; Silva, N.; Costa, E.; Fontes, F.; Marques, M.; Ribeiro, G.; Pimentel, J. Identification of the critically ill patient with augmented renal clearance: Make do with what you have! In Proceedings of the 27th Annual Congress of the European Society of Intensive Care Medicine (ESICM), Barcelona, Spain, 27 September–1 October 2014; Volume 40, p. S110.

54. May, C.; Arora, S.; Parli, S.; Bastin, M.T.; Cook, A. Levetiracetam pharmacokinetics in subarachnoid hemorrhage patients with augmented renal clearance: A monte carlo simulation. In Proceedings of the 2014 Annual Meeting of the American College of Clinical Pharmacy (ACCP), Austin, TX, USA, 12–15 October 2014; Volume 34, pp. e261–e262.
55. Vermis, K.; Steel, E.; Vandenbroucke, J. Prevalence of augmented renal clearance in haematological patients and the impact on vancomycin dosing. In Proceedings of the Journal of Oncology Pharmacy Practice. Conference: 14th Symposium of the International Society of Oncology Pharmacy Practitioners, Montreal, QC, Canada, 2–5 April 2014; Volume 20, p. 7.
56. Weigel, J.; Egal, M.; Lima, A.; Koch, B.; Hunfeld, N.G.; Van Gelder, T.; Mouton, J.W.; Groeneveld, A.B.J. Vancomycin is underdosed in patients with high estimated glomerular filtration rate. In Proceedings of the 27th Annual Congress of the European Society of Intensive Care Medicine (ESICM), Barcelona, Spain, 27 September–1 October 2014; p. S252.
57. Neves, M.; Baptista, J.P.; Rodrigues, L.; Pinho, J.; Teixeira, L.; Pimentel, J. Correlation between estimated glomerular filtration rate and measured renal creatinine clearance in critically ill patients with normal serum creatinine. *Nephrol. Dial. Transplant.* **2013**, *28*, 345.
58. Grootaert, V.; Spriet, I.; Decoutere, L.; Debaveye, Y.; Meyfroidt, G.; Willems, L. Augmented renal clearance in the critically ill: Fiction or fact? *Int. J. Clin. Pharm.* **2012**, *34*, 143.
59. Drust, A.; Troger, U.; MartensLobenhoffer, J.; Tanev, I.; BraunDullaeus, R.C.; BodeBoger, S.M. Therapeutic drug monitoring of meropenem is mandatory for critically ill patients with glomerular hyperfiltration. *Br. J. Clin. Pharmacol.* **2011**, *72*, 18.
60. Ichai, C.; Passeron, C.; Carles, M.; Bouregba, M.; Grimaud, D. Prolonged low-dose dopamine infusion induces a transient improvement in renal function in hemodynamically stable, critically ill patients: A single-blind, prospective, controlled study. *Crit. Care Med.* **2000**, *28*, 1329–1335. [CrossRef] [PubMed]
61. Ichai, C.; Soubielle, J.; Carles, M.; Giunti, C.; Grimaud, D. Comparison of the renal effects of low to high doses of dopamine and dobutamine in critically ill patients: A single-blind randomized study. *Crit. Care Med.* **2000**, *28*, 921–928. [CrossRef] [PubMed]
62. Ljungberg, B.; NilssonEhle, I. Advancing age and acute infection influence the kinetics of ceftazidime. *Scand. J. Infect. Dis.* **1989**, *21*, 327–332. [CrossRef] [PubMed]
63. Sime, F.B.; Udy, A.A.; Roberts, J.A. Augmented renal clearance in critically ill patients: Etiology, definition and implications for beta-lactam dose optimization. *Curr. Opin. Pharmacol.* **2015**, *24*, 1–6. [CrossRef] [PubMed]
64. Carlier, M.; Dumoulin, A.; Janssen, A.; Picavet, S.; Vanthuyne, S.; Van Eynde, R.; Vanholder, R.; Delanghe, J.; De Schoenmakere, G.; De Waele, J.J.; et al. Comparison of different equations to assess glomerular filtration in critically ill patients. *Intensive Care Med.* **2015**, *41*, 427–435. [CrossRef] [PubMed]
65. Sunder, S.; Jayaraman, R.; Mahapatra, H.S.; Sathi, S.; Ramanan, V.; Kanchi, P.; Gupta, A.; Daksh, S.K.; Ram, P. Estimation of renal function in the intensive care unit: The covert concepts brought to light. *J. Intensive Care* **2014**, *2*, 31. [CrossRef] [PubMed]
66. Rybak, M.J. The pharmacokinetic and pharmacodynamic properties of vancomycin. *Clin. Infect. Dis.* **2006**, *42* (Suppl. 1), S35–S39. [CrossRef] [PubMed]
67. Mouton, J.W.; Touzw, D.J.; Horrevorts, A.M.; Vinks, A.A. Comparative pharmacokinetics of the carbapenems: Clinical implications. *Clin. Pharmacokinet.* **2000**, *39*, 185–201. [CrossRef] [PubMed]
68. Binder, L.; Schworer, H.; Hoppe, S.; Streit, F.; Neumann, S.; Beckmann, A.; Wachter, R.; Oellerich, M.; Walson, P.D. Pharmacokinetics of meropenem in critically ill patients with severe infections. *Ther. Drug Monit.* **2013**, *35*, 63–70. [CrossRef] [PubMed]

Pharmacokinetics and Intestinal Metabolism of Compound K in Rats and Mice

Ji-Hyeon Jeon [1], Bitna Kang [2], Sowon Lee [1], Sojeong Jin [2], Min-Koo Choi [2,*] and Im-Sook Song [1,*]

[1] College of Pharmacy and Research Institute of Pharmaceutical Sciences, Kyungpook National University, Daegu 41566, Korea; kei7016@naver.com (J.-H.J.); okjin917@hanmail.net (S.L.)

[2] College of Pharmacy, Dankook University, Cheon-an 31116, Korea; qlcska8520@naver.com (B.K.); astraea327@naver.com (S.J.)

* Correspondence: minkoochoi@dankook.ac.kr (M.-K.C.); isssong@knu.ac.kr (I.-S.S.)

Abstract: We aimed to investigate the plasma concentration, tissue distribution, and elimination of compound K following the intravenous administration of compound K (2 mg/kg) in rats and mice. The plasma concentrations of compound K in mice were much higher (about five-fold) than those in rats. In both rats and mice, compound K was mainly distributed in the liver and underwent biliary excretion. There was 28.4% fecal recovery of compound K in mice and 13.8% in rats, whereas its renal recovery was less than 0.1% in both rats and mice. Relative quantification of compound K and its metabolite protopanaxadiol (PPD) in rat bile and intestinal feces indicated that the metabolism from compound K into PPD occurred in the intestine but not in the plasma. Therefore, PPD detected in the plasma samples could have been absorbed from the intestine after metabolism in control rats, while PPD could not be detected in the plasma samples from bile duct cannulated rats. In conclusion, mice and rats shared common features such as exclusive liver distribution, major excretion pathway via biliary route, and intestinal metabolism to PPD. However, there were significant differences between rats and mice in the plasma concentrations of compound K and the fecal recovery of compound K and PPD.

Keywords: compound K; protopanaxadiol (PPD); pharmacokinetics; biliary excretion; intestinal metabolism

1. Introduction

Compound K, which belongs to the protopanaxadiol (PPD)-type ginsenoside group, was first discovered in 1972 from a hydrolase mixture of ginsenosides (Rb1, Rb2, and Rc) and soil bacteria [1]. Since then, compound K has attracted special attention among the various ginsenosides because it is reported as a major pharmacologically active component that has hepatoprotective, chemo-preventive, anti-diabetic, anti-inflammatory, anti-arthritic, neuroprotective, and immune stimulating effects [1,2]. The therapeutic benefit of compound K has been demonstrated in both in vitro studies and in vivo disease models [1]. Paek et al. [3] investigated the dose-dependent bioavailability of compound K by comparing its oral and intravenous administration in rats. The area under plasma concentration (AUC) of compound K increased linearly following intravenous injection at a dose range of 1–10 mg/kg (dose increase 10-fold; AUC increase 11.6-fold), but the AUC of compound K following oral administration did not increase linearly at a dose range of 5–20 mg/kg (dose increase four-fold; AUC increase 75.8-fold) [3]. The AUC of compound K was significantly increased (23.5-fold) in P-glycoprotein (P-gp) knock-out mice compared to wild-type mice after a single oral dose (10 mg/kg) [4]. Therefore,

P-gp-mediated efflux during intestinal absorption could be a possible explanation for non-linear oral bioavailability of compound K.

The safety, pharmacokinetics, and preliminary efficacy of compound K in tablet form as an anti-rheumatoid arthritis drug are under clinical investigation in China (Study No. NCT03755258) [5]. In this study, Chen et al. [5] investigated the pharmacokinetics of compound K and PPD, a metabolite of compound K, following a single oral administration of a 200 mg compound K tablet. This was the first pharmacokinetic study in humans using pure compound K. The maximum plasma concentration (C_{max}) of compound K was 796.8 ng/mL with a time to reach C_{max} (T_{max}) of 3.6 h. On the other hand, the C_{max} of PPD was 5.7 ng/mL with a T_{max} of 24.5 h. The results suggested that the formation of PPD from compound K occurred slowly. The AUC ratio of PPD to compound K was calculated as 0.04 [5]. They also investigated the effect of high-fat meal on the pharmacokinetics of compound K. The high-fat meal consumption increased C_{max} (2.0-fold) and AUC (2.2-fold) of compound K but decreased T_{max} (3.6 h in fasting group vs. 2.5 h in high-fat meal group, $p < 0.05$) compared with fasting group, suggesting that the high-fat meal accelerated the absorption of compound K [5].

Other pharmacokinetic studies of compound K have been reported in human subjects following oral administration of ginseng product [2,6–9]. The C_{max} of compound K was 41.5 ng/mL in 12 Japanese subjects following a single oral administration of fermented ginseng tablet (274.4 mg total; 2.2 mg as compound K) [6]. The mean C_{max} (254.5 ng/mL) was substantially higher and less variable in subjects who were orally administered fermented Korean red ginseng (3 g total; 10.9 mg as compound K) than the C_{max} (3.2–24.8 ng/mL) in subjects who received non-fermented Korean red ginseng extract (3 g total; 0 mg as compound K) [2,7,9]. The results suggested that the consumption of ginseng product with higher compound K content resulted in higher plasma concentrations of compound K. The compound K in the plasma was absorbed after the metabolism from Rb1, Rb2, Rc, and Rd (major components of red ginseng product) to compound K following oral administration of non-fermented red ginseng product [7,10]. Therefore, the variability in the gut metabolism and intestinal absorption of compound K could be attributed to the variable plasma concentrations of compound K. However, little information is available on the distribution and elimination of compound K. Therefore, the purpose of this study was to investigate the pharmacokinetics of compound K in rats and mice with a focus on tissue distribution, elimination, and metabolism to PPD.

2. Materials and Methods

2.1. Materials

Compound K and 20(S)-protopanaxadiol (PPD) was purchased from the Ambo Institute (Daejeon, Korea). To be used as internal standards (IS), 13C-caffeine was purchased from Sigma-Aldrich Chemical Co. (St. Louis, MO, USA). All other chemicals and solvents were of reagent or analytical grade.

2.2. Animals and Ethical Approval

Male Institute of Cancer Research (ICR) mice (7 or 8-weeks-old, weighing 34–37 g) and male Sprague-Dawley (SD) rats (7 or 8-weeks-old, 230–270 g) were purchased from Samtako Co. (Osan, Korea). The animals were acclimatized for 1 week at an animal facility at Kyungpook National University. Food and water were available ad libitum. All animal procedures were approved by the Animal Care and Use Committee of Kyungpook National University (Approval No. KNU 2018-192, 19 December 2018) and carried out in accordance with the National Institutes of Health guidance for the care and use of laboratory animals. An overview of the study design and methods is provided in Table 1.

Table 1. Overview of the study design and methods.

Study Name	SD Rats	ICR Mice	Remarks
Pharmacokinetics of compound K (n = 4)	• Compound K IV 2 mg/kg • Blood sampling: 0.17–48 h • Feces collection for 48 h • Urine collection for 48 h	• Compound K IV 2 mg/kg • Blood sampling: 0.17–48 h • Feces collection for 48 h • Urine collection for 48 h	• Comparison between rats and mice • PK parameters of compound K • Fecal and urine recovery of compound K and PPD
Tissue distribution of compound K (n = 4)	• Compound K IV 2 mg/kg • Blood and tissue collection: 0.17–24 h • Liver, kidney, brain, heart, lung, spleen, testis	• Compound K IV 2 mg/kg • Blood and tissue collection: 0.17–24 h • Liver, kidney, brain, heart, lung, spleen, testis	• Comparison between rats and mice • Tissue to plasma AUC ratios of compound K
Inhibition of hepatic uptake of compound K (n = 3)	• Compound K IV 2 mg/kg • Rifampin pretreatment PO 20 mg/kg • Blood and liver collection at 0.5 and 2 h	• Compound K IV 2 mg/kg • Rifampin pretreatment PO 20 mg/kg • Blood and liver collection at 0.5 and 2 h	• Comparison between groups with/without rifampin pretreatment • Tissue to plasma concentration ratios of compound K
Biliary excretion of compound K (n = 4)	• Compound K IV 2 mg/kg • Blood sampling: 0.25–8 h • Bile collection: for 12 h		• PK parameters of compound K • Biliary excretion of compound K
Metabolism of compound K (n = 4)	• Compound K IV 2 mg/kg • Bile collection for 0-2 h and 2–12 h • Intestinal feces collection at 2 and 12 h		• PPD quantification in plasma, bile, and intestinal feces samples

IV, intravenous injection; PO, per oral administration, PPD, 20(S)-protopanaxadiol; PK parameters, pharmacokinetic parameters; AUC, area under plasma concentration.

2.3. Pharmacokinetic Study

ICR mice and SD rats received compound K intravenously at a single dose of 2 mg/kg via the tail vein and were returned to the metabolic cage with water and chow ad libitum. Before administration, the compound K was dissolved in a vehicle containing DMSO: saline (2:8, v/v) (vehicle volume, 1 mL/kg for mice and 0.4 mL/kg for rats). Blood samples (approximately 100 μL) were collected at 0, 0.17, 0.5, 1, 2, 4, 8, 24, and 48 h following intravenous injection of compound K with no sign of hemoglobinemia and hemoglobinuria. Blood sampling was performed using a sparse sampling method (time schedule is given in Table 2). The blood samples were centrifuged at 16,000× g for 10 min to separate the plasma. An aliquot (50 μL) of each plasma sample was stored at −80 °C until the analysis. Urine and feces samples were collected from 0–24 h and 24–48 h following the compound K administration. Aliquots (50 μL) of urine and 10% feces homogenates were stored at −80 °C until the analysis.

SD rats were randomly divided into two groups: the non-bile cannulated control group and the bile cannulated group. For the bile cannulated rats, the femoral artery, femoral vein, and bile duct were cannulated with polyethylene tubes (PE-50 and PE-10; Jungdo, Seoul, Korea) under light anesthesia with isoflurane. For the control group, the femoral artery and femoral vein were cannulated with PE-50. Compound K was injected intravenously via the femoral vein at 2 mg/kg. Blood samples (approximately 200 μL) were collected from the femoral artery at 0, 0.25, 0.5, 1, 2, 4, and 8 h after the compound K injection. After each blood sampling, normal saline was injected into the femoral vein to compensate for blood loss. Bile samples were collected every 2 h for a total of 12 h. The blood samples were centrifuged at 16,000× g for 10 min, and 50 μL aliquots of plasma and 50 μL aliquots of bile were stored at −80 °C until the compound K analysis. In the non-bile cannulated rats, the complete contents of the entire gastrointestinal tract were collected using a 10 mL syringe filled with 30 mL pre-warmed saline. The contents were homogenized with tissue homogenizer, and 50 μL aliquots of intestinal fecal homogenates were stored at −80 °C until the analysis.

The 50 μL samples of plasma, urine, 10% fecal homogenates, bile, and intestinal fecal homogenates were each mixed with 60 μL of IS (20 ng/mL 13C-caffeine in water) and 600 μL of methyl *tert*-butyl ether (MTBE). The mixtures were vortexed vigorously for 10 min and centrifuged at 16,000× *g* for 5 min. After centrifugation, the samples were frozen at −80 °C for 2 h. For each sample, the upper layer was transferred to a clean tube and evaporated to dryness under a nitrogen stream. The residue was reconfigured with 200 μL of 80% methanol consisting of 0.1% formic acid, and a 10 μL aliquot was injected into the liquid chromatography–tandem mass spectrometry (LC–MS/MS) system.

Table 2. Blood sampling schedule for the pharmacokinetic study of compound K in mice and rats following intravenous injection of compound K.

Sampling Time (h)	Group 1 (n = 4)	Group 2 (n = 4)	Group 3 (n = 4)	Sampling Method	Anesthesia
0	O			RO-right [1]	O
0.17		O		RO-right	O
0.5			O	RO-right	O
1	O			RO-left [2]	O
2		O		RO-left	O
4			O	RO-left	O
8	O			AA [3]	O
24		O		AA	O
48			O	AA	O

[1] RO-right: retro-orbital blood sampling—right eye under anesthesia with isoflurane; [2] RO-left: retro-orbital blood sampling—left eye under anesthesia with isoflurane; [3] AA: abdominal artery blood sampling.

2.4. Tissue Distribution Study

ICR mice and SD rats received compound K intravenously at a single dose of 2 mg/kg via tail vein and were returned to the metabolic cage with water and chow ad libitum. The animals were euthanized and blood samples (approximately 200 μL) were collected from the abdominal artery at 0.17, 0.5, 2, 4, 8, and 24 h after intravenous injection. The liver, kidney, brain, heart, lung, spleen, and testis were immediately excised, gently washed with ice-cold saline, and weighed. The tissue samples were homogenized with 4 volumes of saline. Aliquots (50 μL) of plasma and 20% tissue homogenates were stored at –80 °C until the analysis of compound K.

To investigate the effect of rifampin (a representative inhibitor of the organic anion-transporting polypeptide (Oatp) transporters [11]) on the hepatic distribution of compound K, ICR mice and SD rats were randomly divided into either control or rifampin groups. The rifampin group was orally administered with rifampin solution (20 mg/kg, dissolved in DMSO: saline = 2:8, *v*/*v*) and the control group received only the vehicle via oral gavage. One hour after rifampin treatment, mice and rats received compound K intravenously at a single dose of 2 mg/kg via tail vein. The animals were euthanized and blood samples (approximately 200 μL) were collected from the abdominal artery at 0.5 and 2 h after intravenous injection. The liver tissues were immediately excised, gently washed with ice-cold saline, and homogenized with 4 volumes of saline. Aliquots (50 μL) of plasma and 20% liver homogenates were stored at −80 °C until the analysis of compound K.

The plasma samples and 20% tissue homogenates samples were each mixed with 60 μL of IS (20 ng/mL 13C-caffeine in water) and 600 μL of MTBE. The mixtures were vortexed vigorously for 10 min and centrifuged at 16,000× *g* for 5 min. After centrifugation, the samples were frozen at −80 °C for 2 h. The upper layer was transferred to a clean tube and evaporated to dryness under a nitrogen stream. The residue was reconfigured with 200 μL of 80% methanol consisting of 0.1% formic acid, and a 10 μL aliquot was injected into the LC-MS/MS system.

2.5. LC-MS/MS Analysis of Compound K

Compound K and PPD concentrations were analyzed using a modified LC-MS/MS method of Jin et al. [8] with an Agilent 6430 triple quadrupole LC-MS/MS system (Agilent, Wilmington, DE, USA). Compound K and PPD were separated using an Eclipse Plus C18 RRHD (1.8 μm particle size, 3.0 × 5.0 mm, Agilent, Wilmington, DE, USA). The mobile phase consisted of 0.1% formic acid in water (8%) and 0.1% formic acid in methanol (92%) at a flow rate of 0.15 mL/min.

Quantification of a separated analyte peak was performed at m/z 645.5 → 203.1 for compound K (T_R (retention time) 6.9 min), m/z 425.3 → 109.1 for PPD (T_R 13.9 min), and m/z 198.2 → 140.1 for 13C-caffeine (IS) (T_R 2.9 min) in the positive ionization mode with collision energy (CE) of 35, 25 and 20 eV, respectively. The analytical data were quantified using Mass Hunter (version B.06.00, Agilent, Wilmington, DE, USA).

The calibration standards and quality control (QC) samples were prepared by spiking a 5 μL aliquot of the working solution with 45 μL aliquot of blank matrix (plasma, liver, kidney, heart, lung, pancreas, brain, testis, and urine). The final concentrations of the compound K and PPD calibration standards for plasma and urine samples were 5, 10, 20, 50, 200, 500, 2000 ng/mL, and the concentrations of QC samples of compound K and PPD were 15, 100, and 1500 ng/mL. The concentrations of calibration standards and QC samples of compound K and PPD for bile and fecal homogenates were 25, 50, 100, 250, 1000, 2500, and 10,000 ng/mL and 75, 500, and 7500 ng/mL, respectively. The concentrations of calibration standards and QC samples of compound K for liver, kidney, heart, lung, pancreas, brain, and testis homogenates were 5, 10, 20, 50, 200, 500, and 2000 ng/mL and 15, 100, and 1500 ng/mL, respectively. The standard calibration curves for compound K and PPD was linear in the concentration range of 5–2000 ng/mL in the plasma, urine, and tissue homogenates samples and in the concentration range of 25–10,000 ng/mL in the bile and feces homogenates samples, respectively. The inter-day and intra-day precision and accuracy (%CV) for compound K and PPD in all biological samples was less than 15%.

2.6. Data Analysis

Pharmacokinetic parameters were estimated using non-compartmental methods (WinNonlin version 2.0, Pharsight Co., Certara, NJ, USA).

All pharmacokinetic parameters are given as the mean ± standard deviation. All statistical analyses were performed using SAS (ver. 9.4; SAS Institute Inc., Cary, NC, USA). A p-value < 0.05 was considered statistically significant.

3. Results

3.1. Comparative Pharmacokinetics of Compound K in Rats and Mice

The plasma concentration-time profile of compound K was compared between the mice and the rats. Since the intestinal absorption of compound K is low and variable [3,4], intravenous injection of compound K was used in this study intead of oral administration. The plasma concentrations of compound K in mice were greater than those in rats (Figure 1). The pharmacokinetic parameters of compound K such as AUC and plasma concentration were about 5–6-fold greater in mice than in rats, while there was no significant difference in the half-life ($T_{1/2}$) and mean residence time (MRT) between rats and mice (Table 3). However, the clearance (CL) and volume of distribution (Vd) values were about five-fold larger in rats than in mice (Table 3). Taken together, the results suggest that the distribution and elimination of compound K differ between rats and mice.

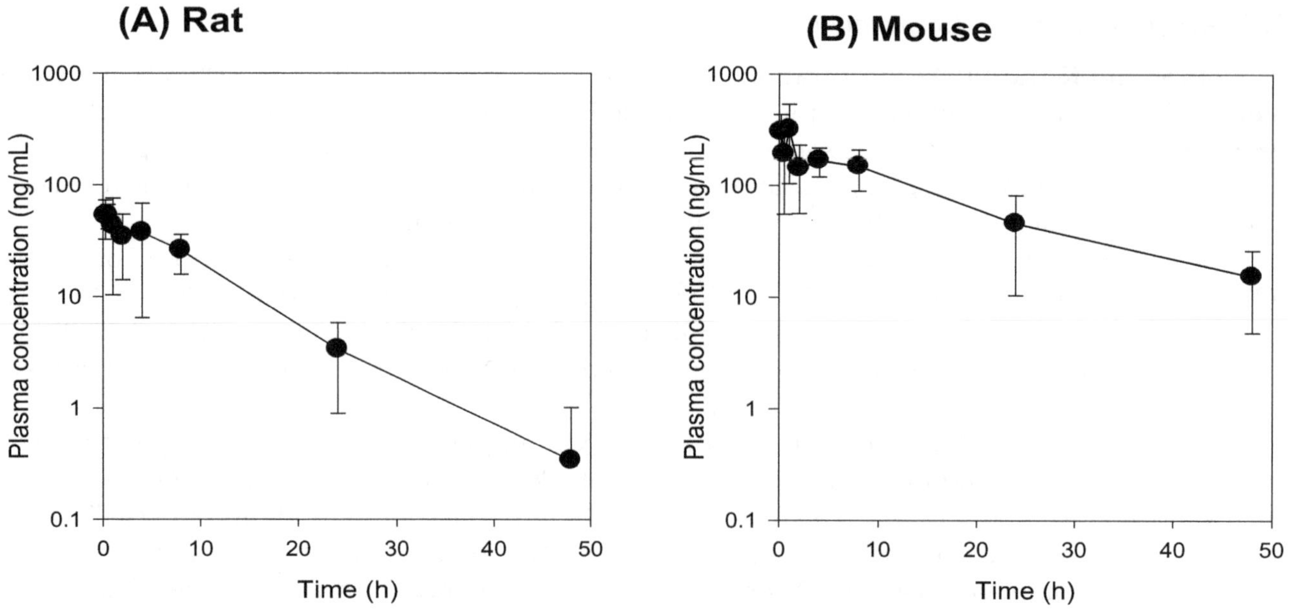

Figure 1. (**A**) Plasma concentration vs. time profile of compound K following intravenous injection of compound K at a single dose of 2 mg/kg in rats (**A**) and mice (**B**). Plasma concentration of compound K (*Y*-axis) was represented using a logarithmic scale. Data expressed as mean± standard deviation from four rats or four mice at different time points.

Table 3. Pharmacokinetic parameters of compound K in rat and mouse.

Characteristics	Parameters	Rat	Mouse
Plasma	C_0 (ng/mL)	75.3 ± 23.3	400 ± 137 *
	$AUC_{48\,h}$ (ng·h/mL)	638.8 ± 298.6	3756.3 ± 1636 *
	AUC_{∞} (ng·h/mL)	670.1 ± 284.1	4025.1 ± 1836 *
	$T_{1/2}$ (h)	7.3 ± 0.4	11.4 ± 1.5
	MRT (h)	8.9 ± 0.4	11.8 ± 2.0
	CL (mL/min/kg)	59.0 ± 21.8	10.4 ± 4.9 *
	Vd (L/kg)	31.8 ± 3.1	7.08 ± 2.6 *
Excretion	$Feces_{48\,h}$ (% of dose)	13.8 ± 7.1	28.4 ± 5.9 *
	$Urine_{48\,h}$ (% of dose)	0.01 ± 0.01	0.02 ± 0.01

$AUC_{48\,h}$ or AUC_{∞}: area under the plasma concentration-time curve from 0 to 48 h or to infinity; C_0: initial plasma concentration; $T_{1/2}$: half-life; MRT: mean residence time; CL: clearance; Vd: Volume of distribution. Data expressed as mean ± standard deviation (n = 4). *: $p < 0.05$ compared with the rat group.

To compare the elimination pathway of compound K, we measured the renal and fecal recovery of compound K following intravenous administration of compound K in both rats and mice. The recovery of compound K from the urine was about 0.02% of the intravenous dose in both mice and rats. In contrast, the fecal recovery of compound K was about 28.4 ± 5.9% in mice and 13.8 ± 7.1% in rats (Table 1). The results suggest that fecal excretion is a major excretion route for compound K in both rats and mice but also that compound K may undergo in vivo metabolism in both rats and mice.

3.2. *Tissue Distribution of Compound K*

To analyze the tissue distribution of compound K, we measured the temporal profile of compound K in various tissues in rats and mice following intravenous administration of compound K. As shown in Figures 2 and 3, the tissue distribution pattern of compound K was comparable in both mice and rats. Compound K was predominantly distributed to the liver in both rats and mice, and the liver to plasma AUC ratio was 11.1 in rats and 16.7 in mice. The AUC ratios of other tissues (i.e., kidney, heart, lung, pancreas, testis, and brain) to plasma, however, were much lower than the liver/plasma AUC ratio for both species (Figures 2B and 3B). These results suggest the involvement of the uptake transport system, which is dominantly expressed in the liver. Previously, Jiang et al. [12] reported the involvement of the Oatp transporters (OATP1B3 in humans and Oatp1b2 in rats) in the hepatic uptake of ginsenosides Rg1, Re, and R1. Therefore, we investigated the effect of rifampin, a representative inhibitor of the Oatp transporter [11], on the liver distribution of compound K to further assess the involvement of the Oatp uptake transporter.

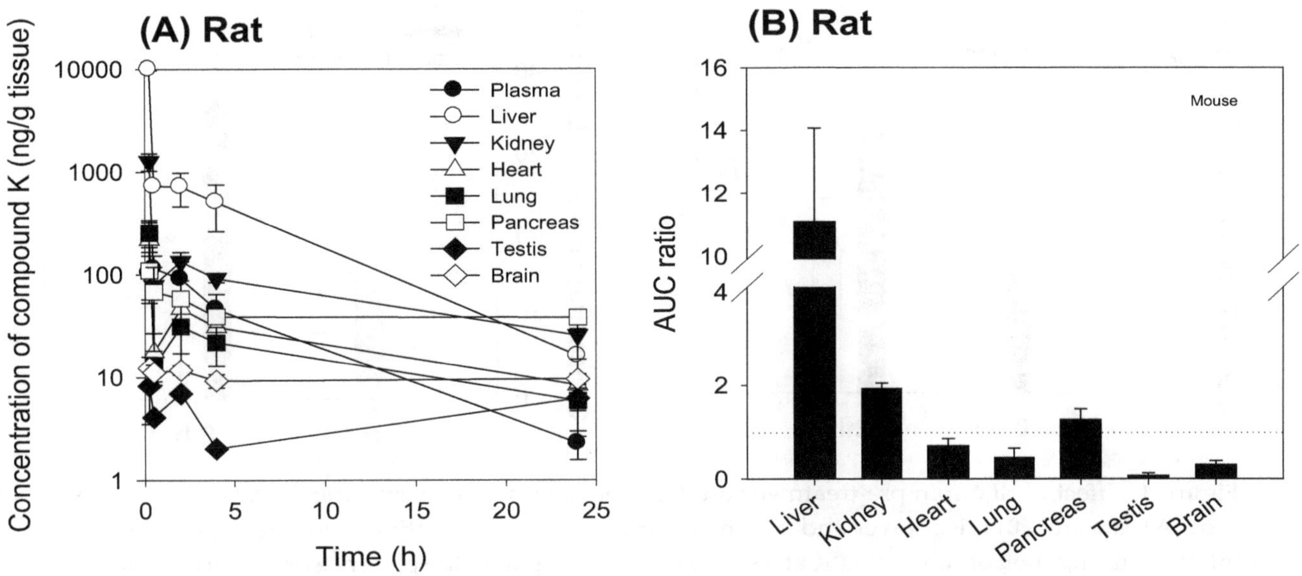

Figure 2. (**A**) Tissue concentration vs. time profile of compound K following intravenous injection of compound K at a single dose of 2 mg/kg in rats. (**B**) AUC ratios ($AUC_{tissue}/AUC_{plasma}$) of compound K in the liver, kidney, heart, lung, pancreas, testis, and brain following intravenous injection (2 mg/kg) in rats. AUC was calculated from the data shown in (**A**) and the dotted line in (**B**) represents unity. Data are expressed as mean± standard deviation from four rats at different time points.

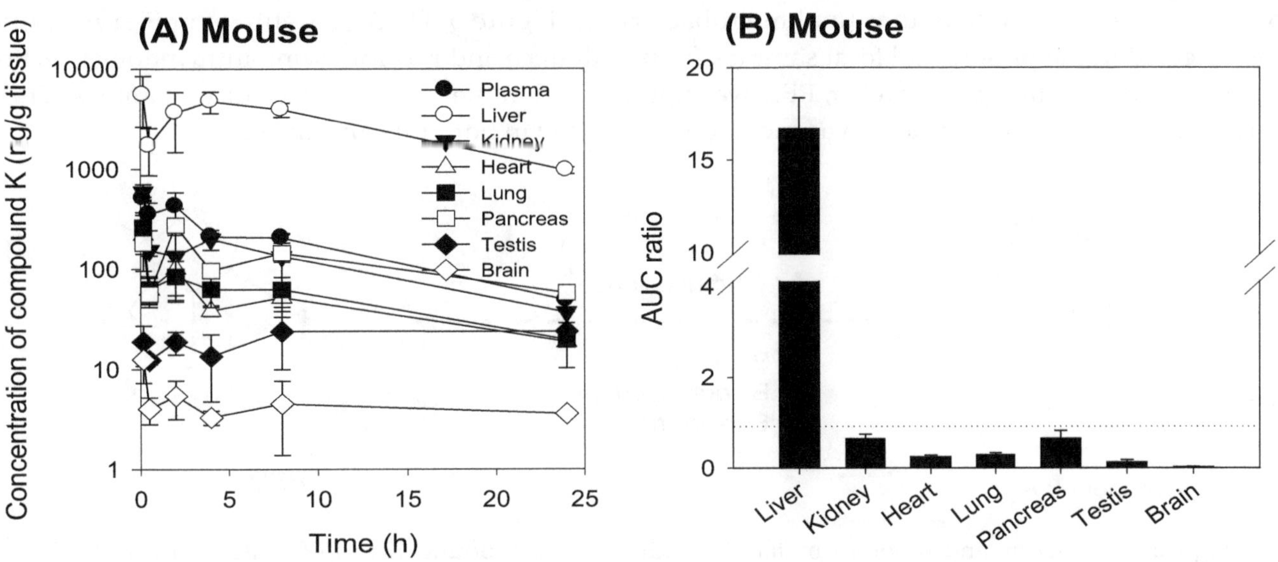

Figure 3. (**A**) Tissue concentration vs. time profile of compound K following intravenous injection of compound K at a single dose of 2 mg/kg in mice. (**B**) AUC ratios of compound K in the liver, kidney, heart, lung, pancreas, testis, and brain to plasma following intravenous injection (2 mg/kg) in mice. AUC was calculated from the data shown in (**A**) and the dotted line in (**B**) represents unity. Data are expressed as mean ± standard deviation from four rats at different time points.

When rifampin was given orally at 1 h prior to compound K injection, the plasma concentration of compound K increased and the liver to plasma concentration ratios decreased when compared to the control group (no rifampin pre-treatment) in both mice and rats (Figure 4). This can be explained by the blocking of Oatp-mediated hepatic uptake of compound K by the rifampin pre-treatment.

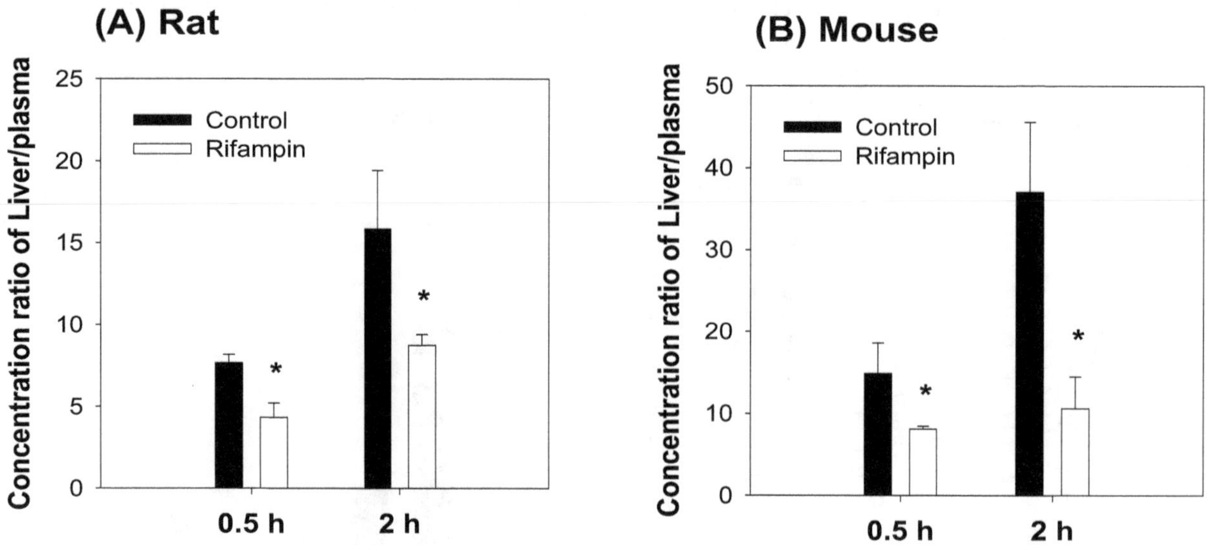

Figure 4. Effect of rifampin pre-treatment on the liver to plasma concentration ratios of compound K in (**A**) rats and (**B**) mice. Liver and plasma compound K concentration were measured following intravenous injection of compound K at a single dose of 2 mg/kg in the presence or absence of rifampin pre-treatment (20 mg/kg, per oral). Data expressed as mean ± standard deviation from four rats or four mice at different time points. *: $p < 0.05$ compared with control group.

3.3. Intestinal Metabolism of Compound K

To understand the metabolism of compound K, we measured PPD levels in the plasma, urine, and feces samples from rats and mice. Previous studies have demonstrated that compound K is metabolized to PPD via β-glucosidase in intestinal microbacterium (Figure 5) [1,13]. As shown in Figure 6, PPD was detected in the plasma and fecal samples from both mice and rats following intravenous injection of compound K (2 mg/kg). However, PPD was not detected in the rat and mouse urine samples. These results suggest that compound K was metabolized to PPD in both rats and mice.

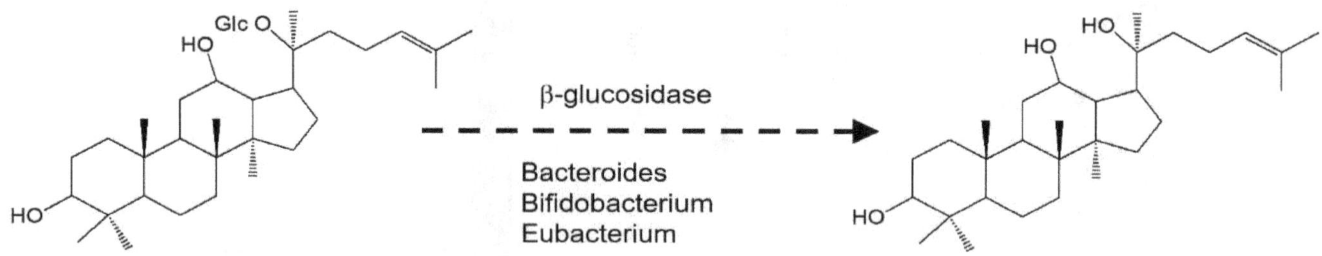

Figure 5. Structure and reported metabolic pathway of compound K to PPD. Glc: glucose; PPD: 20(S)-protopanaxadiol.

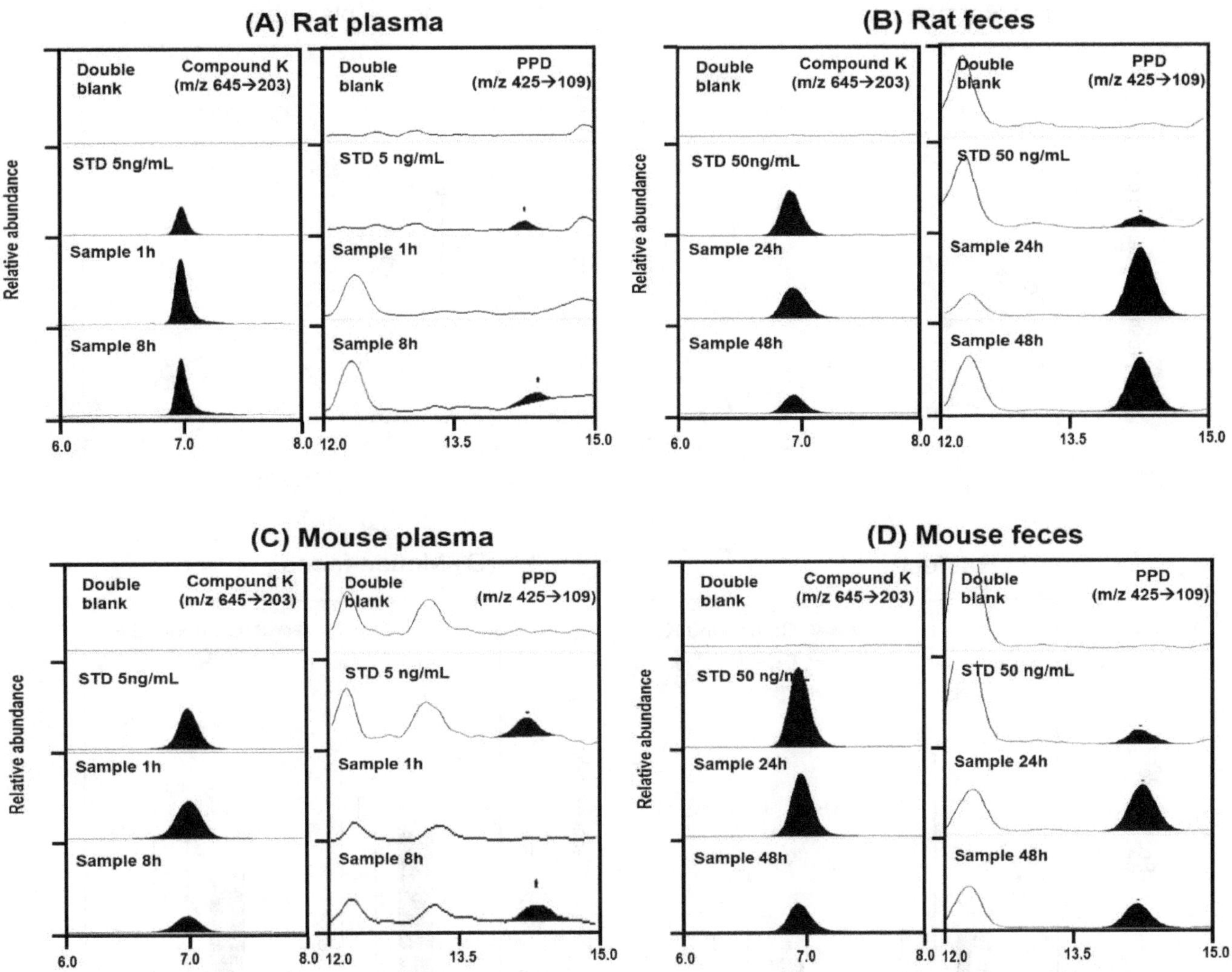

Figure 6. Representative multiple reaction monitoring chromatogram of compound K and PPD in plasma and feces samples collected from rats (**A**,**B**) and mice (**C**,**D**) following intravenous injection of compound K at a dose of 2 mg/kg.

The concentrations of compound K and PPD in plasma and feces samples are shown in Figure 7. Following intravenous injection of compound K, the PPD peak was detected in the mouse plasma samples between 4 and 24 h and in the rat plasma samples between 8 and 24 h (Figure 7A,B), suggesting that the metabolism of compound K to PPD might be slow process. The PPD concentration in the plasma samples at 48 h was below the lower limit of quantification (LLOQ; 5 ng/mL). The metabolic ratio calculated from the PPD to compound K ratio was much greater in rat plasma than in mouse plasma (0.02–0.08 in mouse vs. 0.2–1.6 in rat; Figure 7A,B). Similarly, the ratio of PPD to compound K in the feces samples was also significantly greater in rats than in mice (Figure 7C,D). The recovery of PPD was 3.4-fold higher than that of compound K in rat feces, whereas the recovery of PPD was 1.2-fold higher than that of compound K in mouse feces. As shown in Table 4, compound K and its metabolite PPD were exclusively recovered from feces but not from urine. The higher percentage of PPD recovery in rats compared to mice suggest the higher metabolism of compound K to PPD in rats compared to mice (Figure 1 and Table 3).

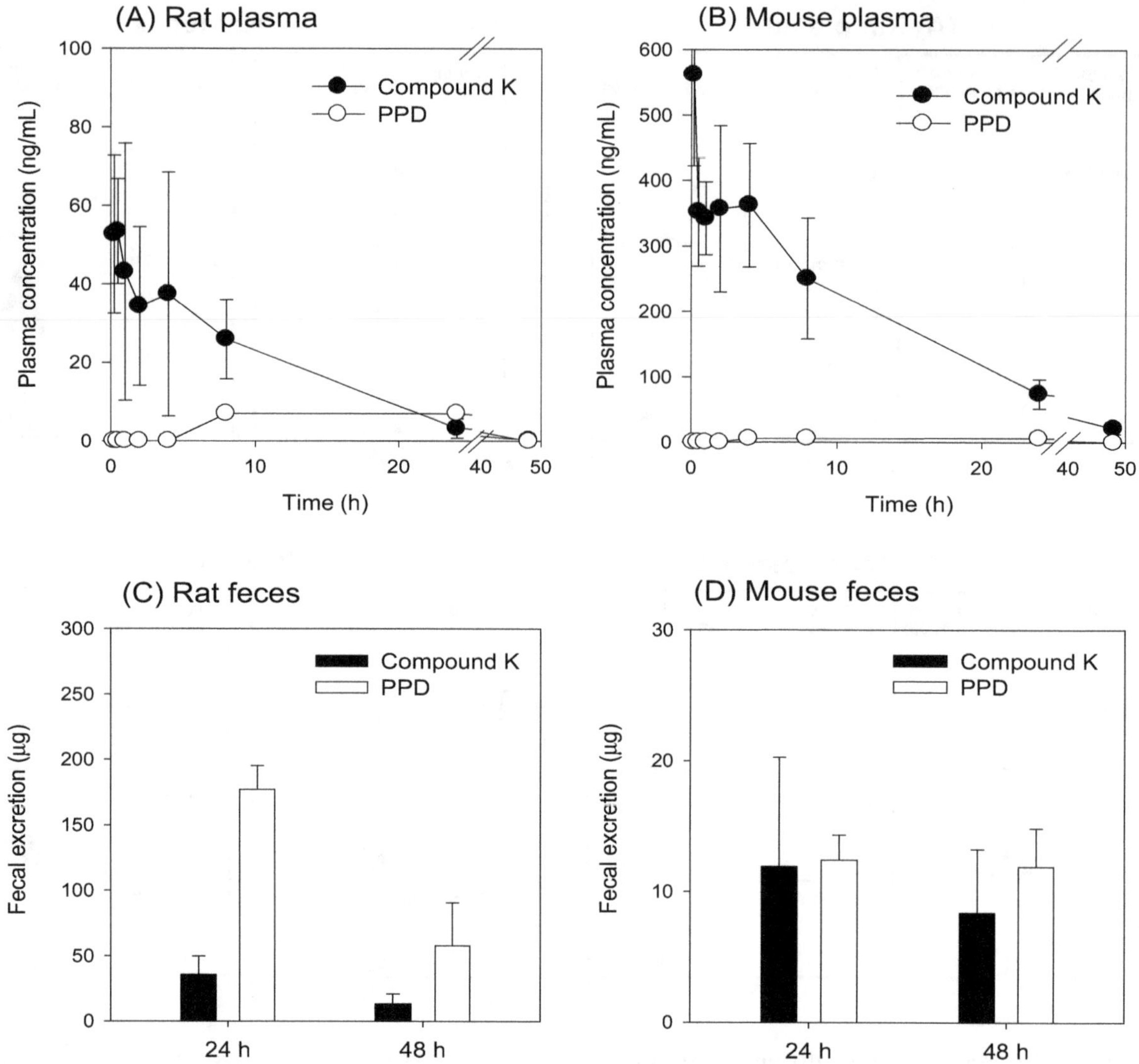

Figure 7. Plasma concentration vs. time profile of compound K and PPD (a metabolite of compound K) following intravenous injection of compound K at a single dose of 2 mg/kg in (**A**) rats and (**B**) mice. Fecal excretion of compound K and PPD following intravenous injection of compound K at a single dose of 2 mg/kg in (**C**) rats and (**D**) mice. Data expressed as mean± standard deviation of four samples for each time point.

Table 4. Recovery of compound K and PPD from urine and feces over the 48 h period following intravenous injection of compound K at a single dose of 2 mg/kg.

Species	Compounds	Recovery$_{48\ h}$ (% of Dose)	
		Feces	Urine
Rat	Compound K	13.8 ± 7.1	0.05 ± 0.03
	PPD	46.6 ± 4.9	ND
Mouse	Compound K	28.4 ± 5.9	0.02 ± 0.01
	PPD	34.4 ± 5.8	ND

ND: Not detected. Data expressed as mean ± standard deviation from four rats and mice per group.

Next, we compared the pharmacokinetic features of compound K between the bile-cannulated rats and the non-bile-cannulated rats. In the bile-cannulated rats, biliary excretion of compound K was very fast and most of the excreted compound K was collected during the 0–2 h period (Figure 8B), which could be due to high and fast distribution of compound K to the liver (Figure 2). Because of the fast distribution to the liver and biliary excretion, the plasma concentration of compound K disappeared rapidly and was best fitted to the one-compartment model. The elimination constant was estimated using 5 points and yielded 0.90 h^{-1} with an r^2 value of 0.92 (Figure 8A). The $T_{1/2}$ was calculated as 0.78 ± 0.11 h in the bile-cannulated rats. In contrast, the AUC value for compound K in the non-bile-cannulated rats was significantly greater than that of the non-bile cannulated control rats (Table 5). The plasma concentration profile of compound K in the control group showed 2-exponential decay. The elimination constant was estimated using 3 points and yielded 0.29 h^{-1} with r^2 value of 0.94 (Figure 9A). As results, $T_{1/2}$ was calculated as 2.40 ± 0.61 h in the non-bile cannulated rats, which is significantly greater than that in bile cannulated rats. The results suggest that the compound K enters into the systemic circulation from other compartments.

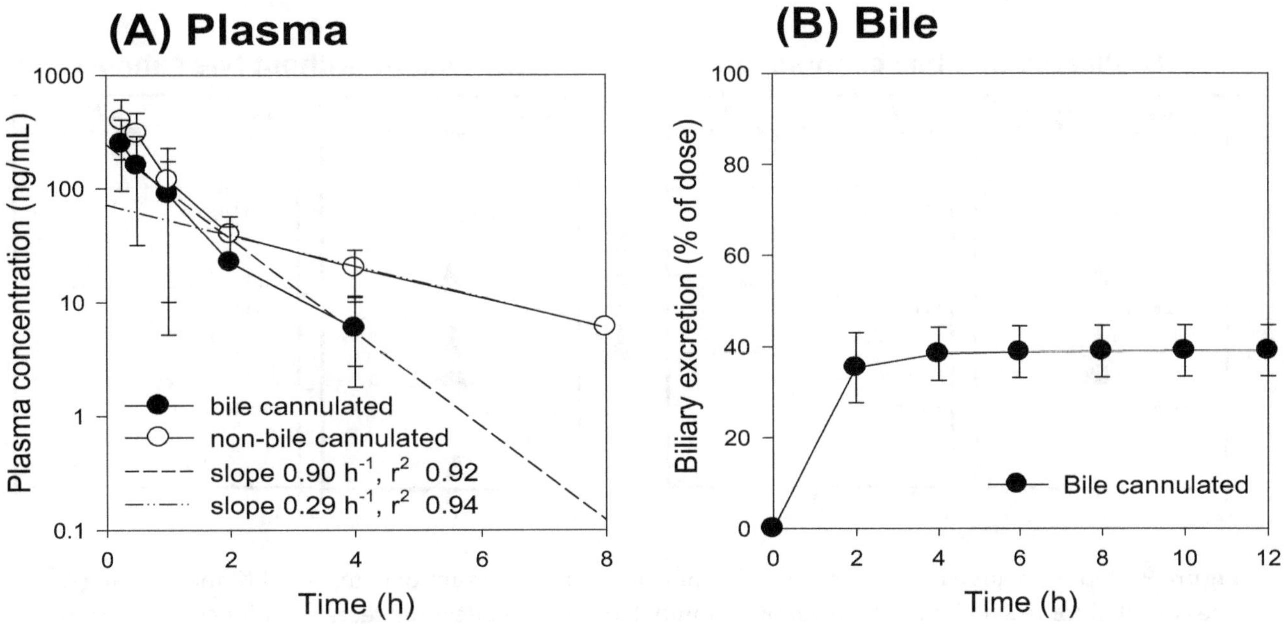

Figure 8. (**A**) Plasma concentration and (**B**) biliary excretion of compound K following intravenous injection at a single dose of 2 mg/kg in the bile-cannulated rats (•) and in the non-bile-cannulated rats (○). Dotted lines represent the regression line of the elimination constant from the plasma concentrations of compound K. Data expressed as mean ± standard deviation from four rats per group.

Table 5. Pharmacokinetic parameters of compound K in rats of bile cannulation and non-bile cannulation.

Characteristics	Parameters	Non-Bile Cannulated Rat	Bile Cannulated Rat
Plasma	C_0 (ng/mL)	451.13 ± 192.5	436.25 ± 325.8
	$AUC_{12\,h}$ (ng·h/mL)	496.38 ± 253.1	211.09 ± 87.32 *
	AUC_∞ (ng·h/mL)	517.19 ± 248.6	234.78 ± 125.6 *
	$T_{1/2}$ (h)	2.40 ± 0.61	0.78 ± 0.11 *
Excretion	$Bile_{12\,h}$ (% of dose)	-	39.1 ± 5.7

C_0: initial plasma concentration; $AUC_{12\,h}$ or AUC_∞: area under the plasma concentration-time curve from 0 to last sampling time or infinity; $T_{1/2}$: half-life. Data expressed as mean ± standard deviation from four rats. *: $p < 0.05$ compared with non-bile cannulated rat group.

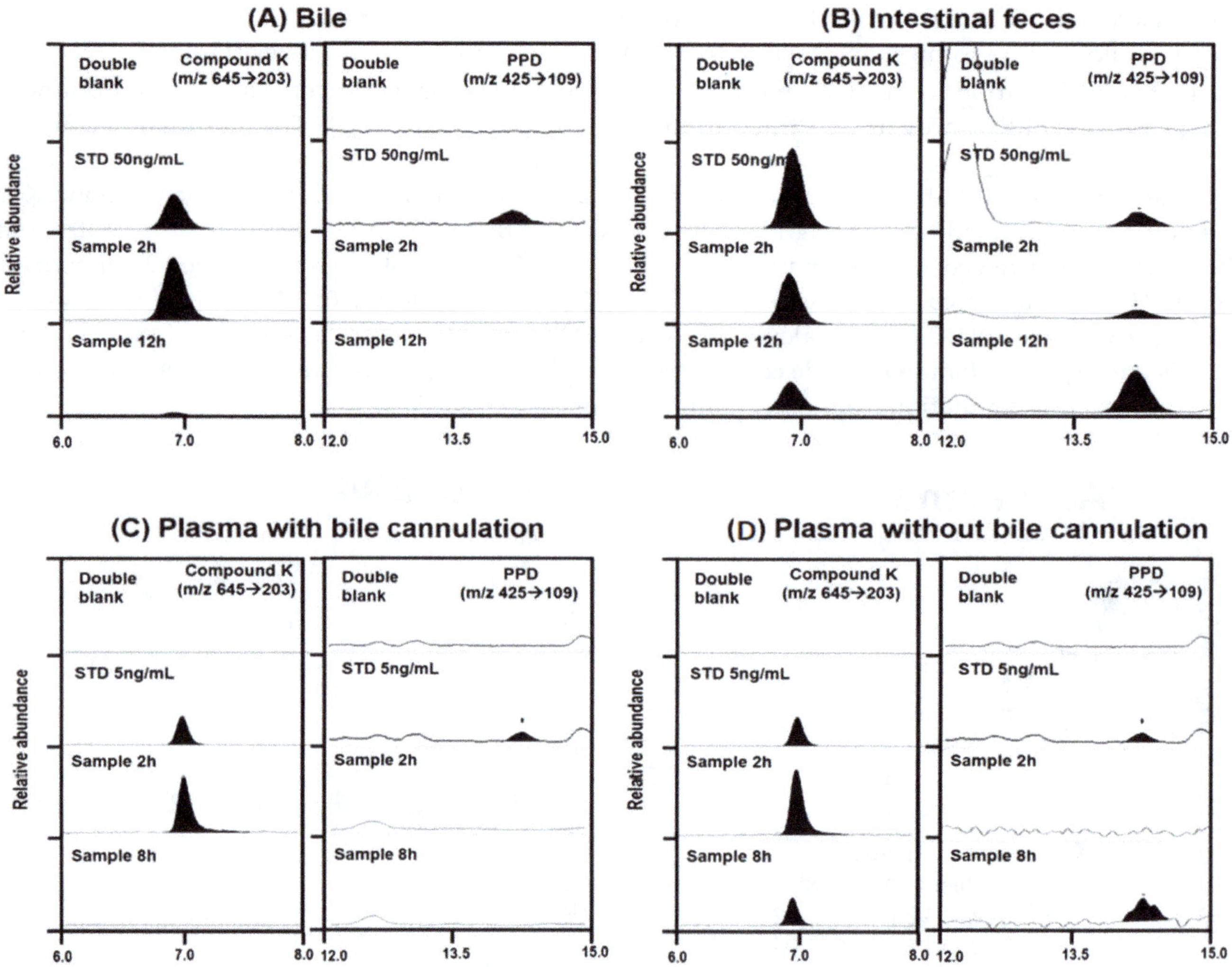

Figure 9. Representative multiple reaction monitoring chromatogram of compound K and PPD in (**A**) bile collected for 0–2 h and 2–12 h from bile cannulated rats, (**B**) intestinal feces samples collected from rats of non-bile cannulation at 2 or 12 h, (**C**) plasma samples taken at 2 and 8 h from bile cannulated rats, and (**D**) plasma samples taken at 2 and 8 h from rats of non-bile cannulation following intravenous injection of compound K (2 mg/kg).

We compared the compound K and PPD levels in the plasma and bile or intestinal feces samples in the bile duct cannulated rats and the control rats (without bile duct cannulation) to determine whether biotransformation from compound K to PPD occurred in the intestine or the plasma. For this, bile samples were collected for 0–2 h and 2–12 h period after administration of compound K from the rats with bile duct cannulation. Since these bile samples were collected directly from the bile duct, the compound K in the sample was distributed to the liver and excreted through the biliary route and, therefore, did not reach the intestinal microbiota. In control group, however, the compound K in the bile sample was excreted via the bile duct, so it reached the intestine and was subjected to further metabolism to PPD. As shown in Figure 8, all of the bile samples collected over a 12 h period from the bile-cannulated rats contained only compound K without PPD (Figure 9A), suggesting no further metabolism of compound K to PPD occurred in the rat plasma, liver, and bile. However, the intestinal fecal samples collected from rats without bile cannulation at 2 and 12 h following intravenous injection of compound K showed peaks for both compound K and PPD, and the amount of PPD was greater in the 12 h samples compared to the 2 h samples (Figure 9B). In addition, PPD was detected in the plasma samples at 8 h in the control rats (Figure 9D), suggesting that the PPD detected in the 8 h sample (which was not present in the 2 h plasma sample) was absorbed from the intestine after metabolism of compound K occurred. These results were consistent with the results from Figure 7A. Contrary to the control group, PPD was not detected in any of the plasma samples collected from bile-cannulated rats (Figure 9C). Taken together, the results suggest slow biotransformation of compound K to PPD in the rat intestine followed by the reabsorption of PPD into the systemic circulation.

4. Discussion

Although much is known about the pharmacological effects of compound K from in vitro studies and in vivo disease models, research on the pharmacokinetics as well as the relationship between the pharmacokinetics and drug response of compound K has been limited. This study aimed to understand the pharmacokinetic features of compound K and to compare its pharmacokinetic behavior in rats and mice, which are often used for disease models. Our study found that biliary excretion of compound K is a major elimination pathway, and fast and extensive liver distribution of compound K was demonstrated in both rats and mice. Oatp transporter-mediated hepatic uptake could be a possible mechanism for the dominant liver distribution compared to other tissues such as kidney, brain, spleen, and testis in both species (Figures 2 and 3), as the hepatic uptake of compound K was significantly inhibited by the pretreatment of rifampin, an Oatp inhibitor (Figure 4). Our results indicate that biotransformation of compound K to PPD occurs in the intestine rather than in the plasma or the liver, based on the comparison between the non-bile-cannulated rats and the bile-cannulated rats (Figure 9). The plasma PPD in rats and mice was then be reabsorbed from the intestine after the metabolism of the excreted compound K (Figures 1 and 9). In addition, the higher plasma AUC and $T_{1/2}$ of compound K in the non-bile cannulated rats compared with those in bile cannulated rats (Table 5) suggests that the excreted compound K was reabsorbed from the intestinal lumen. The $T_{1/2}$ of compound K in non-bile cannulated rats was significantly greater (2.40 ± 0.61 h) than in the bile-cannulated rats (0.78 ± 0.11 h). In addition, the $T_{1/2}$ of compound K in the control rats calculated from the plasma concentration profiles for 48 h was 7.3 ± 0.4 h (Table 3), which is much longer than the $T_{1/2}$ calculated from the plasma concentration profiles for 12 h. Also, the compound K plasma concentrations in the bile-cannulated rats could be fitted to a 1-compartment model while the plasma concentrations in the non-bile cannulated control rats showed 2-exponential decay (Figure 8A). Moreover, the compound K plasma concentrations increased or maintained at 2–4 h after sharply decreasing in the 0–2 h period, and then showed a slow decrease over the 4–48 h time period in both rats and mice (Figure 7A,B). This pattern could be attributable to the continuous reabsorption of compound K. The lipophilicity (LogP value 3.85 for compound K; 5.53 for PPD) and moderate permeability ($0.5–2 \times 10^{-6}$ cm/s for compound K; 1.15×10^{-6} cm/s for PPD) of compound K and PPD in Caco-2 cells also support the possibility of compound K and PPD reabsorption [3,7,14,15].

The features that differed most significantly between the rats and the mice were the higher plasma concentration (C_0 and AUC) of compound K in mice and the greater fecal recovery of PPD in rats. The percent recovery of the parent form (compound K) in mouse feces was much higher than in rat feces (13.8% in rats vs. 28.4% in mice), while the total fecal recovery (sum of compound K and PPD) was similar for both mice and rats (60.4% in rats vs. 62.8% in mice), suggesting that the elimination process of compound K could differ between rats and mice in addition to the difference in Vd between rats and mice. Multiple previous studies have shown that the tri- or four-glycosylated PPD-type ginsenosides (major components in red ginseng; Rb1, Rb2, Rc, and Rd) have been metabolized to compound K (monoglycosylated PPD-type ginsenoside) and further hydrolyzed to PPD, the final metabolite of the PPD-type ginsenosides, in the presence of lactic acid bacteria and gut microbiota [13,16]. Previous studies have reported that Bacteroides sp., Eubacterium sp., and Bifidobacterium sp. could potentially be involved in compound K metabolism and that subjects who have a higher composition of Bacteroides sp., Eubacterium sp., and Bifidobacterium sp. strains showed higher metabolism of Rb1 to compound K [1,10]. Similarly, differences in the composition of the intestinal microbiota in rats and mice could lead to the different rates of metabolism of compound K to PPD. Wang et al. identified the predominant bacterium in human and animal fecal samples [17]. In human fecal samples, 55% of colonies were identified as Bacteroides sp. but Eubacterium sp. and Bifidobacterium sp. were also present in smaller proportions. In mice and rat fecal samples, Bacteroides sp. showed relatively low expression compared to the human samples. Eubacterium sp. and Bifidobacterium sp. also showed lower expression than other species (Clostridium, Fusobacterium, and Peptosreptococcus sp.). The data suggests that there are species-dependent factors that play a role in the gut metabolism of ginsenosides in mice, rats, and humans. Kim et al. [10] reported that human subjects who have a higher proportion Bacteroides sp. in their fecal microbiota showed 6-fold higher metabolic activity of compound K than the subject group that had a smaller proportion of Bacteroides sp. Choi et al. [7] reported that inter-subject variability in gut metabolism of compound K rather than the intestinal absorption of compound K may contribute to the large inter-individual variations in plasma compound K concentrations. Therefore, differences in the gut metabolism of compound K could also explain the variability of the compound K pharmacokinetics between species. In addition, cytochrome P450 3A-mediated metabolism of PPD has been reported in human plasma and urine samples. Multiple oxidized PPD metabolites were identified from human plasma and urine samples, and cytochrome P450 3A is thought to be involved in this process [18,19]. This metabolism of PPD in the liver microsomes could explain the unrecovered portion of compound K and PPD at 48 h following intravenous administration of compound K in this study.

Collectively, the proposed enterohepatic circulation of compound K and PPD (Figure 10) could explain how compound K shows efficacy in vivo despite its fast and exclusive biliary excretion. The distribution of compound K into the liver could be a possible link to the hepatoprotective effect of compound K. However, the therapeutic use of compound K in other tissues and the oral administration of compound K and PPD may be limited because of poor aqueous solubility (33 μg/mL for compound K; <50 ng/mL for PPD) and P-gp-mediated efflux [4,14,15]. The use of nanocrystals for PPD formulation improved oral bioavailability and brain delivery [15]. The use of the metabolism inhibitor piperine [20] in the formulation of PPD and the use of P-gp inhibitor, α-Tocopheryl polyethylene glycol 1000 succinate (TPGS) [21], in the formulation of PPD and compound K enhanced oral absorption and anticancer efficacy of these PPD and compound K [22,23]. These approaches may provide a strategy for developing formulations for compound K and PPD by modulating their pharmacokinetic features.

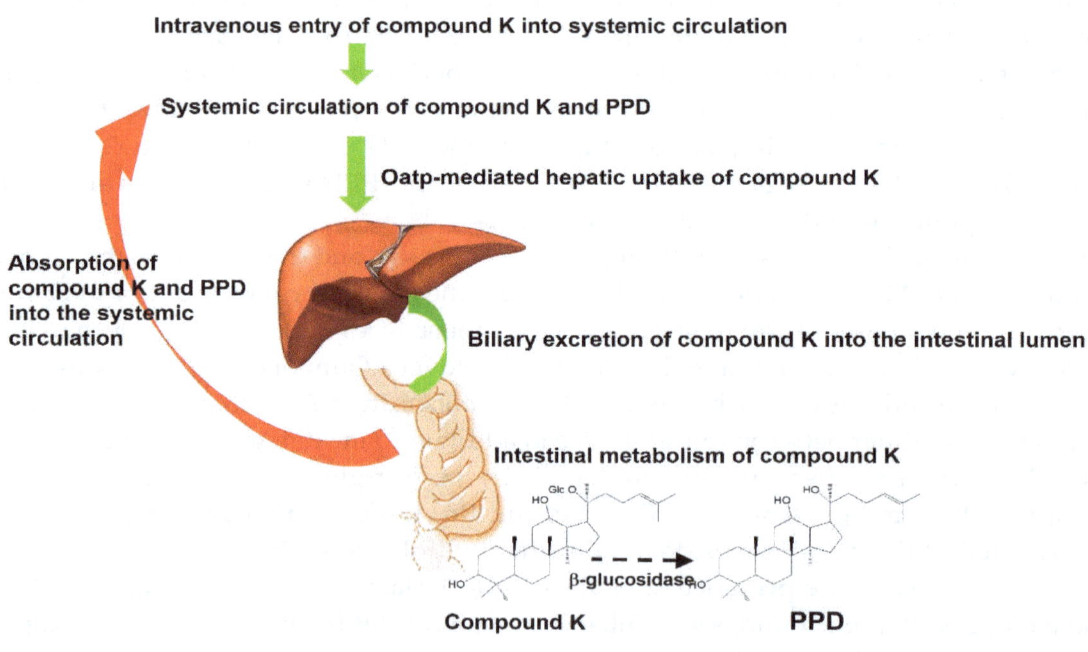

Figure 10. Proposed pharmacokinetic pathway of compound K following intravenous injection. Compound K underwent several steps: (i) intravenous entry of compound K into systemic circulation, (ii) Oatp-mediated hepatic uptake of compound K, (iii) biliary excretion of compound K into the intestinal lumen, (iv) metabolism of compound K into PPD in intestine, and (v) the absorption of compound K and PPD from intestine in blood.

5. Conclusions

This comparative pharmacokinetic and tissue distribution study of compound K in rats and mice demonstrated the following processes (Figure 10). First, the plasma concentration of compound K in mice was significantly greater than that in rats and the fecal recovery of PPD over 48 h in rats was greater than that in mice although the differences in elimination and metabolism between the two species need further investigation. Second, the plasma compound K was quickly distributed into the liver and underwent biliary excretion rather than renal elimination. The distribution of compound K into other major organs (kidney, heart, lung, pancreas, and testis) was much lower than in the liver for both rats and mice. Third, compound K was metabolized into PPD by the intestinal microbiota and the intestinal PPD metabolite was reabsorbed in the systemic circulation of both rats and mice.

Author Contributions: Conceptualization, M.-K.C. and I.-S.S.; Investigation, J.-H.J., B.K., S.L., M.-K.C., S.J. and I.-S.S.; Writing—Original Draft Preparation, J.-H.J. and B.K.; Supervision, M.-K.C. and I.-S.S.; Writing—Review & Editing, M.-K.C. and I.-S.S. All authors have read and agreed to the published version of the manuscript.

References

1. Yang, X.D.; Yang, Y.Y.; Ouyang, D.S.; Yang, G.P. A review of biotransformation and pharmacology of ginsenoside compound K. *Fitoterapia* **2015**, *100*, 208–220. [CrossRef]
2. Choi, I.D.; Ryu, J.H.; Lee, D.E.; Lee, M.H.; Shim, J.J.; Ahn, Y.T.; Sim, J.H.; Huh, C.S.; Shim, W.S.; Yim, S.V.; et al. Enhanced absorption study of ginsenoside Compound K (20-*O*-beta-(D-Glucopyranosyl)-20(S)-protopanaxadiol) after oral administration of fermented red ginseng extract (HYFRG) in healthy Korean volunteers and rats. *Evid. Based Complement. Alternat. Med.* **2016**, *2016*, 3908142. [CrossRef] [PubMed]
3. Paek, I.B.; Moon, Y.; Kim, J.; Ji, H.Y.; Kim, S.A.; Sohn, D.H.; Kim, J.B.; Lee, H.S. Pharmacokinetics of a ginseng saponin metabolite compound K in rats. *Biopharm. Drug Dispos.* **2006**, *27*, 39–45. [CrossRef] [PubMed]
4. Yang, Z.; Wang, J.R.; Niu, T.; Gao, S.; Yin, T.J.; You, M.; Jiang, Z.H.; Hu, M. Inhibition of P-glycoprotein leads to improved oral bioavailability of compound K, an anticancer metabolite of red ginseng extract produced by gut microflora. *Drug Metab. Dispos.* **2012**, *40*, 1538–1544. [CrossRef] [PubMed]
5. Chen, L.L.; Zhou, L.P.; Wang, Y.Q.; Yang, G.P.; Huang, J.; Tan, Z.R.; Wang, Y.C.; Zhou, G.; Liao, J.W.; Ouyang, D.S. Food and sex-related impacts on the pharmacokinetics of a single-dose of ginsenoside compound K in healthy subjects. *Front. Pharmacol.* **2017**, *8*, 636. [CrossRef]
6. Fukami, H.; Ueda, T.; Matsuoka, N. Pharmacokinetic study of compound K in Japanese subjects after ingestion of Panax ginseng fermented by Lactobacillus paracasei A221 reveals significant increase of absorption into blood. *J. Med. Food* **2019**, *22*, 257–263. [CrossRef]
7. Choi, M.K.; Jin, S.; Jeon, J.H.; Kang, W.Y.; Seong, S.J.; Yoon, Y.R.; Han, Y.H.; Song, I.S. Tolerability and pharmacokinetics of ginsenosides Rb1, Rb2, Rc, Rd, and compound K after single or multiple administration of red ginseng extract in human beings. *J. Ginseng Res.* **2018**. [CrossRef]
8. Jin, S.; Jeon, J.H.; Lee, S.; Kang, W.Y.; Seong, S.J.; Yoon, Y.R.; Choi, M.K.; Song, I.S. Detection of 13 ginsenosides (Rb1, Rb2, Rc, Rd, Re, Rf, Rg1, Rg3, Rh2, F1, Compound K, 20(S)-Protopanaxadiol, and 20(S)-Protopanaxatriol) in human plasma and application of the analytical method to human pharmacokinetic studies following two week-repeated administration of red ginseng extract. *Molecules* **2019**, *24*, 2618.
9. Kim, H.K. Pharmacokinetics of ginsenoside Rb1 and its metabolite compound K after oral administration of Korean Red Ginseng extract. *J. Ginseng Res.* **2013**, *37*, 451–456. [CrossRef]
10. Kim, K.A.; Jung, I.H.; Park, S.H.; Ahn, Y.T.; Huh, C.S.; Kim, D.H. Comparative analysis of the gut microbiota in people with different levels of ginsenoside Rb1 degradation to compound K. *PLoS ONE* **2013**, *8*, e62409. [CrossRef]
11. Jeong, H.U.; Kwon, M.; Lee, Y.; Yoo, J.S.; Shin, D.H.; Song, I.S.; Lee, H.S. Organic anion transporter 3- and organic anion transporting polypeptides 1B1- and 1B3-mediated transport of catalposide. *Drug Des. Dev. Ther.* **2015**, *9*, 643–653.
12. Jiang, R.; Dong, J.; Li, X.; Du, F.; Jia, W.; Xu, F.; Wang, F.; Yang, J.; Niu, W.; Li, C. Molecular mechanisms governing different pharmacokinetics of ginsenosides and potential for ginsenoside-perpetrated herb-drug interactions on OATP1B3. *Br. J. Pharmacol.* **2015**, *172*, 1059–1073. [CrossRef] [PubMed]

13. Park, S.E.; Na, C.S.; Yoo, S.A.; Seo, S.H.; Son, H.S. Biotransformation of major ginsenosides in ginsenoside model culture by lactic acid bacteria. *J. Ginseng Res.* **2017**, *41*, 36–42. [CrossRef] [PubMed]
14. Jin, X.; Yang, Q.; Cai, N. Preparation of ginsenoside compound-K mixed micelles with improved retention and antitumor efficacy. *Int. J. Nanomed.* **2018**, *13*, 3827–3838. [CrossRef] [PubMed]
15. Chen, C.; Wang, L.S.; Cao, F.R.; Miao, X.Q.; Chen, T.K.; Chang, Q.; Zheng, Y. Formulation of 20(S)-protopanaxadiol nanocrystals to improve oral bioavailability and brain delivery. *Int. J. Pharm.* **2016**, *497*, 239–247. [CrossRef] [PubMed]
16. Kim, D.H. Gut microbiota-mediated pharmacokinetics of ginseng saponins. *J. Ginseng Res.* **2018**, *42*, 255–263. [CrossRef] [PubMed]
17. Wang, R.F.; Cao, W.W.; Cerniglia, C.E. PCR detection and quantitation of predominant anaerobic bacteria in human and animal fecal samples. *Appl. Environ. Microbiol.* **1996**, *62*, 1242–1247. [CrossRef]
18. Ling, J.; Yu, Y.; Long, J.; Li, Y.; Jiang, J.; Wang, L.; Xu, C.; Duan, G. Tentative identification of 20(S)-protopanaxadiol metabolites in human plasma and urine using ultra-performance liquid chromatography coupled with triple quadrupole time-of-flight mass spectrometry. *J. Ginseng Res.* **2019**, *43*, 539–549. [CrossRef]
19. Hu, Z.; Yang, J.; Cheng, C.; Huang, Y.; Du, F.; Wang, F.; Niu, W.; Xu, F.; Jiang, R.; Gao, X.; et al. Combinatorial metabolism notably affects human systemic exposure to ginsenosides from orally administered extract of Panax notoginseng roots (Sanqi). *Drug Metab. Dispos.* **2013**, *41*, 1457–1469. [CrossRef]
20. Atal, C.K.; Dubey, R.K.; Singh, J. Biochemical basis of enhanced drug bioavailability by piperine: Evidence that piperine is a potent inhibitor of drug metabolism. *J. Pharmacol. Exp. Ther.* **1985**, *232*, 258–262.
21. Song, I.S.; Cha, J.S.; Choi, M.K. Characterization, in vivo and in vitro evaluation of solid dispersion of curcumin containing d-alpha-tocopheryl polyethylene glycol 1000 succinate and mannitol. *Molecules* **2016**, *21*, 31386. [CrossRef] [PubMed]
22. Jin, X.; Zhang, Z.H.; Sun, E.; Tan, X.B.; Li, S.L.; Cheng, X.D.; You, M.; Jia, X.B. Enhanced oral absorption of 20(S)-protopanaxadiol by self-assembled liquid crystalline nanoparticles containing piperine: In vitro and in vivo studies. *Int. J. Nanomed.* **2013**, *8*, 641–652.
23. Yang, L.; Zhang, Z.H.; Hou, J.; Jin, X.; Ke, Z.C.; Liu, D.; Du, M.; Jia, X.B.; Lv, H.X. Targeted delivery of ginsenoside compound K using TPGS/PEG-PCL mixed micelles for effective treatment of lung cancer. *Int. J. Nanomed.* **2017**, *12*, 7653–7667. [CrossRef] [PubMed]

9

Large Volume Direct Injection Ultra-High Performance Liquid Chromatography–Tandem Mass Spectrometry-Based Comparative Pharmacokinetic Study between Single and Combinatory Uses of *Carthamus tinctorius* Extract and Notoginseng Total Saponins

Jinfeng Chen [1], Xiaoyu Guo [1], Yingyuan Lu [1], Mengling Shi [1], Haidong Mu [1], Yi Qian [1], Jinlong Wang [1], Mengqiu Lu [1], Mingbo Zhao [1], Pengfei Tu [1,2], Yuelin Song [2,*] and Yong Jiang [1,*]

1 State Key Laboratory of Natural and Biomimetic Drugs, School of Pharmaceutical Sciences, Peking University, Beijing 100191, China; chenjinfeng0513@163.com (J.C.); guoxiaoyu@bjmu.edu.cn (X.G.); luyingyuan2005@126.com (Y.L.); shimenglingbj@126.com (M.S.); a1538933944@163.com (H.M.); yiqian@163.com (Y.Q.); wang-jinlong@pku.edu.cn (J.W.); mengqiulu@163.com (M.L.); zmb_77@163.com (M.Z.); pengfeitu@bjmu.edu.cn (P.T.)

2 Modern Research Center for Traditional Chinese Medicine, Beijing University of Chinese Medicine, Beijing 100029, China

* Correspondence: syltwc2005@163.com (Y.S.); yongjiang@bjmu.edu.cn (Y.J.)

Abstract: The combination of *Carthamus tinctorius* extract (CTE) and notoginseng total saponins (NGTS), namely, CNP, presents a synergistic effect on myocardial ischemia protection. Herein, comparative pharmacokinetic studies between CNP and CTE/NGTS were conducted to clarify their synergistic mechanisms. A large volume direct injection ultra-high performance liquid chromatography–tandem mass spectrometry (LVDI-UHPLC-MS/MS) platform was developed for sensitively assaying the multi-component pharmacokinetic and in vitro cocktail assay of cytochrome p450 (CYP450) before and after compatibility of CTE and NGTS. The pharmacokinetic profiles of six predominantly efficacious components of CNP, including hydroxysafflor yellow A (HSYA); ginsenosides Rg_1 (GRg_1), Re (GRe), Rb_1 (GRb_1), and Rd (GRd); and notoginsenoside R_1 (NGR_1), were obtained, and the results disclosed that CNP could increase the exposure levels of HSYA, GRg_1, GRe, GRb_1, and NGR_1 at varying degrees. The in vitro cocktail assay demonstrated that CNP exhibited more potent inhibition on CYP1A2 than CTE and NGTS, and GRg_1, GRb_1, GRd, quercetin, kaempferol, and 6-hydroxykaempferol were found to be the major inhibitory compounds. The developed pharmacokinetic interaction-based strategy provides a viable orientation for the compatibility investigation of herb medicines.

Keywords: *Carthamus tinctorius* extract; notoginseng total saponins; comparative pharmacokinetic study; large volume direct injection; compatibility mechanism

---

1. Introduction

Myocardial ischemia-induced infarction is one of the leading causes of human death worldwide. The benefits of either *Carthamus tinctorius* extract (CTE) or notoginseng total saponins (NGTS) towards myocardial ischemia injury on rats have been well defined, and more interestingly, previous studies have demonstrated that better cardio-protective effects were observed when using their combination preparation (CNP) [1–3]. However, the underlying synergetic mechanisms of CTE and NGTS combination, their pharmacokinetic (PK) interactions in particular, still remain unclear.

It is widely accepted that the drug–drug interactions (DDIs) and herb–herb interactions (HHIs) can cause changes of pharmacokinetic profiles, which result in the possible improvement of drug efficacy and in the decrease of side effects, or vice versa [4,5]. However, most of the literature has merely focused on the pharmacokinetic profile variations of these primary components between individual dosing and combined use, but has overlooked the reasons responsible for the changed pharmacokinetic behaviors, which may be caused, at least in part, by cytochrome p450 (CYP450)- and/or transporter-mediated HHIs [6]. Therefore, the objective of this study was to gain insight into the synergistic actions between CTE and NGTS by determination of the pharmacokinetic profiles of six major active components from CTE and NGTS, as well as their CYP450-based synergetic mechanisms. An in vitro cocktail assay, which is an efficient and widely favored approach for CYP450-mediated HHIs, was employed to pursue the factors accounting for the different pharmacokinetic patterns before and after compatibility.

Our previous pharmacological evaluations optimized a relatively low dosage CNP for the anti-myocardial ischemia effect [2]. Furthermore, the cocktail method usually suffers from extensive CYP450 crossover within the probe substrates [7]. Therefore, the emerging demand is to develop a sensitive and efficient method for reliable detection and determination of the trace ingredients for the PK and cocktail studies. Attempts were made herein to propose and apply a large volume direct injection ultra-high performance liquid chromatography–tandem mass spectrometry (LVDI-UHPLC-MS/MS) method for direct and sensitive multiple-component PK and cocktail studies.

2. Materials and Methods

2.1. Plant Materials

Notoginseng total saponins (NGTS), containing ginsenoside Rg_1 (GRg_1, A_1, 26.6%), ginsenoside Rb_1 (GRb_1, A2, 32.5%), ginsenoside Rd (GRd, A3, 6.6%), ginsenoside Re (GRe, A4, 4.1%), and notoginsenoside R_1 (NGR_1, A5, 6.2%), prepared according to the Monograph of NGTS recorded in Chinese Pharmacopoeia [8], was purchased from Yunnan Plant Pharm. Co., Ltd. (Yunnan, China). Besides NGR_1, GRg_1, GRe, GRb_1, and GRd (Han et al., 2010), the remaining amount of around 25% ginsenosides in NGTS were further clarified as previously described [9]. *Carthamus tinctorius* extract, containing hydroxysafflor yellow A (HSYA; A9, 8.0%) and kaempferol-3-*O*-rutinoside (A11, 0.2%) was prepared following the protocol described in a previous report [1]. The chemical structures of the main components contained in CNP are shown in Figure 1. The chemical profiling based on LC–MS (Figure S1) and the detail chemical composition information were reported in our previous research papers [10]. The detailed information of other chemicals and reagents is shown in the Supplementary Materials section.

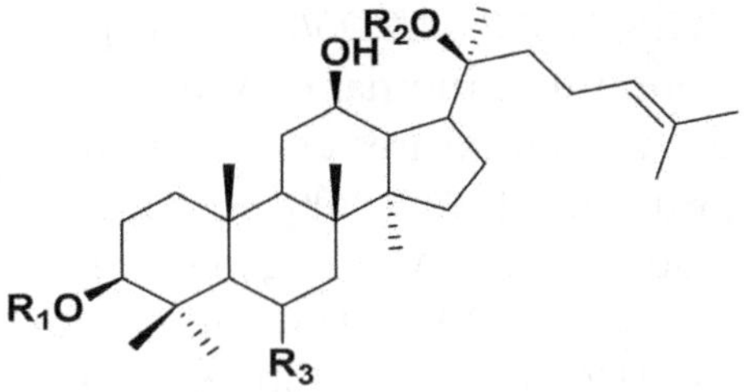

Compound	R_1	R_2	R_3
GRg_1(A1)	H	Glc	OGlc
GRb_1 (A2)	Glc^2-Glc	Glc^6-Glc	H
GRd (A3)	Glc^2-Glc	Glc	H
GRe (A4)	H	Glc	$OGlc^2$-Rha
NGR_1 (A5)	H	Glc	OGlc

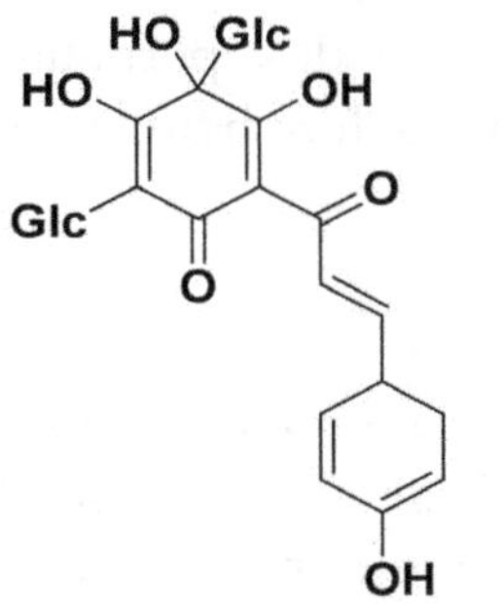

HSYA (A9)

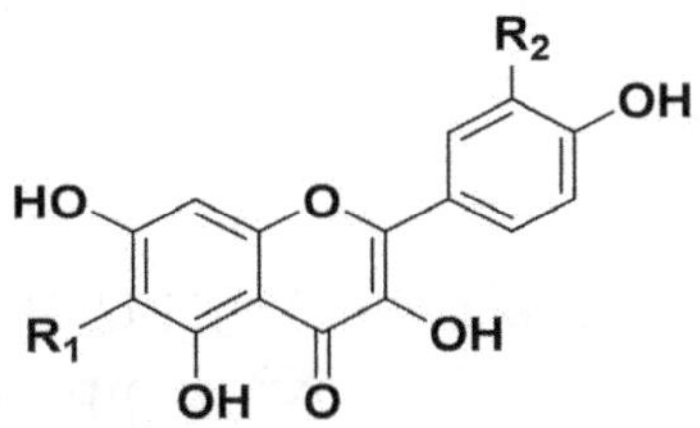

Compound	R_1	R_2
Quercetin (A16)	H	OH
Kaempferol (A17)	H	H
6-Hydoxykaempferol (A18)	OH	H

Figure 1. The chemical structures of the main components contained in the combination of *Carthamus tinctorius* extract and notoginseng total saponins (CNP).

2.2. Animals and Rat Liver Microsomes

Male Sprague-Dawley (SD) rats (12–14 weeks, 200–240 g) were provided by the Experimental Animal Center, Peking University Health Science Center. All animal experimental protocols were approved by the Biomedical Ethical Committee of Peking University Health Science Center (SYXK (Jing) 2016-0041, 23 December 2016). The animal experiments were carried out in accordance with the National Institutes of Health guide for the care and use of laboratory animals (NIH Publications no. 8023, revised 1978).

Pooled SD rat liver microsome (RLM, 20 mg/mL, LM-DS-02M, BDVH) were purchased from the Research Institute for Liver Diseases (Shanghai, China) Co. Ltd.

2.3. Plasma Pharmacokinetic Studies

CTE, NGTS, and CNP powders were dissolved using saline, and were orally dosed at 50 mg·kg^{-1}, 60 mg·kg^{-1}, and 50 mg·kg^{-1} CTE + 60 mg·kg^{-1} NGTS, respectively, whereas saline was administered to the vehicle group. Six rats were used in each group, and all rats fasted overnight but had free access to water prior to treatment. A terminal sampling design was used to collect blood samples at 0 (pre-dose), 0.08, 0.16, 0.25, 0.5, 1, 2, 3, 4, 6, 8, 12, 24, 48, 72, and 96 h. At each time, 0.5 mL of blood was collected in the heparin sodium tubes. Plasma was separated by centrifugation at 4000 rpm for 10 min and stored below −80 °C until bioanalysis. Oasis PRiME HLB SPE cartridges (1 cc/30 mg, Waters, Milford, MA, USA) were used to process the plasma samples (Supplementary Materials).

2.4. Incubation Procedure and CYP450 Activity Assay

The effects of CTE, NGTS, CNP, and 18 representative compounds (A1–A18, Supplementary Materials) on CYP450 activities were investigated using a pool of SD RLM following the procedure in [11]. Incubations were conducted at 37 ± 1 °C in 200 μL of incubation mixtures containing RLM (0.2 mg/mL), phosphate buffer saline (PBS) (pH 7.4, 0.1 mM), $MgCl_2$ (5 mM), nicotinamide adenine dinucleotide phosphate (NADPH) (1 mM), and CYP450 probe substrates (90/1.07/18/0.13/0.02/3.6/90 μM of phenacetin/omeprazole/tolbutamide/dextromethorphan/midazolam/chlorzoxazone/ bupropion, respectively). CYP450 inhibitors (triethylenethiophosphoramide/sulfaphenazole/ticlopidine/furafylline/

ketoconazole/quinidine/4-methylpyrazole for CYP2B6/2C9/2C19/1A2/3A4/2D6/2E1, respectively) were added as the positive control, and blank solvents (PBS containing methanol and/or dimethyl sulfoxide (DMSO)) were used as the negative control. The incubation mixtures also contained eight concentrations for CTE (2.5–200 μg/mL), NGTS (2.5–200 μg/mL), CNP (2.5–200 μg/mL), A1–A17 (5–200 μM), and A18 (0.25–10 μM). Reactions were initiated by adding the NADPH-generating system and terminated after 15 min by 200 μL of cold methanol containing 105 nM hydroxybupropion-[D_6] (OHBUP-[D_6]) and 5 nM 4′-hydroxydiclofenac-[$^{13}C_6$] (OHDIC-[$^{13}C_6$]) as internal standards (ISs). The mixture was placed in an ice bath for 30 min, and the precipitated protein was removed by centrifugation (12,000 rpm for 10 min at 4 °C) three times. Then an aliquot of 100 μL supernatant was diluted with 100 μL ultrapure water, and centrifuged at 12,000 rpm for 10 min, before being subjected to LVDI-UHPLC-MS/MS analysis.

2.5. LVDI-UHPLC-MS/MS Analysis

The generic layout of instrumentation setup of the LVDI-UHPLC-MS/MS was conducted on a Shimadzu UHPLC system consisting of two LC-20ADXR pumps, a DGU-20A3R degasser, and a CBM-20A controller (Kyoto, Japan) with a SCIEX 4500 QTRAP mass spectrometer mounted with an electron spray ionization (ESI) interface as well as an electronic 6-port/2-channel valve (Foster City, CA, USA). Analyst software package (version 1.6.2, SCIEX) was implemented to control and synchronize the entire system, and also for data acquisition and processing. A single analytical run was fragmented into two phases, namely, loading and elution phases, by switching the electronic valve (Figure 2). At the loading phase, the valve was maintained at A-channel. The specimen aliquot of large volume delivered from the auto-sampler was captured onto a guard column. Meanwhile, the pumps were responsible for delivering the mobile phase at a high flow rate, aiming to dilute the sample solvent, thus facilitating the candidate constituents to concentrate on the pre-guard column. Then, the valve was automatically switched to the B-channel to trigger the elution phase. The trapped components were flushed from the pre-guard column into an analytical column, and underwent multiple reaction monitoring (MRM) analysis on the optimized LC gradients. The detailed information of LVDI-UHPLC-MS/MS analysis for pharmacokinetic and cocktail studies is shown in the Supplementary Materials section.

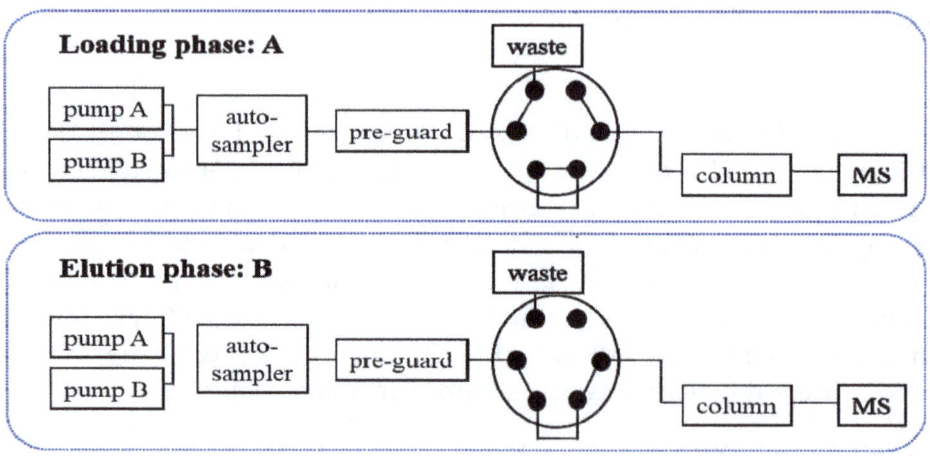

Figure 2. Connectivity sketch of the six-port/two-channel switching valve controlling the large volume direct injection ultra-high performance liquid chromatography–tandem mass spectrometry (LVDI-UHPLC-MS/MS) system. At the loading phase, the valve was maintained at A-channel. The sample delivered from the auto-sampler was captured onto a pre-guard column. Meanwhile, the pumps delivered the mobile phase at a high flow rate. Then, the valve was automatically switched to the B-channel to trigger the elution phase. The trapped components were flushed from the pre-guard column into an analytical column.

2.6. Method Validations

Method validations for the pharmacokinetic and cocktail assays, in terms of specificity, linearity, and sensitivity; precision and accuracy; recovery and matrix effect; and stability, were individually carried out by following the U.S. Food and Drug Administration (FDA) Guidance on Bioanalytical Method Validation and Drug Interaction Studies [12].

2.7. Data Processing

Calibration data were fitted to linear calibration curves using $1/x^2$ weighting. For the PK study, the half-time ($T_{1/2}$), maximum plasma concentration (C_{max}), time to reach the maximum concentration (T_{max}), and area under concentration-time curve (AUC) were determined by non-compartmental method using Drug and Statistics 3.0 (DAS 3.0, Mathematical Pharmacology Professional Committee of China, Shanghai, China). For the cocktail assay, the activity is expressed as the percentage of activity remaining comparing with that of a control sample containing no inhibitor. Substrate inhibition data were analyzed using GraphPad Prism 6 (version 6.01; San Diego, CA, USA) in logistic regression. All the data were described as mean ± standard deviation (SD). Normality assumptions were tested by the Kolmogorov–Smirnov statistic setting $p = 0.10$ as the limit for rejection of the null hypothesis of normality. If the distribution of the data was normal with equal variances, a two-sided test was performed at the 5% level of significance. The Welch's correction was then applied when the underlying variances were not equal. When the assumption of normality must be rejected, the Mann-Whitney test, a non-parametric equivalent of the independent-measures t-test, was used.

3. Results

3.1. Injection Solvent Optimization

It is well known that the sample solvent and volume have large effects on the peak asymmetry and column efficiency [13]. Herein, we established a LVDI-UHPLC-MS/MS method, assisted by injection solvent optimization, for sensitive bioassays of the pharmacokinetic interactions and cocktail analysis of CTE and NGTS. Considering the solubility and the sample pretreatment methods (Supplementary Materials) of the target analytes, the mixed standard solution of the six reference compounds was diluted with methanol (MeOH)/water (H_2O) in a ratio of 20% increment ranging from 100% H_2O to 100% MeOH for the PK study, and all the six standards of the PK study showed the highest responses when using 40% or 60% aqueous MeOH as the injection solvent. The CYP450 probe substrates and their corresponding metabolites for the in vitro cocktail assay were chosen according to the FDA guide [14]. Likewise, the six metabolites for the cocktail assay showed the best chromatograms when the 25% aqueous MeOH was served as the sample solvent, with exception of 1′-hydroxymidazolam, for which 50% aqueous MeOH was selected as the injection solvent (Figure S2).

3.2. Optimization of the Loading Phase for the LVDI-UHPLC-MS/MS-Based Method

The instrument stability of the LVDI-UHPLC-MS/MS setup was first investigated, and the results indicated the LVDI-UHPLC-MS/MS could meet the demands of quantitation (Table S3). An analytical run of the LVDI-UHPLC-MS/MS-based method was fragmented into a loading phase and an elution phase. The gradient condition for the elution phase turned out to be the same as that of the regular UHPLC-MS/MS analysis. Thus, the optimization works were concentrated on the loading phase, including the flow rate, mobile phase, and dilution time. According to the optimized gradient programs of the elution phases, both PK and cocktail studies employed water as the mobile phase for their loading phase after evaluating the solvents ramped from 0% to 20% aqueous acetonitrile. The flow rate of the loading phase for the PK study was finally optimized as 3.0 mL·min^{-1} after assays of 0.4, 1.0, 2.0, and 3.0 mL·min^{-1} flow rates. Because the higher the flow rate, the lower the signal responses of paracetamol and 6-hydroxychlorzoxazone, the cocktail assay finally chose 0.4 mL·min^{-1} as the flow rate of the loading phase. It turned out that the dilution time did not have a profound effect on the total chromatogram by comparing 0.5, 1, and 2 min. Thus, the shortest time, 0.5 min, was chosen to promote the analytical efficiency. The corresponding bioanalytical method validations were carried out by following the FDA guidance [12], and the results demonstrated that the newly developed LVDI-UHPLC-MS/MS-based methods enabled reliable detection and precise determination of the multiple-component in PK and cocktail studies. The lower limits of quantitation (LLOQ) of most analytes (except Rb_1 and Rd) were lower than 60 pg/mL.

3.3. Comparative Multiple-Component PK Studies

Considering the bioavailability improvement of active ingredients is a key point of traditional Chinese medicine compatibility, we executed a multiple-component PK study. HSYA, GRb_1, GRd, GRe, GRg_1, and NGR_1 were the primary circulating compounds and the main cardio-protective components in CNP [15,16], and thus were chosen as the PK markers. Meanwhile, the optimized injection solvent and LVDI-UHPLC-MS/MS method were integrated to achieve a much more sensitive method for reliable quantification of these components in vivo. After validation (Figure 3, Tables S4–S7), the developed method was first applied to characterize the pharmacokinetic characters of HSYA, GRb_1, GRd, GRe, GRg_1, and NGR_1 in rat plasma. Their plasma concentrations versus time profiles are displayed in Figure 4 and Table S8. The combination group showed greater C_{max} and $AUC_{0\text{-}t}$ values (Table 1) of HSYA, GRg_1, GRb_1, NGR_1, and GRe over the individual extract groups. Exceptionally, GRd exhibited considerable $AUC_{0\text{-}t}$ and C_{max} between NGTS and CNP dosing groups, whereas significantly different $T_{1/2}$ values, which indicated the combination use of CTE and NGTS, may have accelerated the elimination processes of GRd. The reason may have been due to the hydrolysis of GRb_1 to GRd in vivo [17], resulting in a more complicated PK behavior of GRd than other compounds in CNP.

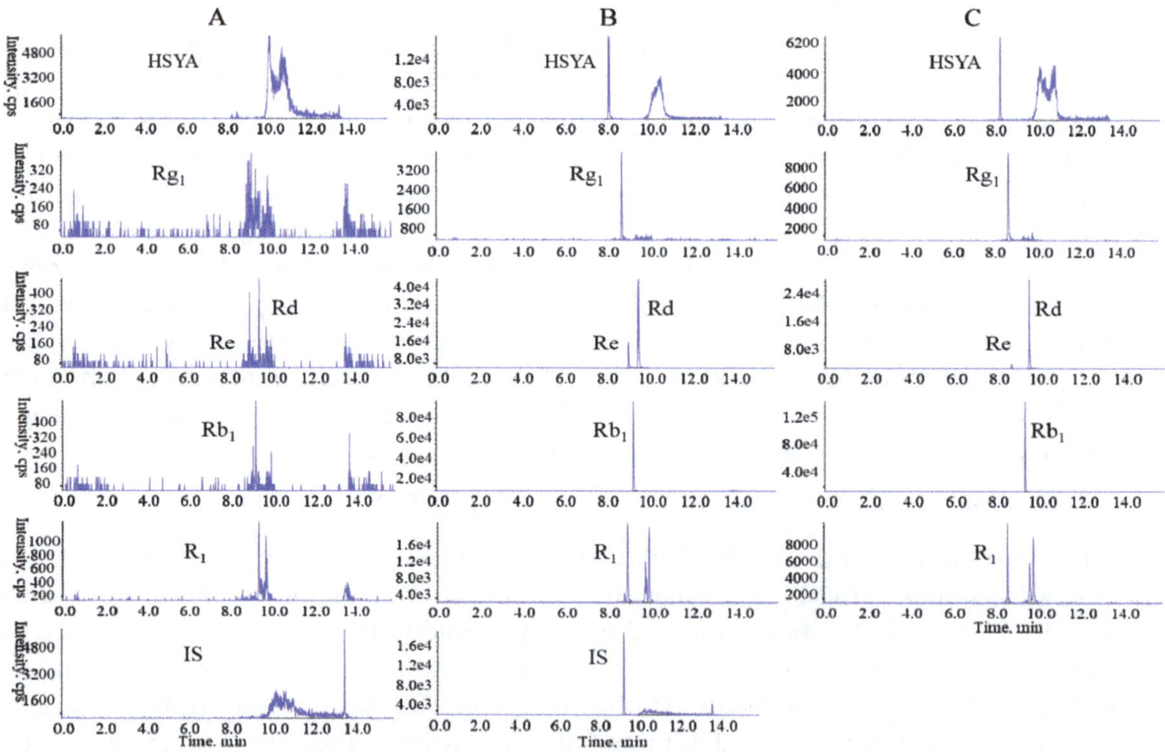

Figure 3. Representative multiple reaction monitoring (MRM) chromatograms of target analytes in rat plasma in a positive mode: (**A**) blank plasma; (**B**) blank plasma spiked with six chemical standards and internal standards (IS); (**C**) plasma sample collected at 2 h following oral administration of extract CNP (*Carthamus tinctorius* extract (CTE) 50 mg/kg + notoginseng total saponins (NGTS) 60 mg/kg) to rats.

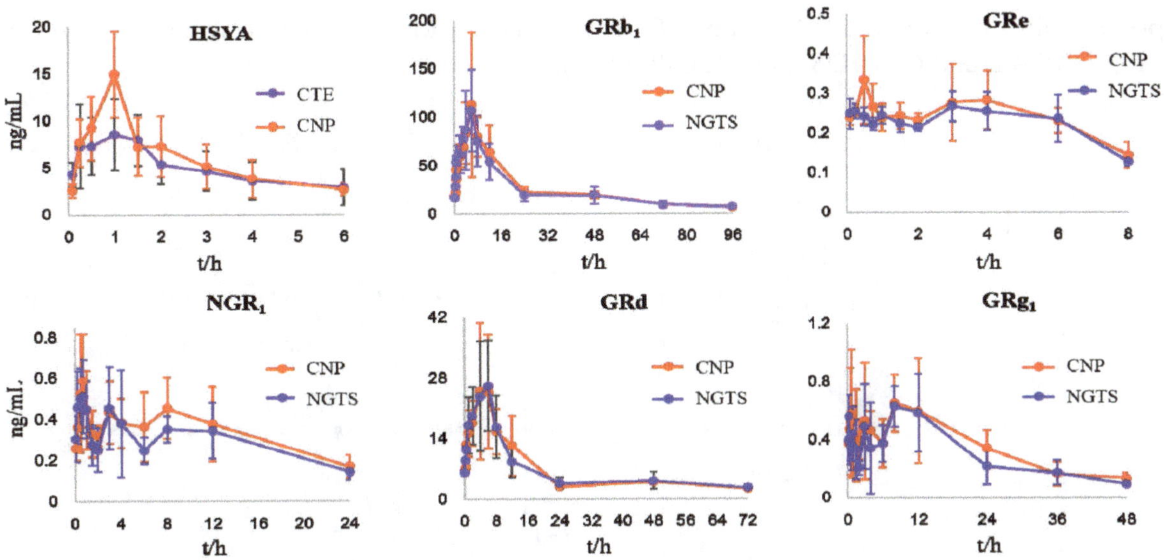

Figure 4. Mean plasma concentration-time profiles of the six analytes in rats after oral administration of CTE, NGTS, and CNP. Each point represents the mean ± SD (n = 6).

Table 1. Pharmacokinetic parameters of hydroxysafflor yellow A (HSYA), ginsenoside Re (GRe), ginsenoside Rb1 (GRb_1), ginsenoside Rd (GRd), ginsenoside Rg_1 (GRg_1), and notoginsenoside R_1 (NGR_1) after oral administration of CTE, NGTS, and CNP to rats. Each point represents the mean ± SD (n = 6).

Analyte	Group	$t_{1/2}$ (h)	T_{max} (h)	C_{max} ($ng{\cdot}mL^{-1}$)	AUC_{0-t} ($ng{\cdot}h{\cdot}mL^{-1}$)	$AUC_{0-\infty}$ ($ng{\cdot}h{\cdot}mL^{-1}$)
HSYA	CTE	2.01 ± 0.34	0.88 ± 0.54	12.16 ± 3.09	33.05 ± 10.70	33.85 ± 10.78
	CNP	1.68 ± 0.79	1.17 ± 0.41	15.17 ± 4.39	38.33 ± 8.42	38.94 ± 8.60
NGR_1	NGTS	10.53 ± 3.06	1.15 ± 1.06	0.64 ± 0.18	6.30 ± 2.41	8.14 ± 3.60
	CNP	12.36 ± 4.48	1.04 ± 0.97	0.79 ± 0.18	8.12 ± 1.53	11.49 ±3.54
GRb_1	NGTS	36.89 ± 9.65	5.50 ± 1.80	113.08 ± 41.78	2317.66 ± 682.70	2808.87 ± 617.99
	CNP	34.47 ± 8.45	6.33 ± 3.45	129.00 ± 65.97	2472.33 ± 394.72	2816.01 ± 563.44
GRd	NGTS	42.75 ± 8.84 *	4.50 ± 1.76	29.43 ± 10.69	460.90 ± 117.22	618.90 ± 157.23
	CNP	27.79 ± 6.94	6.33 ± 3.44	31.07 ± 16.78	459.04 ± 51.04	549.10 ± 50.09
GRg_1	NGTS	11.68 ± 2.09 *	4.71 ± 3.71	0.78 ± 0.13	13.99 ± 5.03	16.72 ± 3.93
	CNP	15.11 ± 8.89	5.38 ± 4.66	1.04 ± 0.34	16.69 ± 3.42	20.23 ± 3.35
GRe	NGTS	5.25 ± 2.27	2.60 ± 0.89*	0.29 ± 0.04*	1.82 ± 0.19	2.90 ± 0.60
	CNP	5.99 ± 3.86	0.80 ± 0.41	0.39 ± 0.08	1.93 ± 0.19	3.33 ± 1.13

*: $p < 0.05$, versus the combination group. T_{max}: the time of peak concentration; $t_{1/2}$: half-life; C_{max}: the peak or maximum concentration; AUC: area under concentration-time curve. For abbreviations of analytes A6–A18, please refer to the Supplementary Materials section.

3.4. CYP450-Mediated Herb–Herb Interactions

To investigate the possible HHIs between NGTS and CTE, an in vitro cocktail assay involving seven probe substrates was conducted, with the assistance of LVDI-UHPLC-MS/MS method to avoid CYP450 crossovers (Figure 5, Tables S9–S11). The incubation system was optimized in the aspects of substrate choice, enzyme concentration, incubation time, and substrate concentration (Figures S3–S4, Table S12), following the guidance of the FDA [14]. According to the half inhibiting concentration (IC_{50}) values of CTE, NGTS, and CNP (Table 2), CTE showed weak inhibition on CYP1A2, CYP2D6, and CYP2C9 and moderate inhibition on CYP2B6 and CYP2E1, whereas NGTS presented much more potent inhibitions on all these detected CYP450s than CTE (Table 2). After combination, CNP showed more potent inhibition on CYP1A2 than CTE and NGTS, and more potent inhibition on CYP2C9, CYP2C19, CYP3A4, and CYP2D6 than CTE (Table 2).

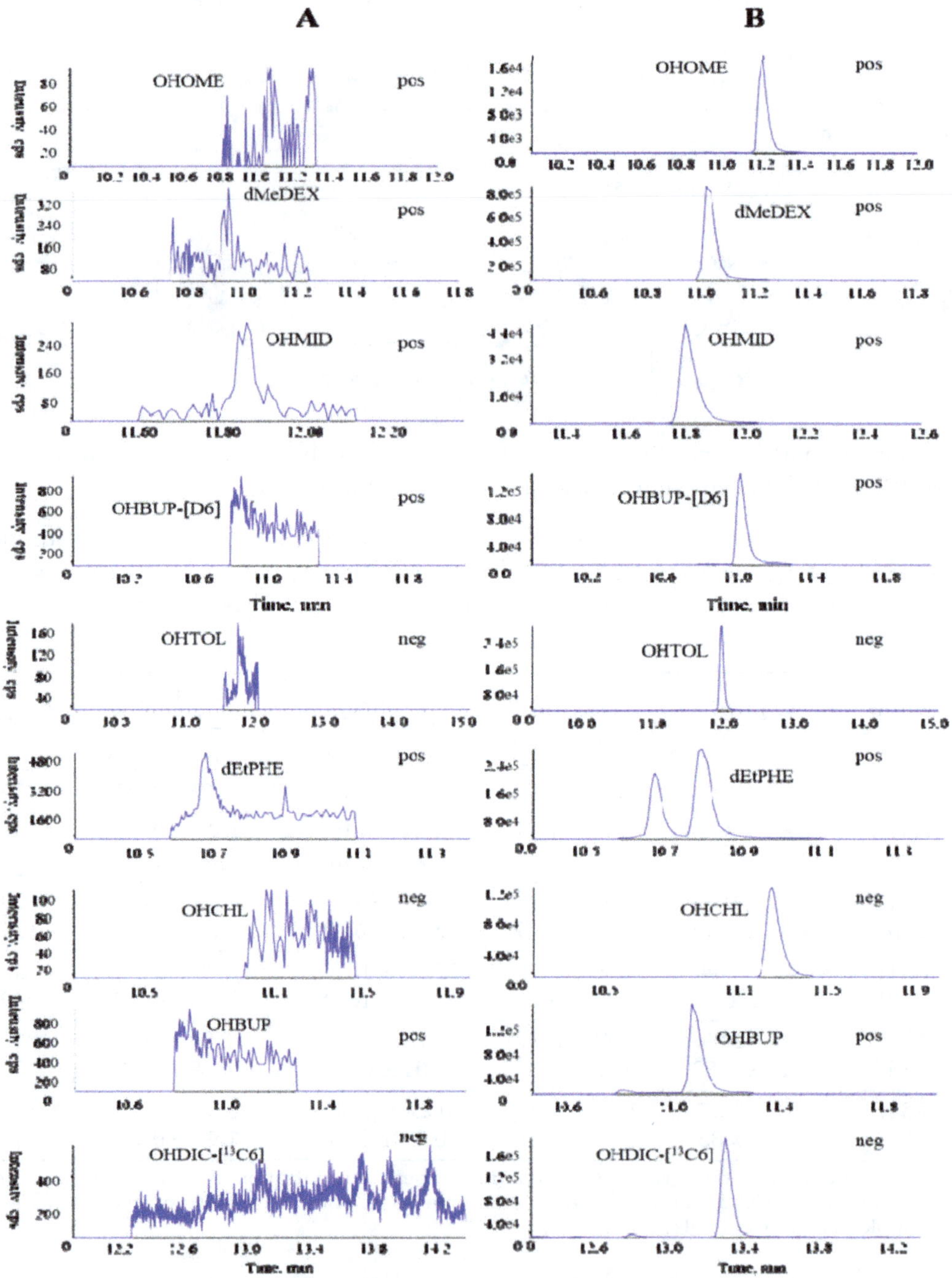

Figure 5. Representative MRM chromatograms of all probe metabolites and two ISs in the incubated rat microsomal sample with no substrate cocktails: (**A**) blank microsomal sample, (**B**) blank microsomal sample spiked with seven chemical standards and two ISs monitored in a polarity switching mode.

Table 2. IC_{50} values of CTE, NGTS, CNP and the 18 representative compounds for inhibiting cytochrome p450 (CYP450) isozymes.

No.	IC_{50} (μg·mL^{-1}/μM) #						
	CYP2C9	CYP2E1	CYP2C19	CYP2D6	CYP2B6	CYP1A2	CYP3A4
CNP	21.66 ± 1.15	31.85 ± 1.15	62.95 ± 1.17	25.27 ± 0.25	52.19 ± 2.24	26.36 ± 6.98	91.77 ± 5.16
CTE	183.30 ± 17.98	35.47 ± 2.98	>200	126.17 ± 17.63	58.09 ± 13.41	138.60 ± 14.36	>200
NGTS	*9.32 ± 0.56*	16.12 ± 2.59	40.85 ± 6.98	*12.23 ± 4.25*	43.90 ± 7.91	60.68 ± 2.26	106.27 ± 14.00
GRg_1 (A1)	36.49 ± 1.32	34.08 ± 1.76	78.12 ± 5.25	55.73 ± 6.08	*11.02 ± 0.87*	*13.09 ± 8.24*	39.25 ± 4.57
GRb_1 (A2)	17.57 ± 2.03	27.96 ± 2.39	16.80 ± 2.52	17.06 ± 1.29	120.83 ± 10.89	*5.84 ± 0.14*	30.04 ± 2.47
GRd (A3)	73.01 ± 3.71	43.46 ± 3.06	71.36 ± 14.28	64.81 ± 11.68	>200	*4.36 ± 2.31*	61.43 ± 14.32
GRe (A4)	>200	25.59 ± 3.03	50.53 ± 15.39	>200	39.40 ± 4.81	94.41 ± 4.52	75.11 ± 7.24
NGR_1 (A5)	154.47 ± 16.65	121.70 ± 8.96	107.59 ± 29.58	20.42 ± 3.45	>200	112.07 ± 7.72	84.59 ± 1.79
A6	55.84 ± 3.40	40.76 ± 1.65	53.67 ± 0.22	19.46 ± 2.83	114.70 ± 3.04	52.77 ± 1.93	26.45 ± 1.39
A7	80.47 ± 1.05	*13.59 ± 0.60*	18.50 ± 1.60	31.02 ± 4.17	177.17 ± 4.21	153.27 ± 8.73	126.70 ± 4.24
A8	*1.21 ± 0.51*	*9.06 ± 1.85*	111.26 ± 21.57	*10.54 ± 1.11*	>200	>200	34.38 ± 9.16
A9 (HSYA)	*0.17 ± 0.02*	*0.73 ± 0.15*	49.33 ± 3.28	*0.14 ± 0.06*	>200	>200	*9.42 ± 2.26*
A10	39.06 ± 0.09	>200	>200	>200	>200	>200	>200
A11	24.92 ± 4.96	*5.45 ± 1.37*	>200	64.55 ± 7.71	17.33 ± 0.96	53.17 ± 6.12	16.18 ± 4.30
A12	>200	>200	>200	98.56 ± 12.30	>200	>200	>200
A13	93.00 ± 2.56	*10.22 ± 0.65*	48.91 ± 4.36	37.12 ± 8.85	21.02 ± 2.31	*13.35 ± 2.27*	58.52 ± 0.66
A14	>200	>200	>200	>200	>200	>200	>200
A15	>200	>200	>200	>200	>200	127.47 ± 6.55	>200
A16	*13.48 ± 2.41*	20.29 ± 4.13	46.35 ± 7.05	31.11 ± 3.91	68.48 ± 9.88	41.22 ± 3.18	73.74 ± 13.64
A17	*14.92 ± 4.24*	32.46 ± 5.79	70.38 ± 1.18	59.17 ± 1.01	>200	21.46 ± 4.50	117.00 ± 6.77
A18	*2.13 ± 0.64*	*4.27 ± 1.30*	*1.79 ± 0.52*	*0.98 ± 0.38*	*4.42 ± 1.31*	*0.12 ± 0.01*	*2.48 ± 0.48*

#: Values were obtained from triplicate tests, and presented as mean ± SD. The units of IC_{50} values for CTE, NGTS, and CNP are μg·mL^{-1}, whereas for the 18 single components are μM. Potent inhibitors (IC_{50} < 15 μM for 1A2, 2C9, 2C19, 2D6, 2B6, and 3A4) are presented in italic. For abbreviations of analytes A6–A18, please refer to the Supplementary Materials section.

To identify the major CNP components responsible for the inhibition, 18 representative components from CNP were evaluated by the cocktail assays. The results (Table 2) showed that HSYA and ginsenosides showed high or moderate inhibition activities on the seven CYP450 isozymes. Although flavonoid glycosides showed moderate or weak inhibition activities, or even no inhibition activities (IC_{50} values of >200 μM, Table 2), the flavonoid aglycones quercetin (A16), kaempferol (A17), and 6-hydoxykaempferol (A18), in contrast, exhibited potent inhibitory activities against the seven CYP450 isozymes. In particular, 6-hydroxykaempferol (A18) showed remarkably stronger inhibitory activities on the seven CYP450 isozymes (IC_{50} < 5 μM, Table 2). In conclusion, the ginsenosides GRg_1 (A1), GRb_1 (A2), and GRd (A3), and the flavonoids 6-hydoxykaempferol-3-*O*-glucoside (A6), kaempferol-3-*O*-glucoside (A7), anhydroxysafflor yellow B (AHSYB, A8), hydroxysafflor yellow A (HSYA, A9), 6-hydroxykaempferol-3,6-di-*O*-glucoside (A13), quercetin (A16), kaempferol (A17), and 6-hydroxykaempferol (A18) were presented as being the intensive inhibitors to different CYP450s ($IC_{50} \leq 15$ μM). Among them, GRg_1 (A1), GRb_1 (A2), GRd (A3), quercetin (A16), kaempferol (A17), and 6-hydroxykaempferol (A18) were the main active components of CNP for the inhibition of CYP1A2.

3.5. Discussion

Herbal pair, the most fundamental and simplest form of Chinese herbal medicine formula, has been favored for centuries because of its better therapeutic outcomes and fewer side effects [18]. Herein, we primarily aimed to clarify the compatibility mechanisms between NGTS and CTE from PK interactions. Given the low dosage, more efforts were paid onto the detection and quantification of trace CNP-derived components in vivo. We found the injection solvent extensively affected the chromatographic performances. Increasing the injection volume could advance the sensitivity owing to the subjection of larger amounts of analytes [19]. However, the solvent effect might be initiated by directly injecting large volume of solution onto the chromatographic column without any additional treatment. Increasing the flow rate of the mobile phase could guarantee the dilution of the injection solvent and retention of the target analytes, which should be a practical choice to minimize, or even avoid the solvent effect. However, a rapid flow rate gave rise to a higher back pressure. Therefore, the evaporation–reconstitution step often involved loading the sufficient quantity of sample onto the column for LC–MS analysis. Fortunately, the electronic six-port/two-channel valve mounted on the QTRAP system can be applied as a viable solution to split the back pressure. Therefore, LVDI-UHPLC-MS/MS method was proposed. With the LVDI-UHPLC-MS/MS method, the sample can be directly injected into LC-MS analysis without any evaporation–reconstitution step, which is time-consuming and risks crucial chemical degradation during the evaporation procedure. Under the assistance of the injection solvent optimization, the validated LVDI-UHPLC-MS/MS-based method turned out to be extremely sensitive, accurate, and qualified for the bioassay measurement.

The pharmacokinetic results of HSYA, GRg_1, GRe, GRb_1, and NGR_1 indicated that after combination, the absorption of these active components was increased inferred from their higher C_{max} and $AUC_{0\text{-}t}$ values over that of the individual extract groups (Table 1). The increment of C_{max} and $AUC_{0\text{-}t}$ values suggested that CYP450-mediated HHIs between CTE and NGTS may primarily account for the compatibility mechanisms of CTE and NGTS. An in vitro cocktail assay was then carried out to find the clues being responsible for HHIs between CTE and NGTS. The results showed CNP exhibited more potent inhibition on CYP1A2 (Table 2), the key enzyme involved in the oxidation reactions of most xenobiotics [20], compared with CTE and NGTS. In order to search for the single components contained in CNP responsible for the inhibition of CYP1A2 and other CYP450s, 18 main components from CNP were evaluated for their inhibition on CYP450s.

The results showed that GRg_1 (A1), GRb_1 (A2), GRd (A3), 6-hydoxykaempferol-3-*O*-glucoside (A6), kaempferol-3-*O*-glucoside (A7), anhydroxysafflor yellow B (AHSYB, A8), hydroxysafflor yellow A (HSYA, A9), 6-hydroxykaempferol-3,6-di-*O*-glucoside (A13), quercetin (A16), kaempferol (A17), and 6-hydroxykaempferol (A18) were the main active components for the CYP450 inhibition, and GRg_1

(A1), GRb_1 (A2), GRd (A3), quercetin (A16), kaempferol (A17), and 6-hydroxykaempferol (A18) were the main active components for CYP1A2 inhibition.

To further discuss the possibility of in vivo interaction between CTE and NGTS, the inhibitions of GRg_1, GRb_1, GRd, HSYA, NGR_1, and GRe to CYP450s at their C_{max} levels were calculated by their respective "dose–response curve". The results (Table S13) showed GRg_1, GRb_1, GRd, HSYA, NGR_1, and GRe could not significantly inhibit CYP450s at their C_{max} levels, which is in accordance with the results that the combination use of CTE and NGTS can only increase the system exposures of these components to some extent.

4. Conclusions

In conclusion, the findings gained from the comparative pharmacokinetic investigations revealed there were pharmacokinetic interactions between CTE and NGTS, which may explain the integrative mechanisms of CNP and provide the experimental data and theoretical basis for further development and clinical applications of CNP. The developed LVDI-UHPLC-MS/MS method and pharmacokinetic interaction-based strategy provide a viable orientation for the compatibility investigation of herb medicines.

Supplementary Materials:
Figure S1. The total ion current chromatogram (TIC) of CTE; the corresponding chemical composition information was reported in previous research (Chen, et al., 2014; Analyst 139, 6474–6485). Figure S2. The optimization of sample solvents for the pharmacokinetic analysis (A) and the cocktail assay (B) (n = 3). Figure S3. Kinetic profiles for the enzymatic turnover of CYP450-mediated probe reactions. Figure S4. Inhibition curves of the seven positive inhibitors obtained from the substrate cocktail incubation. Table S1. Multiple reaction monitoring transitions and fragmentation parameters of six standards and IS1 for PK analysis. Table S2. Multiple reaction monitoring transitions and fragmentation parameters of seven metabolites and two internal standards (IS2 and IS3) for cocktail assay. Table S3. The instrument stability of the LVDI-UHPLC-MS/MS setup. Table S4. Regression equations, linear ranges, and low limits of quantification (LLOQ) of the six standards in rat plasma for the PK study. Table S5. Intra- and inter-day precisions and determination accuracies of six standards for the pharmacokinetic study. Table S6. Extract recoveries and matrix effects of six target constituents in rat plasma samples for the PK study. Table S7. Stability of the six CNP constituents in rat plasma samples for the PK study. Table S8. Plasma concentration time of the six target constituents after oral administration of CTE, NGTS, and CNP. Table S9. Regression equations, linear ranges, and LLOQs of the seven metabolites for the cocktail analysis. Table S10. Intra- and inter-day precisions and determination accuracies of the seven metabolites for cocktail analysis. Table S11. Extract recoveries and matrix effects of seven target constituents and two ISs for the cocktail analysis. Table S12. Michaelis constant (Km) determined for the enzymatic reaction of the probe substrates and the inhibition IC_{50} values were measured for the positive inhibitors of seven CYP450s. Table S13. Responses (% control) of HSYA, GRb_1, GRd, GRe, GRg_1, and NGR_1 at their C_{max} levels in the rat plasma.

Author Contributions: Conceptualization, P.T. and Y.J.; data curation, J.C.; funding acquisition, X.G. and Y.J.; investigation, J.C., Y.L., M.S., H.M., Y.Q., J.W., and M.L.; methodology, J.C., X.G., Y.L., M.S., and M.Z.; project administration, Y.J.; resources, P.T. and Y.J.; supervision, Y.J.; visualization, J.C.; writing—review and editing, J.C., Y.S., and Y.J. All authors have read and agreed to the published version of the manuscript.

References

1. Han, S.Y.; Li, H.X.; Ma, X.; Zhang, K.; Ma, Z.Z.; Jiang, Y.; Tu, P.F. Evaluation of the anti-myocardial ischemia effect of individual and combined extracts of Panax notoginseng and *Carthamus tinctorius* in rats. *J. Ethnopharmacol.* **2013**, *145*, 722–727. [CrossRef] [PubMed]
2. Meng, Y.; Du, Z.; Li, Y.; Wang, L.; Gao, P.; Gao, X.; Li, C.; Zhao, M.; Jiang, Y.; Tu, P.; et al. Integration of metabolomics with pharmacodynamics to elucidate the anti-myocardial ischemia effects of combination of notoginseng total saponins and safflower total flavonoids. *Front. Pharmacol.* **2018**, *9*, 667. [CrossRef] [PubMed]
3. Han, S.Y.; Li, H.X.; Bai, C.C.; Wang, L.; Tu, P.F. Component analysis and free radical-scavenging potential of Panax notoginseng and *Carthamus tinctorius* extracts. *Chem. Biodivers.* **2010**, *7*, 383–391. [CrossRef] [PubMed]
4. Zhou, D.; Andersson, T.B.; Grimm, S.W. In vitro evaluation of potential drug-drug interactions with ticagrelor: Cytochrome P450 reaction phenotyping, inhibition, induction, and differential kinetics. *Drug Metab. Dispos.* **2011**, *39*, 703–710. [CrossRef] [PubMed]

5. Dong, L.C.; Fan, Y.X.; Yu, Q.; Ma, J.; Dong, X.; Li, P.; Li, H.J. Synergistic effects of rhubarb-gardenia herb pair in cholestatic rats at pharmacodynamic and pharmacokinetic levels. *J. Ethnopharmacol.* **2015**, *175*, 67–74. [CrossRef] [PubMed]
6. Wang, L.; Zhang, D.; Raghavan, N.; Yao, M.; Ma, L.; Frost, C.E.; Maxwell, B.D.; Chen, S.Y.; He, K.; Goosen, T.C.; et al. In vitro assessment of metabolic drug-drug interaction potential of apixaban through cytochrome P450 phenotyping, inhibition, and induction studies. *Drug Metab. Dispos.* **2010**, *38*, 448–458. [CrossRef] [PubMed]
7. Spaggiari, D.; Geiser, L.; Daali, Y.; Rudaz, S. A cocktail approach for assessing the in vitro activity of human cytochrome P450s: An overview of current methodologies. *J. Pharm. Biomed. Anal.* **2014**, *101*, 221–237. [CrossRef] [PubMed]
8. Pharmacopoeia Committee. *Pharmacopoeia of the Peoples's Republic of China*; Part 1; Medical Science and Technology Press: Beijing, China, 2015; pp. 393–394.
9. Chen, J.; Guo, X.; Song, Y.; Zhao, M.; Tu, P.; Jiang, Y. MRM-based strategy for the homolog-focused detection of minor ginsenosides from notoginseng total saponins by ultra-performance liquid chromatography coupled with hybrid triple quadrupole-linear ion trap mass spectrometry. *RSC Adv.* **2016**, *6*, 96376–96388. [CrossRef]
10. Chen, J.; Tu, P.; Jiang, Y. HPLC fingerprint-oriented preparative separation of major flavonoids from safflower extract by preparative pressurized liquid chromatography. *J. Chin. Pharm. Sci.* **2014**, *23*, 6. [CrossRef]
11. Walsky, R.L.; Boldt, S.E. In vitro cytochrome P450 inhibition and induction. *Curr. Drug Metab.* **2008**, *9*, 928–939. [CrossRef] [PubMed]
12. U.S. Food and Drug Administration. Bioanalytical Method Validation Guidance for Industry. 2018. Available online: https://www.fda.gov/regulatory-information/search-fda-guidance-documents/bioanalytical-method-validation-guidance-industry (accessed on 18 February 2020).
13. Tsimidou, M.; Macrae, R. Reversed-phase chromatography of triglycerides-theoretical and practical aspects of the influence of injection solvents. *J. Chromatogr. Sci.* **1985**, *23*, 155–160. [CrossRef] [PubMed]
14. U.S. Food and Drug Administration. Clinical Drug Interaction Studies-Study Design, Data Analysis, and Clinical Implications Guidance for Industry. 2017. Available online: https://www.fda.gov/regulatory-information/search-fda-guidance-documents/clinical-drug-interaction-studies-cytochrome-p450-enzyme-and-transporter-mediated-drug-interactions (accessed on 18 February 2020).
15. Chen, J.F.; Song, Y.L.; Guo, X.Y.; Tu, P.F.; Jiang, Y. Characterization of the herb-derived components in rats following oral administration of *Carthamus tinctorius* extract by extracting diagnostic fragment ions (DFIs) in the $MS^{(n)}$ chromatograms. *Analyst* **2014**, *139*, 6474–6485. [CrossRef] [PubMed]
16. Liu, H.; Yang, J.; Du, F.; Gao, X.; Ma, X.; Huang, Y.; Xu, F.; Niu, W.; Wang, F.; Mao, Y.; et al. Absorption and disposition of ginsenosides after oral administration of *Panax notoginseng* extract to rats. *Drug Metab. Dispos.* **2009**, *37*, 2290–2298. [CrossRef] [PubMed]
17. Hu, Z.; Yang, J.; Cheng, C.; Huang, Y.; Du, F.; Wang, F.; Niu, W.; Xu, F.; Jiang, R.; Gao, X.; et al. Combinatorial metabolism notably affects human systemic exposure to ginsenosides from orally administered extract of *Panax notoginseng* roots (Sanqi). *Drug Metab. Dispos.* **2013**, *41*, 1457–1469. [CrossRef] [PubMed]
18. Ung, C.Y.; Li, H.; Cao, Z.W.; Li, Y.X.; Chen, Y.Z. Are herb-pairs of traditional Chinese medicine distinguishable from others? Pattern analysis and artificial intelligence classification study of traditionally defined herbal properties. *J. Ethnopharmacol.* **2007**, *111*, 371–377. [CrossRef] [PubMed]
19. Song, Y.; Zhang, N.; Jiang, Y.; Li, J.; Zhao, Y.; Shi, S.; Tu, P. Simultaneous determination of aconite alkaloids and ginsenosides using online solid phase extraction hyphenated with polarity switching ultra-high performance liquid chromatography coupled with tandem mass spectrometry. *RSC Adv.* **2015**, *5*, 6419–6428. [CrossRef]
20. Rendic, S.; Guengerich, F.P. Survey of human oxidoreductases and cytochrome p450 enzymes involved in the metabolism of xenobiotic and natural chemicals. *Chem. Res. Toxicol.* **2015**, *28*, 38–42. [CrossRef] [PubMed]

10

Regulation of Hepatic UGT2B15 by Methylation in Adults of Asian Descent

Steffen G. Oeser [1], Jon-Paul Bingham [1] and Abby C. Collier [2,*]

[1] Molecular Biosciences and Bioengineering, University of Hawaii, Manoa, 1955 East-West Rd. #218, Honolulu, HI 96822, USA; steffengo@gmail.com (S.G.O.); jbingham@hawaii.edu (J.-P.B.)

[2] Faculty of Pharmaceutical Sciences, 2405 Wesbrook Mall, University of British Columbia, Vancouver, BC V6T1Z3, Canada

* Correspondence: abby.collier@ubc.ca

Abstract: The hepatic uridine 5′-diphosphate-glucuronosyl transferases (UGTs) are critical for detoxifying endo- and xenobiotics. Since UGTs are also dynamically responsive to endogenous and exogenous stimuli, we examined whether epigenetic DNA methylation can regulate hepatic UGT expression and differential effects of ethnicity, obesity, and sex. The methylation status of UGT isoforms was determined with Illumina Methylation 450 BeadChip arrays, with genotyping confirmed by sequencing and gene expression confirmed with quantitative reverse transcriptase polymerase chain reaction (q-RT-PCR). The UGT1A3 mRNA was 2-fold higher in females than males ($p < 0.05$), while UGT1A1 and UGT2B7 mRNA were significantly higher in Pacific Islanders than Caucasians (both $p < 0.05$). Differential mRNA or methylation did not occur with obesity. The methylation of the UGT2B15 locus cg09189601 in Caucasians was significantly lower than the highly methylated locus in Asians ($p < 0.001$). Three intergenic loci between UGT2B15 and 2B17 (cg07973162, cg10632656, and cg07952421) showed higher rates of methylation in Caucasians than in Asians ($p < 0.001$). Levels of UGT2B15 and UGT2B17 mRNA were significantly lower in Asians than Caucasians ($p = 0.01$ and $p < 0.001$, respectively). Genotyping and sequencing indicated that only UGT2B15 is regulated by methylation, and low UGT2B17 mRNA is due to a deletion genotype common to Asians. Epigenetic regulation of UGT2B15 may predispose Asians to altered drug and hormone metabolism and begin to explain the increased risks for adverse drug reactions and some cancers in this population.

Keywords: glucuronidation; obesity; sex; polymorphisms

---

1. Introduction

The uridine 5′-diphosphate-glucuronosyl transferases (UGTs, E.C. 2.4.1.17) primarily eliminate xeno- and endobiotics in humans through conjugating them with a polar sugar [1]. Alone, or in conjunction with other enzymes, the UGTs are involved in the clearance of more than 90% of clinically relevant drugs from the body [2]. Based on nucleotide sequence analysis, 22 human UGT proteins have been identified in 4 families, with the UGT1A and UGT2B subfamilies being most critical for hepatic metabolism [3–5].

The UGT enzymes are genetically polymorphic, with over 200 variant alleles described for the UGT1 and UGT2 subfamilies that can influence enzymatic function, cellular trafficking, or gene expression, modifying individual drug and endobiotic exposure [6]. Additional variants have also been identified, but have not been characterized for function. Moreover, although some of these single nucleotide polymorphisms (SNPs) are functional, changes in total glucuronidation also tend to occur when many polymorphisms are inherited together as a haplotype [6].

In addition to genetic factors, UGT enzymes are known to be regulated by environmental, xenobiotic, and endobiotic exposure, but at present there is limited information regarding epigenetic regulation, such as the effects of methylation. Methylation of UGT1A1 has been associated with colon cancer and with altered drug disposition in cancer [7,8]. More recently, a link between DNA methylation and the regulation of UGT1A1 protein expression and activity in healthy human livers has been presented [9]. This latter study implies that epigenetics are not merely a disease-state effect in UGT disposition, but may be intimately involved in modifying basal UGT enzyme expression. Therefore, examining epigenetic modifications that alter mRNA levels of UGT enzymes in common demographics, such as sex, ethnicity, and obesity, may help determine how glucuronidation varies in mixed populations. This can help determine demographic contributions to the hepatic disposition of compounds.

If glucuronidation is dysregulated or differs inherently between members of mixed populations, it is important to understand the mechanisms for these changes. These mechanisms may present druggable targets in themselves for preventing or mitigating disease and could be exploited to prevent adverse drug reactions. Moreover, epigenetic mechanisms may provide insight into the differential susceptibility of some ethnicities to diseases and syndromes, including cancer. The purpose of this study was to determine the differential methylation of all hepatic UGT isoforms in a well-characterized cohort of human livers and investigate whether hepatic methylation of UGTs is associated with sex, ethnicity, or obesity.

2. Materials and Methods

2.1. Tissue Availability and Collection

Liver samples (n = 24) were collected from the Hawaii Human Biorepository, which collects samples with informed consent from non-surviving organ donors' families, and with permission for future experimentation. The characteristics of this set of livers were as follows: Median age 52 $\pm$ 13 (range: 20–69), Males n = 15 and Females n = 9, Ethnicity: Caucasian n = 9 (38%), Asian n = 11 (33%), and Pacific Island (PI) n = 4 (16%). Three unknowns were excluded from analysis; moreover, one each of Caucasian and Asian were excluded from the methylation analysis due to poor sample quality. "Asian" in this study is reflective of Japanese, Chinese, or Korean ethnicity. The Body Mass Index (BMI) ranged from normal (20.8 kg/m^2) to morbidly obese (52.4 kg/m^2) with a median of 30.7 $\pm$ 8.5. For analysis, samples were grouped into two discrete categories, normal weight (NW) and overweight (OW), which corresponded to BMI ranges of 18.5–24.9 kg/m^2 and above 25 kg/m^2, respectively. These studies were approved by the Hawaii Institutional Review Board for Human Subjects (CHS #21144).

2.2. Liver Samples

Tissue samples (1 cm) were extracted from the anterior portion of the right lobe closest to the inferior vena cava from frozen livers. All livers were collected and archived (flash frozen) within 6 h of brain death, and these tissues were from livers that had never been thawed. None of the livers was diseased. Tissues samples were disrupted on liquid nitrogen using a mortar and pestle and stored at −80 °C until nucleic acid extraction.

2.3. DNA and RNA Extraction

DNA, RNA, and protein were extracted from 20 mg of disrupted liver sample according to the manufacturer's instructions (Qiagen AllPrep DNA/RNA/Protein Mini kit, Valencia, CA, USA). Nucleic acid purity was examined using a Nanodrop spectrophotometer (ThermoFisher Scientific, Wilmington, DE, USA), and quality was examined with a Bioanalyzer (Agilent, Palo Alto, CA, USA). To further purify DNA, ethanol precipitation was performed and the pellet re-dissolved in nuclease free water.

2.4. DNA Methylation Analysis

The Illumina Infinium Methylation Assay (Illumina Inc., San Diego, CA, USA) was performed as per the manufacturer's instructions. This assay covers 99% of RefSeq genes and 95% of Cytosine-guanine (CpG) islands in the human genome. The entire genome was interrogated and examined, but results with respect to UGT genes were the focus of this study. All CpG interrogation sites associated with all UGT genes were analyzed, but only significant results are presented. The DNA samples (1 μg) were first treated with sodium bisulfite using a Zymo Research Bisulfite conversion kit (Zymo Irvine, CA, USA) to deaminate un-methylated cytosine to produce uracil. Extraction, analysis, and visualization of the methylation data were performed using the Illumina Genome Studio software (version 2011.1) with methylation and genome viewer plug-ins (version 1.9.0, Illumina, San Diego, CA, USA). Differential methylation analysis was performed for grouped data utilizing the Illumina custom error model, resulting in a differential methylation score (diffscore) that provides directionality to the p-value. The diffscore was converted to an adjusted p-value with the formula: $p\text{-value} = 1/((10^{|\text{DiffScore}|})/10)$.

2.5. Gene Expression via Quantitative Reverse Transcriptase Polymerase Chain Reaction (q-RT-PCR)

Total RNA (1 μg) was converted to cDNA using a qScript™ cDNA synthesis kit from Quanta Biosciences (Gaithersburg, MD, USA) according to the protocol provided. After mixing, reaction was incubated using the following conditions: 5 min at 25 °C, 30 min at 42 °C, 5 min at 85 °C, and then held at 4 °C for at least 5 min. From the resulting 20 μL reaction, 4 μL of cDNA product was then combined with forward and reverse qPCR primers (Table 1) to a final concentration of 500 nM. This reaction was then combined with an equal volume of 2× Roche Power SYBR Green Master Mix containing ROX. Samples were cycled on an Applied Biosystems 7900HT qPCR machine (ABI, Foster City, CA, USA) as follows: 2 min at 50 °C, 10 min at 95 °C, then 40 cycles of 15 s at 95 °C, and 1 min at 60 °C. Additionally, a dissociation step was performed at the end of the run, utilizing a +1 °C ramp rate per second from 60 °C to 95 °C with continuous detection, to ensure that only a single product was formed. Data for q-RT-PCR were displayed utilizing Applied Biosystems SDS software version 2.1 (ABI, Foster City, CA, USA). All mRNA expression C_T values were normalized against Beta-Glucuronidase (GUSB) before relative quantitation. Resulting C_T values were analyzed and converted to fold change differences using the $\Delta\Delta C_T$ method for relative quantitation [10].

Table 1. Uridine 5′ diphosphate-glucuronosyl transferases (UGT) primer sequences used to produce quantitative polymerase chain reaction (qPCR) results for gene expression analysis. The isoform examined, forward and reverse primer sequences, as well as publication source (reference number) are listed. Primers were from references. GUSB: Beta-Glucuronidase.

UGT	Forward Primer Sequence (5′-3′)	Reverse Primer Sequence (5′-3′)
1A1	AATAAAAAAGGACTCTGCTATGCT	ACATCAAAGCTGCTTTCTGC
1A3	TGTTGAACAATATGTCTTTGGTCTA	ACCACATCAAAGGAAGTAGCA
1A4	GAACAATGTATCTTTGGCCC	ACCACATCAAAGGAAGTAGCA
1A6	CATGATTGTTATTGGCCTGTAC	TCTGTGAAAAGAGCATCAAACT
1A8	GAAAGCACAAGTACGAAGTTTG	GGGAGGGAGAAATATTTGGC
1A9	TGGAAAGCACAAGTACGAAGTATATA	GGGAGGGAGAAATATTTGGC
1A10	GAAAGCACAGGCACAAAGTATA	GGGAGGGAGAAATATTTAGCAAC
2B4	TCTTTCGATCCAACAGCC	CATCTCTTAACCGCTGCTTGATA
2B7	GGAGAATTTCTCATGCAACAGA	CAGAACTTTCTATTATGTCACCAAATATTG
2B11	AGTAACATGACAGCAGAAAGGGCCAAT	AGACCTAAGGCATCTGGTTTATTCCCG
2B15	CTTCTGAAAATCTCGATAGATGGAT	CATCTTTACAGACTTGTTACTGTAGTCAT
2B17	TTTATGAAAAGTTCGATAGATGGAC	CATCTTCACAGACTTTATATTATAGTCAG
GUSB	AGCCAGTTCCTCATCAATGG	GGTAGTGGCTGGTACGGAAA

2.6. Genotyping of the UGT2B17 Deletion

The presence or absence of the UGT2B17 gene deletion was determined. The C and J primer pairs (Table 2) were combined into a duplex reaction, generating a 316 bp fragment from within the UGT2B17 gene or an 884 bp fragment spanning the deletion breakpoint, respectively. Upon electrophoresis, individuals homozygous for the presence of UGT2B17 (Ins/Ins) show a single 316 bp product, individuals homozygous for the deletion show a single 884 bp product (Del/Del), and heterozygotes (Ins/Del) show both products with a reduction after the 316 bp fragment [11]. The PCR for the C and J primer pairs was carried out in 25 μL reactions containing 22.5 μL of Platinum Blue PCR Supermix (Invitrogen, Grand Island, NY, USA), 100 pmol each of forward and reverse primer, and 30 ng of genomic DNA. The cycle conditions were 94 °C for 3 min, 35 cycles of 94 °C for 30 s, 60 °C for 30 s, 72 °C for 3 min, and then finishing with a 4 °C hold.

Table 2. Primer sequences for PCR reactions to characterize single nucleotide polymorphisms (SNPs) and deletions. The UGT isoform being examined, region of amplification, primer name, direction, and sequence as well as the resulting amplicon size are shown. UTR: untranslated region.

UGT	Region	Primer	Orientation	Sequence (5′-3′)	Amplicon (bp)
2B17	Gene	C	Forward	CCTGGAAGAGCTTGTTCAGA	316
2B17	Gene	C	Reverse	CTGCATCTTCACAGAGCTTT	316
2B17	Deletion	J	Forward	TGCACAGAGTTAAGAAATGGAGAGATGTG	884
2B17	Deletion	J	Reverse	GATCATCCTATATCCTGACAGAATTCTTTTG	884
2B15	Promoter	A	Forward	GGTCCCACTTCTTCAGATCAT	3368
2B15	Promoter	A	Reverse	GAGAGAAGGAAGAAGCCAGAAG	3368
2B15	Promoter	B	Forward	ACATAGGAAGGAGGGAACAGA	3224
2B15	Promoter	B	Reverse	TTCCTGCTGAGGGTTTGAAG	3224
2B15	UTR	D	Forward	TGGTGTGGATGTCCTTTCTG	2567
2B15	UTR	D	Reverse	GGCAGGAGAATGACTTGACTAC	2567
2B15	UTR	E	Forward	CTGCAGGTCTGTTGGAATTTG	2401
2B15	UTR	E	Reverse	GCAGTTGTAGTCCTAGCTTCTC	2401

2.7. UGT2B15 Polymerase Chain Reaction (PCR) Amplification for Promoter Region

The primers for the promoter region were designed utilizing Primer-BLAST software [12]. The A primer pair listed in Table 3 was used to amplify a 3368 bp region of the UGT2B15 promoter, and after ethanol precipitation to clean-up the PCR product, primer pair B was used to amplify that product to produce a final, specific, 3224 bp fragment for sequencing (Table 2). PCR for both reactions was carried out in a 10 μL reaction volume consisting of 9 μL of Platinum Blue PCR Supermix (Invitrogen, Grand Island, NY, USA), 1 pmol each of forward and reverse primer, and 20 ng of DNA. The cycle conditions were 94 °C for 3 min, 25 cycles of 94 °C for 30 s, 45 °C for 30 s, 72 °C for 3.5 min, and then finishing with a 4 °C hold. For SNP examination, samples were cleaned via ethanol precipitation and cycle sequenced utilizing the B forward PCR primer in addition to the sequencing primers for the promoter region listed in Table 3.

Table 3. Sequencing primers used to obtain the sequence data for the PCR reactions. The UGT isoform being examined, region of amplification, primer name, binding DNA strand, and sequence are shown.

UGT Isoform	Region	Primer #	Strand	Sequence (5′-3′)
2B17	Gene	1	−	CTGGTCCCACTTCTTCAGAT
2B15	Promoter	2	+	GTTTGCAGATTTTTAATGAGGCA
2B15	Promoter	3	+	CTCCTAGGATTTGGCACCAG
2B15	Promoter	4	+	TTCTCTAATTTGACTCAGCTTCACA
2B15	Promoter	5	−	CTCAGCCCACCTGCAACC
2B15	Promoter	6	−	CCCCCTCTCCAGAATACACA
2B15	Promoter	7	−	TATCGTGGTGCAAGTAATGTCTTC
2B15	Promoter	8	−	TTATCCAATGGCTGTATTCTGTG
2B15	Promoter	9	+	ACTTTCCCACCGAAAATTCC
2B15	Promoter	10	+	TGCGTGGCAACTGTGATATT

Table 3. *Cont.*

UGT Isoform	Region	Primer #	Strand	Sequence (5′-3′)
2B15	Promoter	11	−	CAGGAAAAAGGAAATCCTCCA
2B15	Promoter	12	−	CTTTCGTGTGTAACTTTTGGATT
2B15	UTR	13	+	GAGGTTACTGCTGTCTCTTTGT
2B15	UTR	14	+	TGGTGTGGATGTCCTTTCTG
2B15	UTR	15	−	CCCTGGATCGAGCAGTCTTC
2B15	UTR	16	−	GACCAACCAATGAAGCCCCT

2.8. UGT2B15 PCR Amplification for 3′ Untranslated Regulatory Region

The primers for the untranslated regulatory region were designed utilizing the Primer-BLAST software [12]. The D primer pair listed in Table 3 was used to amplify 2567 bp of the UGT2B15 3′ untranslated regulatory region and after ethanol precipitation to clean-up the PCR product, primer pair E was used to amplify that product to produce a 2401 bp region for sequencing (Table 3). PCR for both reactions was carried out in a 10 µL reaction volume consisting of 9 µL of Platinum Blue PCR Supermix (Invitrogen, Grand Island, NY, USA), 1 pmol each of forward and reverse primer, and 20 ng of DNA. The cycle conditions were 94 °C for 3 min, 25 cycles of 94 °C for 30 s, 49 °C for 30 s, 72 °C for 3.5 min, and then finishing with a 4 °C hold. Samples were cleaned via ethanol precipitation and cycle sequenced utilizing the E forward PCR primer in addition to the listed sequencing primers for the untranslated regulatory region in Table 3. Products (300 ng) were electrophoresed on 2% (*w*/*v*) Tris-buffered EDTA (TBE) agarose gel and sized compared to a DNA ladder (Thermo Fisher, Wilmington, DE, USA) with imaging on a Typhoon Scanner 9410 (GE Healthcare, Chicago, IL, USA).

2.9. Cycle Sequencing

Each sample was sequenced in duplicate, combining 7.5 ng of PCR template with 2.5 pmol of sequencing primer in a total volume of 5 µL in a 96-well polypropylene half-skirted sequencing plate (Applied Biosystems, Foster City, CA, USA). Each 5 µL reaction was then mixed with 1.5 µL of nuclease free water, 1.5 µL of 5X Applied Biosystems Sequencing Buffer, and 2 µL of BigDye® Terminator v3.1 Ready Reaction Enzyme Mix (Life Technologies, Grand Island, NY, USA). Samples were mixed, sealed, and sequenced under the following cycling conditions: 96 °C for 1 min followed by 25 cycles of 96 °C for 10 s, 50 °C for 5 s, and 60 °C for 4 min and terminating with a 4 °C hold until samples were ready for purification.

Samples were cleaned according to the BigDye® Terminator v3.1 protocol and sequenced utilizing the Applied Biosystems DNA Analyzer 3730xl Sequencer (Foster City, CA, USA). Resulting chromatograms were examined via 4Peaks software v1.7.2 (Mek & Tosj, Amsterdam, The Netherlands), and sequences were extracted and examined for SNPs using Aliview to align and trim the sequences (Uppsala University, Uppsala, Sweden).

The resulting sequences were then entered into the BLAST program and aligned to the UGT2B15 gene (Genbank ID: NC_0000012.4). Sequences were examined and nucleotide calls recorded for each sample at each position where a known or suspected SNP exists (indicated in the BLAST program in the SNP annotation database).

2.10. Statistical Analyses

Statistical analysis was performed using the GraphPad Prism Program version 5.02 (Graph Pad, San Diego, CA, USA). Normality of the data was checked using D'Agostino–Pearson's test and variance verified using the Bartlett's test. A one-way analysis of variance (ANOVA) with Bonferroni's post-hoc comparison was used if the data were found to be normally distributed; alternatively, the Kruskal–Wallis one-way ANOVA was performed with Dunn's post hoc analysis. For binary data sets (sex), student's *t*-tests were performed with $\alpha = 0.05$.

3. Results

3.1. Summary of Methylation Beta Values for All UGT-Associated Loci

Inspection of the methylation status of all the UGT loci demonstrated that for UGT1A isoforms, most of the loci were generally moderately or hyper-methylated, but significant differential methylation was not occurring between samples. However, for UGT2B isoforms, at least four loci have differential methylation occurring with a clear splitting pattern between samples. These loci are associated with UGT2B15 (cg09189601) and both UGT2B15 and 2B17 (cg07973162, cg10632656, and cg07952421, Figure 1). No significant differences in methylation patterns were attributed to age, sex, or BMI for any of the four differentially methylated loci associated with UGT2B15 and UGT2B17.

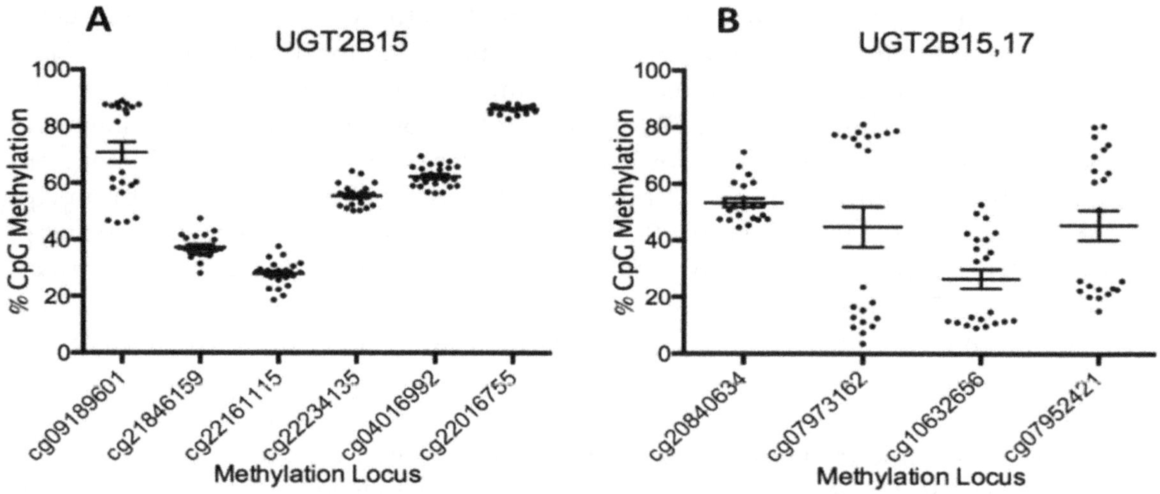

Figure 1. Grouped data showing the methylation beta values (y-axis) for each sample at a particular Cytosine-Guanine (CG) locus (x-axis) UGT2B15 (**A**) and UGT2B15/17 (**B**). Because UGT2B15/2B17 were formed by a gene duplication event, they also share common loci. Values above 70% are generally considered to be fully methylated on both strands and values below 30% are typically un-methylated on both strands with intermediate values indicating that only one of the two strands are methylated.

The only difference attributed to differential methylation was ethnicity (Figure 2). For locus cg09189601, which is associated with UGT2B15 only, we observed hyper-methylation (90%) in Asians (n = 8) compared to the moderate methylation (50–60%) in Caucasians (n = 10, p < 0.0001), which would imply less transcription of UGT2B15 in Asians. In contrast, at loci cg07973162, cg10632656, and cg07952421 hepatic UGT2B15 and 2B17 were hypo-methylated in Asians (<20%) compared to the more highly methylated (40–80%) Caucasian samples (p < 0.0001 for all loci).

The Pacific Island cohort in our study (PI, n = 4) displayed two samples that reflected Asian methylation patterns and two samples that reflected Caucasian patterns. Due to a limited sample size and the split nature of their methylation pattern, no significant differences in methylation patterns were determined. The ethnic makeup of our PI group was ≥50% (i.e., at least one parent PI) to define ethnicity. However, for Asian and Caucasian populations 100% (i.e., both parents of this race) defined ethnicity, hence we cannot rule out admixed genetic information in PI from other ethnic groups, and this likely explains the splitting observed. Notably, intermarriage of PI/Caucasian and PI/Asian is common in Hawaii.

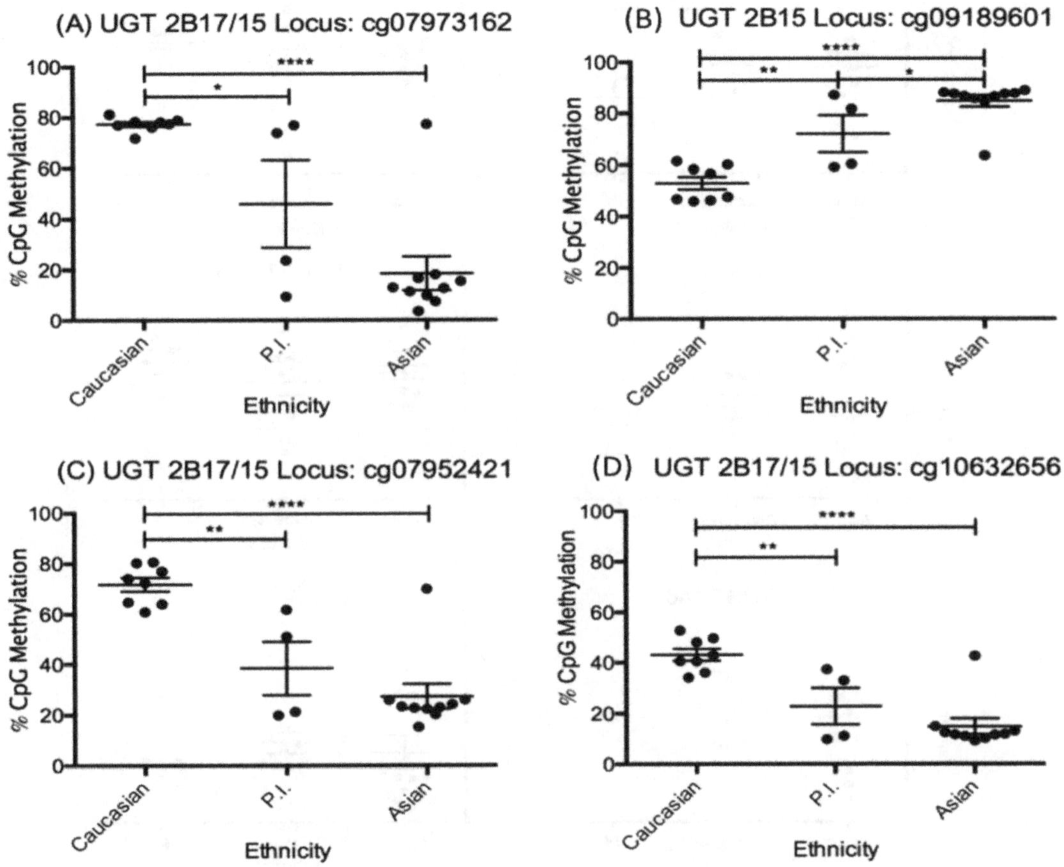

Figure 2. Graphs showing beta values (β) for differentially methylated loci associated with UGT2B15 and 2B17, grouped according to ethnicity with separate columns for Caucasians (n = 8), Pacific Islanders (PI, n = 4) and Asians (n = 10). The UGT isoform and the specific loci where the methylation is taking place are listed in the title for each individual graph such that loci cg07973162 (**A**), cg10632656 (**B**), cg07952421 (**C**), and cg09189601 (**D**) show different patterns of methylation between Asians, PI and Caucasians for UGT2B15 and UGT2B17. Statistical significance is listed for p-values ≤0.05 (*), ≤0.01 (**), and ≤0.0001 (****). As compared to PCR, two samples (one Caucasian and one Asian) were lost to analysis due to low sample quality.

3.2. The mRNA Expression of UDP-Glucuronosyl Transferase (UGT) Isoforms in This Liver Cohort

To determine differences in UGT mRNA expression and confirm methylation effects, we performed q-RT-PCR on all hepatic UGT1A and 2B isoforms. Obesity was not associated with any significant differences in mRNA levels for any UGT1A or 2B isoforms. Only UGT1A3 showed significant differences in mRNA levels with sex, where females had 2-fold higher mRNA expression than males (p = 0.02, data not shown).

Ethnicity was associated with significant differences in mRNA abundance for UGT1A1, where Caucasians had significantly lower mRNA levels than PI (higher ΔC_T, p = 0.03, Figure 3). Caution should be exercised with these data, as the number of samples in the PI group is fairly low for statistical comparison.

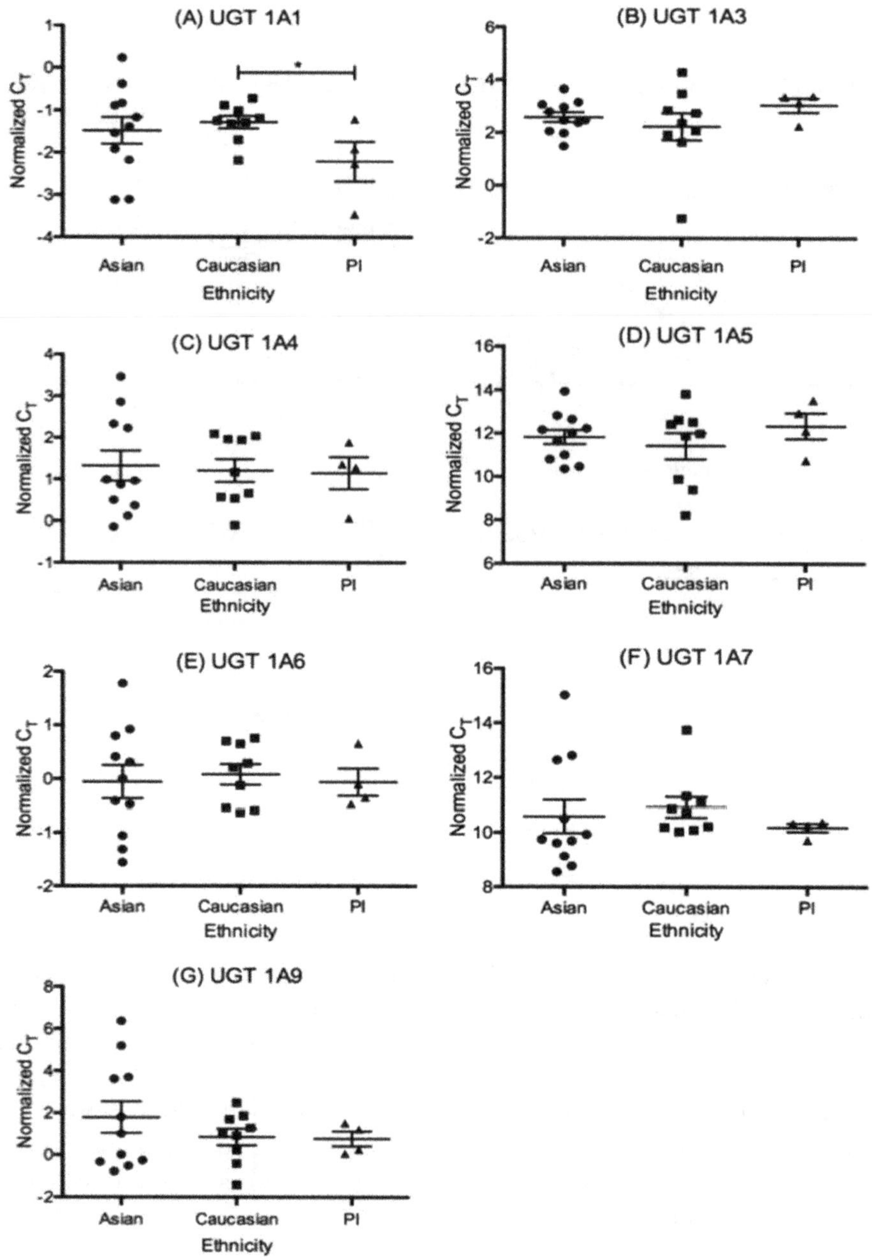

Figure 3. The quantitative PCR $\Delta\Delta C_T$ values in Asian (A, n = 11), Caucasian (C, n = 9), and Pacific Islander (PI, n = 4) ethnicities for all liver-specific UGT1A isoforms examined. Statistical significance is listed for p-values ≤ 0.05 (*) Note that higher $\Delta\Delta C_T$ means lower level of mRNA. (**A**–**G**) represent results for each individual UGT1A subfamily isoform.

Gene expression data for UGT2B samples demonstrated significantly lower UGT2B7 mRNA levels in Caucasians (higher ΔC_T) as compared to PI (p = 0.038, Figure 4). When mRNA expression of UGT2B15 (Figure 4) was determined across the three ethnicities, Asians show significantly lower mRNA expression than Caucasians (p = 0.02) and approached significance for PI (p = 0.08). Finally, for UGT2B17 (Figure 4), Asians exhibited significantly lower mRNA levels than Caucasians (p = 0.001) and approached significance as compared to PI (p = 0.08). These data translate to a 3-fold significant downregulation in UGT2B15 in Asians as compared to Caucasians and PI. For UGT2B17, there is no fold change between Caucasians and PI, but there is a 1500-fold downregulation between Caucasians and the three Asian samples that produced gene expression data for this isoform.

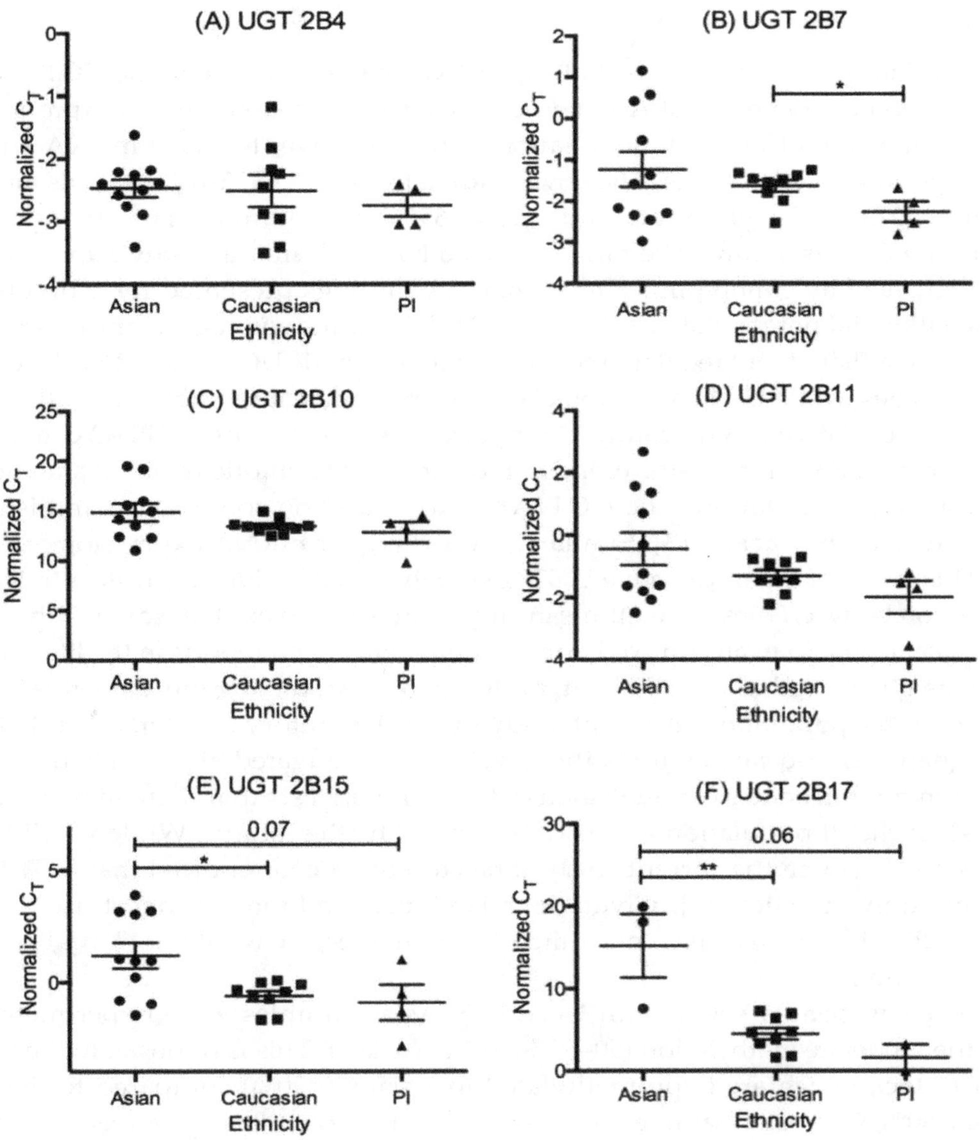

Figure 4. The quantitative PCR ΔC_T values in Asian (A, n = 11), Caucasian (C, n = 9), and Pacific Islander (PI, n = 4) ethnicities for all examined UGT2B isoforms in liver. Statistical significance is listed for p-values ≤ 0.05 (*), ≤ 0.01 (**), and p values approaching significance (<0.1). Note that a higher ΔC_T means a lower level of mRNA. (**A**–**F**) represent results for each individual UGT2B subfamily isoform.

3.3. UGT2B15 and UGT2B17 Genetic Analysis

Comparison of SNP data to mRNA levels demonstrates that the decreased expression for UGT2B15 in these samples is not caused by any of the known UGT2B15 SNPs in the areas interrogated. Deletion genotyping of UGT2B17 demonstrated that eight of nine Asian samples and two of the PI samples have the UGT2B17 Del/Del genotype. Caucasian samples had at least one copy of the UGT2B17 gene, with three Ins/Ins, four Ins/Del, and two samples that failed genotyping. The two PI samples that did not have the deletion are of Ins/Del genotype. These genotyping results are consistent with the q-RT-PCR data for UGT2B17, where Asian samples had either an absent, or an extremely low, expression of UGT2B17. The deletion polymorphism is the major cause for this low UGT2B17 gene expression for the Asian samples and also explains the hypo-methylated CpG loci in the UGT2B15/2B17 intergenic region that reside within the deletion.

4. Discussion

The critical finding of this study is that the mRNA expression of hepatic UGT2B15 is partially regulated by methylation in people of Asian descent, causing decreased mRNA expression. Moreover, while UGT2B17 showed differential methylation in Asians, lower levels of mRNA are caused by a deletion genotype and not epigenetics. The novel finding from the UGT2B17 studies is that methylation of the three loci cg07973162, cg07952421, and cg10632656 in the Illumina platform is predictive of the deletion genotype. This is because the range targeted by the Illumina methylation assay covers the deletion, as confirmed by genotyping. Other than the findings presented for individuals of Asian descent, methylation did not regulate UGT1A or UGT2B isoforms with age, ethnicity, obesity, or sex in this cohort. Finally, although not regulated by methylation, hepatic UGT1A3 mRNA levels were higher in females than males, while UGT1A1 mRNA levels were significantly higher in PI than Caucasians.

Because females showed significantly higher mRNA expression of UGT1A3 compared to males, this may have implications for sex-differences in drug and endobiotic metabolism and disposition if it is indicative of protein levels. The UGT1A3 isoform acts on some drugs and is an important metabolic pathway for bile acids [13]. Similarly, PI had higher mRNA expression of UGT1A1 than Caucasians. This is one of the most active UGTs in the liver, with wide substrate affinity. Differences in UGT expression between these two ethnic groups may begin to explain some of the differences in drug and chemical response in an admixed population. There are no reports in the literature indicating disproportionate glucuronidation in PIs, but, rather than contradicting our data, this is due to a lack of study in this ethnic population. A recent study by our laboratory has demonstrated that morbid obesity in pregnancy is associated with higher levels of unconjugated bilirubin in the blood of obese PI women and in their neonates (unpublished data). This suggests that there may be ethnic-specific effects on UGT in the PI population and is deserving of further study. While we did not find any associations with obesity in the current study, it has recently been reported that UGT2B17 can vary with obesity but only in males [14]. Given the mixed male and female cohort used, as well as the deletion of UGT2B17 in approximately one third of our samples, we would not have been empowered to confirm this finding.

For the locus associated solely with UGT2B15, Asian samples were hyper-methylated (90%) compared to the moderate methylation (50–60%) in Caucasians. This is opposite to the three common UGT2B15/2B17 loci, which are hypo-methylated in Asians (<20%) compared to the more highly methylated (40–80%) Caucasian samples. Taken together, these results imply a regulatory mechanism by which both UGT2B15 and 2B17 are methylated simultaneously at the intergenic region and UGT2B15 is modified at another site to modulate its glucuronidation separately. Because these two isoforms are the result of a gene duplication event in the recent past, this complex differential regulation is empirically sensible. The mRNA expression patterns are not concordant with methylation data that is typically observed in connection with gene promoters, which was expected because methylation occurs within intergenic areas for UGT2B15 and UGT2B17. In general, regulatory methylation occurs at hypo-methylated sites commonly located in CpG islands within 1.5 kb of the transcription start site of a gene, while hyper-methylated sites tend to be located in the distal intergenic and gene body regions [15–17]. Another potential explanation for this is that the liver is highly enriched in 5 hmC and the bisulfite technique does not discriminate between 5 mC and 5 hmC. Since these two CpG modifications have opposing effects, this may also explain why mRNA levels are not concordant with traditional methylation patterns. Finally, methylation patterns presenting with a beta value of 50% could represent an admixed cell population where half the cells are methylated and half are not. This is highly unlikely to be the case in our study, since the cells in the small 1–2 g pieces of human liver would be exposed to the same endo- and xenobiotic stimuli and concordance between a majority of the UGT-related CpG sites was high.

In addition to epigenetic mechanisms, functional and clinically relevant polymorphisms in UGT2B15 and 2B17 that affect drug and chemical disposition exist. This includes the UGT2B15*2 polymorphism, where reduced lorazepam and S-oxazepam clearance occurs [18,19], as well as the

UGT2B17*2 and UGT2B17 deletion genotypes, which both reduce MK-7246 and exemestane clearances, potentially leading to toxic accumulation [20,21]. Polymorphisms may also increase activity, such as with UGT2B15*4, which has a C > A nucleotide change in the coding region, increasing UGT2B15 catalysis [18,19]. Polymorphisms in UGT2B15 and 2B17 have been implicated in modifying the clearance of a wide range of drugs, reviewed in: [22]. Here, an analogy can be made with methylation because if Asians have differential methylation patterns compared to Caucasians for UGT2B15, they may also have altered glucuronidation capacity.

In addition to drugs and chemicals, UGT2B15 and 2B17 have been investigated in relation to risks for cancer and other endocrine diseases [23]. This is especially true with regard to the UGT2B17 deletion phenotype, which is more prevalent in the Asian population [24] and is particularly important because UGT2B17 is more active than UGT2B15 for testosterone glucuronidation [25,26]. Polymorphisms in both of these genes have been shown to alter steroid metabolism and also are predictors of fat mass in men [27]. Most studies indicate that genetic polymorphisms affecting UGT2B15 and/or 2B17 are risk factors for prostate cancer [28–31]. Although lifestyle and environmental factors account for some prostate cancer in Asians, these only account for a small proportion of the relative risk [32]. These prior research efforts have elucidated many of the biological effects of UGT2B15 and UGT2B17 polymorphisms, but the impact of epigenetic methylation has not previously been established. Our study implies that hyper-methylation of UGT2B15 in Asians may affect androgen disposition as compared to the Caucasian population and is a promising avenue for investigating some of the altered risk for androgen-related cancers in these populations.

Although this study contained only a relatively small sample size, making interactions between environment, genotype, and demographics difficult to establish, the numbers of samples for ethnicities, sex, and obesity were well-balanced. This is bolstered by our findings from the samples of PI ethnicity, where UGT genotypes showed commonality with Asians for two of the samples and for Caucasians with the other two samples. Since most of the PI participants were of mixed heritage ($\geq$50% PI, admixed with either Asian or Caucasian), these findings fit the rules of heritability. Moreover, a strong Asian linkage is not surprising, as PI are theorized to have originated in Asia and mixed extensively with Melanesians both depositing and accumulating genes into their genomes during colonization of the Pacific Islands [33], which has been further corroborated by both Y chromosome and mitochondrial DNA analyses [34]. Finally, our work is complemented by recent data demonstrating that hepatic UGT1A1 can be regulated during early human development by histone modification [35], a novel and interesting finding that supports the concept that UGTs can be regulated at the transcriptional level through genetic mechanisms. Having said this, we believe that future work in this area will need to encompass protein-level studies with Western blot of UGT2B15 and/or activity studies to confirm if these results found at the mRNA levels also follow through to the levels of enzyme proteins and their function.

A secondary finding here is that deletion of UGT2B17 is entirely predicted by methylation status, allowing for genotyping of the (Del/Del) allele via a methylation assay when all three UGT2B15/2B17 loci (cg07973162, cg07952421, and cg10632656) are hypo-methylated (<20%) due to the deletion of UGT2B17. In these samples, this occurred entirely within the Asian population of samples, which agrees with published research showing that this deletion is prevalent in Asian populations [24]. The deletion was also mirrored perfectly by the elimination of mRNA expression for UGT2B17. While it is currently very expensive to use methylation technologies, as the cost progressively reduces the validation of this finding may present an alternative avenue to sequencing or genotyping for determining the UGT2B17 deletion genotype.

5. Conclusions

In summary, methylation may be a mode of regulatory control for UGT2B15 in Asians, which likely acts in conjunction with SNP modification, reducing the enzyme's expression. Impairment of UGT2B15 is of clinical significance with respect to risks for prostate cancer [29] and renal disorders [36] as well as drug metabolism. As this is a small sample size, a larger cohort will be needed to confirm these findings, although with a signal-to-noise ratio as high as we observed we expect the findings to be reproducible. Elucidating the genetic and environmental regulation of UGT2B15 and 2B17 can be useful for predicting susceptibility to cancer and adverse drug reactions, but more work on the precise mechanisms of UGT2B15 methylation, the interplay of methylation and SNPs, as well as the effects on drug and hormone handling in vivo are needed to tease out the clinical significance of these findings.

Acknowledgments: All of the authors are grateful to Maarit Tirikainen for her assistance in running the Illumina chips at the University of Hawaii Cancer Research Center Genomics Facility. The Hawaii Biorepository is supported by the National Institutes of Health National Institute for Research Resources and the National Institute for Minority Health and Health Disparities Grant MD007601. The studies were supported in part by NSERC 17-03808.

Author Contributions: Steffen G. Oeser, Jon-Paul Bingham, and Abby C. Collier conceived and designed the experiments; Steffen G. Oeser performed the experiments; Steffen G. Oeser and Abby C. Collier analyzed the data; and Steffen G. Oeser, Jon-Paul Bingham, and Abby C. Collier wrote the paper.

References

1. Miners, J.O.; Mackenzie, P.I. Drug glucuronidation in humans. *Pharmacol. Ther.* **1991**, *51*, 347–369. [CrossRef]
2. Rowland, A.; Miners, J.O.; Mackenzie, P.I. The UDP-glucuronosyltransferases: Their role in drug metabolism and detoxification. *Int. J. Biochem. Cell Biol.* **2013**, *45*, 1121–1132. [CrossRef] [PubMed]
3. Mackenzie, P.I.; Bock, K.W.; Burchell, B.; Guillemette, C.; Ikushiro, S.; Iyanagi, T.; Miners, J.O.; Owens, I.S.; Nebert, D.W. Nomenclature update for the mammalian UDP glycosyltransferase (UGT) gene superfamily. *Pharmacogenet. Genom.* **2005**, *15*, 677–685. [CrossRef]
4. Miners, J.O.; Smith, P.A.; Sorich, M.J.; McKinnon, R.A.; Mackenzie, P.I. Predicting human drug glucuronidation parameters: Application of in vitro and in silico modeling approaches. *Ann. Rev. Pharmacol. Toxicol.* **2004**, *44*, 1–25. [CrossRef] [PubMed]
5. Izukawa, T.; Nakajima, M.; Fujiwara, R.; Yamanaka, H.; Fukami, T.; Takamiya, M.; Aoki, Y.; Ikushiro, S.; Sakaki, T.; Yokoi, T. Quantitative analysis of UDP-glucuronosyltransferase (UGT) 1A and UGT2B expression levels in human livers. *Drug Metab. Dispos.* **2009**, *37*, 1759–1768. [CrossRef] [PubMed]
6. Zhou, J.; Koszik, F.; Brunner, P.; Stingl, G. "Overrepresentation of T17 cells in the peripheral blood of psoriatic patients is not confined to the skin-homing T cell subset". *J. Dermatol. Sci.* **2014**, *75*, 190–193. [CrossRef] [PubMed]
7. Belanger, A.S.; Tojcic, J.; Harvey, M.; Guillemette, C. Regulation of UGT1A1 and HNF1 transcription factor gene expression by DNA methylation in colon cancer cells. *BMC Mol. Biol.* **2010**, *11*, 9. [CrossRef] [PubMed]
8. Gagnon, J.F.; Bernard, O.; Villeneuve, L.; Tetu, B.; Guillemette, C. Irinotecan inactivation is modulated by epigenetic silencing of UGT1A1 in colon cancer. *Clin. Cancer Res.* **2006**, *12*, 1850–1858. [CrossRef] [PubMed]
9. Yasar, U.; Greenblatt, D.J.; Guillemette, C.; Court, M.H. Evidence for regulation of UDP-glucuronosyltransferase (UGT) 1A1 protein expression and activity via DNA methylation in healthy human livers. *J. Pharm. Pharmacol.* **2013**, *65*, 874–883. [CrossRef] [PubMed]
10. Livak, K.J.; Schmittgen, T.D. Analysis of relative gene expression data using real-time quantitative PCR and the 2(-delta delta c(t)) method. *Methods* **2001**, *25*, 402–408. [CrossRef] [PubMed]
11. Wilson, W., 3rd.; Pardo-Manuel de Villena, F.; Lyn-Cook, B.D.; Chatterjee, P.K.; Bell, T.A.; Detwiler, D.A.; Gilmore, R.C.; Valladeras, I.C.; Wright, C.C.; Threadgill, D.W.; et al. Characterization of a common deletion polymorphism of the UGT2B17 gene linked to UGT2B15. *Genomics* **2004**, *84*, 707–714. [PubMed]
12. Ye, J.; Coulouris, G.; Zaretskaya, I.; Cutcutache, I.; Rozen, S.; Madden, T.L. Primer-blast: A tool to design target-specific primers for polymerase chain reaction. *BMC Bioinform.* **2012**, *13*, 134. [CrossRef] [PubMed]
13. Trottier, J.; Verreault, M.; Grepper, S.; Monte, D.; Belanger, J.; Kaeding, J.; Caron, P.; Inaba, T.T.; Barbier, O. Human UDP-glucuronosyltransferase (UGT) 1A3 enzyme conjugates chenodeoxycholic acid in the liver. *Hepatology* **2006**, *44*, 1158–1170. [CrossRef] [PubMed]
14. Zhu, A.Z.; Cox, L.S.; Ahluwalia, J.S.; Renner, C.C.; Hatsukami, D.K.; Benowitz, N.L.; Tyndale, R.F. Genetic and phenotypic variation in UGT2B17, a testosterone-metabolizing enzyme, is associated with BMI in males. *Pharmacogenet. Genom.* **2015**, *25*, 263–269. [CrossRef] [PubMed]
15. Gutknecht, N.; van Gogswaardt, D.; Conrads, G.; Apel, C.; Schubert, C.; Lampert, F. Diode laser radiation and its bactericidal effect in root canal wall dentin. *J. Clin. Laser Med. Surg.* **2000**, *18*, 57–60. [PubMed]

16. Wagner, J.R.; Busche, S.; Ge, B.; Kwan, T.; Pastinen, T.; Blanchette, M. The relationship between DNA methylation, genetic and expression inter-individual variation in untransformed human fibroblasts. *Genome Biol.* **2014**, *15*, R37. [CrossRef] [PubMed]
17. Jones, P.A. Functions of DNA methylation: Islands, start sites, gene bodies and beyond. *Nat. Rev. Genet.* **2012**, *13*, 484–492. [CrossRef] [PubMed]
18. Court, M.H.; Duan, S.X.; Guillemette, C.; Journault, K.; Krishnaswamy, S.; Von Moltke, L.L.; Greenblatt, D.J. Stereoselective conjugation of oxazepam by human UDP-glucuronosyltransferases (UGTs): S-oxazepam is glucuronidated by UGT2B15, while R-oxazepam is glucuronidated by UGT2B7 and UGT1A9. *Drug Metab. Dispos.* **2002**, *30*, 1257–1265. [CrossRef] [PubMed]
19. He, X.; Hesse, L.M.; Hazarika, S.; Masse, G.; Harmatz, J.S.; Greenblatt, D.J.; Court, M.H. Evidence for oxazepam as an in vivo probe of UGT2B15: Oxazepam clearance is reduced by UGT2B15 D85Y polymorphism but unaffected by UGT2B17 deletion. *Br. J. Clin. Pharmacol.* **2009**, *68*, 721–730. [CrossRef] [PubMed]
20. Sun, D.; Chen, G.; Dellinger, R.W.; Sharma, A.K.; Lazarus, P. Characterization of 17-dihydroexemestane glucuronidation: Potential role of the UGT2B17 deletion in exemestane pharmacogenetics. *Pharmacogenet. Genom.* **2010**, *20*, 575–585. [CrossRef] [PubMed]
21. Wang, Y.H.; Trucksis, M.; McElwee, J.J.; Wong, P.H.; Maciolek, C.; Thompson, C.D.; Prueksaritanont, T.; Garrett, G.C.; Declercq, R.; Vets, E.; et al. Ugt2B17 genetic polymorphisms dramatically affect the pharmacokinetics of MK-7246 in healthy subjects in a first-in-human study. *Clin. Pharmacol. Ther.* **2012**, *92*, 96–102. [CrossRef] [PubMed]
22. Stingl, J.C.; Bartels, H.; Viviani, R.; Lehmann, M.L.; Brockmoller, J. Relevance of UDP-glucuronosyltransferase polymorphisms for drug dosing: A quantitative systematic review. *Pharmacol. Ther.* **2014**, *141*, 92–116. [CrossRef] [PubMed]
23. Belanger, A.; Pelletier, G.; Labrie, F.; Barbier, O.; Chouinard, S. Inactivation of androgens by UDP-glucuronosyltransferase enzymes in humans. *Trends Endocrinol. Metab.* **2003**, *14*, 473–479. [CrossRef] [PubMed]
24. Nadeau, G.; Bellemare, J.; Audet-Walsh, E.; Flageole, C.; Huang, S.P.; Bao, B.Y.; Douville, P.; Caron, P.; Fradet, Y.; Lacombe, L.; et al. Deletions of the androgen-metabolizing UGT2B genes have an effect on circulating steroid levels and biochemical recurrence after radical prostatectomy in localized prostate cancer. *J. Clin. Endocrinol. Metab.* **2011**, *96*, E1550–E1557. [CrossRef] [PubMed]
25. Sten, T.; Finel, M.; Ask, B.; Rane, A.; Ekstrom, L. Non-steroidal anti-inflammatory drugs interact with testosterone glucuronidation. *Steroids* **2009**, *74*, 971–977. [CrossRef] [PubMed]
26. Sten, T.; Bichlmaier, I.; Kuuranne, T.; Leinonen, A.; Yli-Kauhaluoma, J.; Finel, M. Udp-glucuronosyltransferases (UGTs) 2B7 and UGT2B17 display converse specificity in testosterone and epitestosterone glucuronidation, whereas UGT2A1 conjugates both androgens similarly. *Drug Metab. Dispos.* **2009**, *37*, 417–423. [CrossRef] [PubMed]
27. Swanson, C.; Mellstrom, D.; Lorentzon, M.; Vandenput, L.; Jakobsson, J.; Rane, A.; Karlsson, M.; Ljunggren, O.; Smith, U.; Eriksson, A.L.; et al. The uridine diphosphate glucuronosyltransferase 2B15 D85Y and 2B17 deletion polymorphisms predict the glucuronidation pattern of androgens and fat mass in men. *J. Clin. Endocrinol. Metab.* **2007**, *92*, 4878–4882. [CrossRef] [PubMed]
28. Gauthier-Landry, L.; Belanger, A.; Barbier, O. Multiple roles for UDP-glucuronosyltransferase (UGT) 2B15 and UGT2B17 enzymes in androgen metabolism and prostate cancer evolution. *J. Steroid Biochem. Mol. Biol.* **2014**, *145*, 187–192. [CrossRef] [PubMed]
29. Kpoghomou, M.A.; Soatiana, J.E.; Kalembo, F.W.; Bishwajit, G.; Sheng, W. UGT2B17 polymorphism and risk of prostate cancer: A meta-analysis. *ISRN Oncol.* **2013**, *201*. [CrossRef] [PubMed]
30. Park, J.; Chen, L.; Shade, K.; Lazarus, P.; Seigne, J.; Patterson, S.; Helal, M.; Pow-Sang, J. Asp85tyr polymorphism in the UDP-glucuronosyltransferase (UGT) 2B15 gene and the risk of prostate cancer. *J. Urol.* **2004**, *171*, 2484–2488. [CrossRef] [PubMed]
31. MacLeod, S.L.; Nowell, S.; Plaxco, J.; Lang, N.P. An allele-specific polymerase chain reaction method for the determination of the D85Y polymorphism in the human UDP-glucuronosyltransferase 2B15 gene in a case-control study of prostate cancer. *Ann. Surg. Oncol.* **2000**, *7*, 777–782. [CrossRef] [PubMed]
32. Whittemore, A.S.; Kolonel, L.N.; Wu, A.H.; John, E.M.; Gallagher, R.P.; Howe, G.R.; Burch, J.D.; Hankin, J.; Dreon, D.M.; West, D.W.; et al. Prostate cancer in relation to diet, physical activity, and body size in blacks, whites, and Asians in the United States and Canada. *JNCI* **1995**, *87*, 652–661. [CrossRef] [PubMed]

33. Kayser, M.; Brauer, S.; Weiss, G.; Underhill, P.A.; Roewer, L.; Schiefenhovel, W.; Stoneking, M. Melanesian origin of Polynesian Y chromosomes. *Curr. Biol.* **2000**, *10*, 1237–1246. [CrossRef]
34. Kayser, M.; Brauer, S.; Cordaux, R.; Casto, A.; Lao, O.; Zhivotovsky, L.A.; Moyse-Faurie, C.; Rutledge, R.B.; Schiefenhoevel, W.; Gil, D.; et al. Melanesian and Asian origins of Polynesians: mtDNA and Y chromosome gradients across the Pacific. *Mol. Biol. Evol.* **2006**, *23*, 2234–2244. [CrossRef] [PubMed]
35. Nie, Y.; Meng, X.; Liu, J.; Yan, L.; Wang, P.; Bi, H.; Kan, Q.; Zhang, L. Histone modifications regulate the developmental expression of human hepatic UDP-glucuronosyltransferase 1A1. *Drug Metab. Dispos.* **2017**, *45*, 1372–1378. [CrossRef] [PubMed]
36. Deshmukh, N.; Petroczi, A.; Barker, J.; Szekely, A.D.; Hussain, I.; Naughton, D.P. Potentially harmful advantage to athletes: A putative connection between UGT2B17 gene deletion polymorphism and renal disorders with prolonged use of anabolic androgenic steroids. *Subst. Abuse Treat. Prev. Policy* **2010**, *5*, 7. [CrossRef] [PubMed]

11

Disposition, Metabolism and Histone Deacetylase and Acetyltransferase Inhibition Activity of Tetrahydrocurcumin and Other Curcuminoids

Júlia T. Novaes [1,†], Ryan Lillico [1,†], Casey L. Sayre [2], Kalyanam Nagabhushanam [3], Muhammed Majeed [3], Yufei Chen [1], Emmanuel A. Ho [4], Ana Luísa de P. Oliveira [1], Stephanie E. Martinez [5], Samaa Alrushaid [1], Neal M. Davies [6,*] and Ted M. Lakowski [1,*]

1. The Rady Faculty of Health Sciences, College of Pharmacy, Pharmaceutical Analysis Laboratory, University of Manitoba, Winnipeg, MB R3E 0T5, Canada; juliatnovaes@gmail.com (J.T.N.); umLillic@myumanitoba.ca (R.L.); umche355@myumanitoba.ca (Y.C.); analuisapoliv@gmail.com (A.L.d.P.O.); umalrush@myumanitoba.ca (S.A.)
2. College of Pharmacy, Roseman University of Health Sciences, South Jordan, UT 84096, USA; csayre@roseman.edu
3. Sabinsa Corporation, 20 Lake Drive, East Windsor, NJ 08520, USA; kalyanam@sabinsa.com (K.N.); mmjd52@hotmail.com (M.M.)
4. Faculty of Science, School of Pharmacy, University of Waterloo, Kitchener, ON N2G 1C5, Canada; emmanuel.ho@uwaterloo.ca
5. Department of Veterinary Clinical Sciences, College of Veterinary Medicine, Washington State University, Pullman, WA 99164-6610, USA; smartinez@vetmed.wsu.edu
6. Faculty of Pharmacy and Pharmaceutical Sciences, University of Alberta, Edmonton, AB T6G 2R3, Canada

* Correspondence: ndavies@ualberta.ca (N.M.D.); ted.lakowski@umanitoba.ca (T.M.L.)

† These Authors contributed equally to this work.

Abstract: Tetrahydrocurcumin (THC), curcumin and calebin-A are curcuminoids found in turmeric (*Curcuma longa*). Curcuminoids have been established to have a variety of pharmacological activities and are used as natural health supplements. The purpose of this study was to identify the metabolism, excretion, antioxidant, anti-inflammatory and anticancer properties of these curcuminoids and to determine disposition of THC in rats after oral administration. We developed a UHPLC–MS/MS assay for THC in rat serum and urine. THC shows multiple redistribution phases with corresponding increases in urinary excretion rate. In-vitro antioxidant activity, histone deacetylase (HDAC) activity, histone acetyltransferase (HAT) activity and anti-inflammatory inhibitory activity were examined using commercial assay kits. Anticancer activity was determined in Sup-T1 lymphoma cells. Our results indicate THC was poorly absorbed after oral administration and primarily excreted via non-renal routes. All curcuminoids exhibited multiple pharmacological effects in vitro, including potent antioxidant activity as well as inhibition of CYP2C9, CYP3A4 and lipoxygenase activity without affecting the release of TNF-α. Unlike curcumin and calebin-A, THC did not inhibit HDAC1 and PCAF and displayed a weaker growth inhibition activity against Sup-T1 cells. We show evidence for the first time that curcumin and calebin-A inhibit HAT and PCAF, possibly through a Michael-addition mechanism.

Keywords: curcumin; tetrahydrocurcumin; calebin-A; UHPLC–MS/MS; pharmacokinetics; antioxidant; anti-inflammatory; anticancer; HDAC; HAT

1. Introduction

Turmeric from *Curcuma longa* is a popular spice known to contain curcuminoids and has been used traditionally as a natural health product [1]. There are many compounds of the curcuminoid family that are thought to produce its effects, the most studied being curcumin (**1**) (Figure 1) [2]. Curcumin is a deep yellow, poorly water-soluble substance that has been claimed to exhibit a variety of effects including antioxidant, anti-inflammatory, antiviral, antifungal, antibacterial, anticancer, antidiabetic and neuroprotective properties [3]. The effects elicited by curcumin are thought to be partly a result of its activity inhibiting the histone lysine acetyltransferases (HATs) p300/CBP [4] as well as histone deacetylases (HDACs) such as HDAC1 [5]. Inhibition of enzymes that catalyze lysine acetylation are known to have a variety of effects on gene expression and such activity confers a potential epigenetic mechanism to curcumin that has led to its exploration as an anticancer medication. Indeed, several HDAC inhibitors are already in use alone or in combination for the treatment of cancer and several groups have thought to exploit curcumin for its HDAC inhibition activity. This activity has been shown to suppress some DNA damage repair pathways and may be used to increase the effectiveness of existing cancer treatments [6]. Despite its poor bioavailability, curcumin has even been shown to suppress medulloblastoma growth in vivo through its HDAC inhibition activity [7]. Inhibition of HAT is currently being explored as a new class of cancer treatment, but despite promising results, no HAT inhibitors are currently approved; therefore, the anticancer potential of the HAT inhibition of curcumin has not been explored as much as its HDAC inhibition activity [8]. Curcumin is thought to exhibit its HAT inhibition activity by a Michael-addition reaction, alkylating the active-site cysteines of HAT [9].

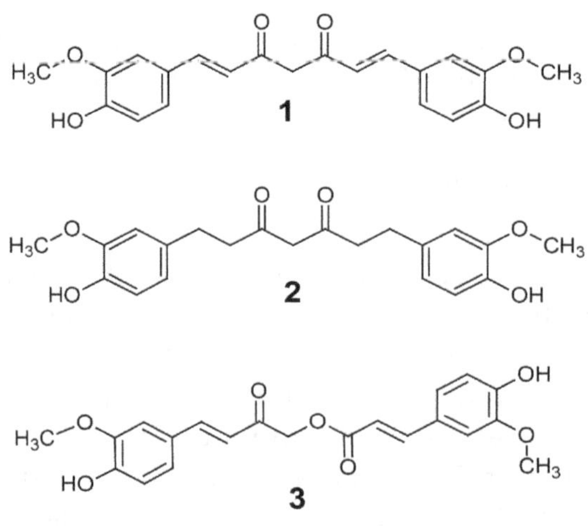

Figure 1. The structures of curcuminoids curcumin (**1**), tetrahydrocurcumin (THC) (**2**) and calebin-A (**3**). Both THC and curcumin are shown in the keto tautomer.

Another important consequence of inhibiting HAT activity is the repression of genes important in the inflammatory response. For example, some HAT inhibitors have been shown to inhibit the NF-κB pathway [10,11]. Recently, HAT inhibitors having a similar mechanism of inhibition to curcumin [9] have been shown to reduce expression of COX2, yielding anti-inflammatory and analgesic effects [12]. Although a great deal of attention has been paid to curcumin, there are many other curcuminoid-type compounds in turmeric that have potential pharmacological activities, such as tetrahydrocurcumin (THC) (**2**) and calebin-A (**3**) (Figure 1) [2].

Calebin-A has been studied for its antioxidant, anti-inflammatory and anticancer effects that have been demonstrated in vitro by inhibition of cyclooxygenase and lipoxygenase; it may also have cytochrome P450 inhibitory activity, as it appears to interact with CYP2D6 and CYP1A2 [2]. It has also been shown to inhibit dipeptidyl peptidase-4 (DPP-4), which is a membrane glycoprotein and serine exopeptidase that is implicated in type 2 diabetes mellitus through its activity inhibiting incretin release, including GLP-1 [13]. Inhibitors of DPP-4, such as gliptins, are currently used clinically as hypoglycemic agents. Calebin-A has potential as an adjuvant for cancer therapy, increasing the effectiveness of currently used cancer treatments, as it has been shown to directly inhibit P-glycoprotein and has been co-administered with vincristine to treat multidrug-resistant human gastric cancer cells. Furthermore, calebin-A also appears to modulate the mitogen-activated protein-kinase pathway. These data suggest the calebin-A may be an effective cancer treatment [1], however, a major drawback is that it has an extremely low oral bioavailability, much like curcumin [2].

THC is another curcuminoid found in turmeric that is produced by the reduction of curcumin [14]. It can be synthesized in the laboratory by hydrogenation of curcumin, yielding a colorless substance. THC can also be produced in vivo through Phase I metabolism in the liver by hepatic reductases, and as a result, after oral administration it is found as free THC and conjugated as glucuronides. Like curcumin and calebin-A, THC is also thought to have several biological activities; among the most studied are its antioxidant properties. In fact, the antioxidant role of THC has been studied as a potential preventative treatment for cardiovascular disease by reducing the formation of atherosclerotic lesions. THC has also been studied for its anti-inflammatory activity, both as a treatment for arthritis and cancer [14]. Like calebin-A and curcumin, THC is an inhibitor of P-glycoprotein, and because of this, THC has been explored as a potential way to overcome multidrug resistance in cancer [15].

THC has a number of attractive properties not shared with curcumin that may make it superior. For example, THC is significantly more stable under physiological pH and temperature conditions than curcumin [16]. Moreover, it is slightly more soluble in water, making it much easier to formulate into an acceptable dosage form than curcumin which, as stated above, has had longstanding issues with its near-insolubility in water and a number of other common solvents.

Currently, there are few studies in the literature about curcuminoids, apart from curcumin. Considering the depth of study of curcumin as a treatment for cancer among other diseases, the fact that curcumin is metabolized to THC, and the fact that THC has therapeutic potential in its own right, it is necessary to describe the pharmacological effects and pharmacokinetic characteristics of THC. In this study we developed a bioanalytical assay to quantify THC in urine and serum using ultra-high-performance liquid chromatography–mass spectrometry (UHPLC–MS/MS) to characterize its pharmacokinetics in rats after oral (PO) administration. We also identify the HDAC and HAT activities, as well as the antioxidant, anti-inflammatory and cell viability activities of THC compared to curcumin and calebin-A. As far as we know, this is the first study to dose rats with THC and measure serum and urine concentrations of THC.

2. Materials and Methods

2.1. Chemicals and Reagents

Tetrahydrocurcumin, curcumin and calebin-A were provided by Sabinsa Corporation® (Piscataway, NJ, USA). Sulfaphenazole, ketoconazole, α-naphthoflavone, quinidine, DMSO, PEG-400 and β-glucuronidase type IX A (β-glucuronidase) were purchased from Sigma-Aldrich (St. Louis, MO, USA). Analytical-grade formic acid and HPLC-grade acetonitrile were purchased from Fisher Scientific. Ultrapure water from a Milli-Q® system (Millipore, Billerica, MA, USA) was used for mobile phase. The antioxidant activity kit, cyclooxygenase-1 and -2 inhibitor screening kits, lipoxygenase inhibitor screening kit, HDAC1 and PCAF inhibitor screening kits were purchased from Cayman Chemical Company (Ann Arbor, MI, USA). Vivid® CYP2C9 green screening kit, Vivid® CYP3A4 green screening kit, Vivid® CYP1A2 blue screening kit and Vivid® CYP2D6 blue screening kit were bought from Life Technologies™ (Carlsbad, CA, USA). Human CXCL9/MIG, Human TNF-α, Human IFN-γ and Human CXCL10/IP-10 DuoSet® ELISA kits, solutions and reagents were purchased from R & D Systems® (Minneapolis, MN, USA). CellTiter 96® AQueous One Solution Cell Proliferation Assay (MTS) was purchased from Promega (Madison, WI, USA). Heat-inactivated fetal bovine serum was purchased from Gibco® by Life Technologies™ and Roswell Park Memorial Institute (RPMI) 1640 medium and Penicillin Streptomycin solution were purchased from Corning.

2.2. UHPLC–MS/MS Analysis and Conditions

THC was analyzed using the Shimadzu Nexera UHPLC coupled to a Shimadzu LCMS 8040 triple quadrupole mass spectrometer (Shimadzu, Kyoto, Japan). Chromatography was performed using a Waters Acquity UPLC BEH C18 column under isocratic conditions with 45% aqueous acetonitrile in 0.1% formic acid at a flow rate of 0.4 mL/min. THC and the internal standard (curcumin) were measured using Multiple Reaction Monitoring (MRM) in positive mode using the transitions m/z 373.3 > 137.1 and m/z 369.3 > 177.1, respectively. Data analysis was performed with the LabSolutions software version 5.72 (Shimadzu, Kyoto, Japan).

2.3. Animals

Surgically-modified, exposed jugular vein-catheterized (polyurethane-silastic blended catheter), adult male CD Sprague-Dawley rats (250–300 g) were purchased from Charles River Laboratories (St. Constant, QC, Canada). Rats received free access to food (Purina Rat Chow 5001) and water in the animal facility for at least 3 days before use. Rats were housed in temperature-controlled rooms with a 12 h light/dark cycle. Animal ethics approval was obtained from University of Manitoba Office of Research Ethics and Compliance (protocol 11-064) and a minimal number of rats were utilized to answer the hypothesis tested.

2.4. Pharmacokinetic Study

THC was provided as a dry powder from Sabinsa Corporation® and this was dissolved in a mixture of DMSO 2% and 98% PEG-400. Each rat was placed in a separate metabolic cage and fasted for 12 h prior to dosing with free access to water. On the day of experiment, the animals (N = 3) received a single dose of THC by oral gavage (500 mg/kg) in a volume not exceeding 1 mL. Animals had free access to water pre- and post-dosing, and food (Purina Rat Chow 5001) was provided 2 hours post-dosing. A series of blood samples (0.3 mL) were collected at 0, 15 and 30 min, and 1, 2, 4, 6, 12, 24, 48 and 72 h post-dose. At 72 h after administration, the animals were euthanized and exsanguinated. Immediately after each blood collection time point (except the terminal point), the cannula was flushed with 0.3 mL of 0.9% saline to replenish the collected blood volume. The dead volume of the cannula was replaced with sterile heparin/50% dextrose catheter lock solution (SAI Infusion Technologies, Strategic Applications, Lake Villa, IL, USA) to maintain the patency of the cannula as advised in the technical sheet supplied with the animals from Charles River. Following centrifugation of blood samples at 15,000 rpm for 5 min, serum was collected and placed into 2 mL tubes at −20 °C until further analysis. Urine samples were collected at 0, 2, 6, 12, 24, 48 and 72 h post-dose and placed in 15 mL tubes. The exact urine volume of each sample was recorded then stored at −20 °C until further analysis.

2.5. Standard Solutions and Standard Curve Preparation

Stock solutions of THC and curcumin were prepared in acetonitrile and calibration standards were prepared from these stocks in blank urine and serum into a series of concentrations: 0.005, 0.01, 0.05, 0.1, 0.5, 1.0, 5.0 and 10.0 μg/mL. Briefly, 100 μL of serum or urine, 50 μL of internal standard (curcumin 1 μg/mL) and the corresponding concentration of THC stock solution were combined and vortexed in a 2 mL microtube. Ice-cold acetonitrile (1 mL) was added to precipitate serum proteins from solution and the same was done in urine for consistency. These solutions were vortexed, centrifuged and the supernatants were collected and evaporated to dryness by a stream of nitrogen gas. The pellet was reconstituted with 50 μL of 45% aqueous acetonitrile (ACN) with 0.1% formic acid (F.A.) and injected into the UHPLC–MS/MS. The accuracy was measured from three standard curves on three separate days and precision measured with 4 quality control (QC) samples at the low, mid and high range of the curve. The accuracy and precision of the assay were 89.2 ± 10% and 95.1 ± 4.9%, respectively.

2.6. Serum and Urine Sample Preparation

Serum and urine samples (100 μL) were treated with 20 μL of 500 U/mL β-glucuronidase, vortexed and incubated at 37 °C for 2 h to release any glucuronide conjugates. 50 μL of internal standard (curcumin 1 μg/mL) was added, vortexed and rapidly, 1 mL of cold acetonitrile was added to precipitate the proteins present in both samples. Urine and serum samples were vortexed and centrifuged at 15,000 rpm for 5 min. The supernatants were collected and evaporated to dryness by nitrogen gas. Samples were reconstituted with 50 μL of mobile phase (45% ACN, 0.1% F.A.) and vortexed. The samples were transferred to HPLC vials and 10 μL was injected into the UHPLC system for each sample.

2.7. Cytochrome P450 Inhibition Determination

CYP2C9, CYP3A4, CYP1A2 and CYP2D6 assays were performed to assess metabolism and inhibition of human P450 isozymes involved using Vivid® CYP450 screening kits and CYP450 BACULOSOMES® Plus Reagents. CYP450 BACULOSOMES® Plus Reagents express only one CYP450 enzyme, preventing metabolism by other CYP450s. For CYP2C9, the substrate was BOMF and the positive control inhibitor sulfaphenazole; for CYP3A4, DBOMF was the substrate and ketoconazole the positive control inhibitor; for CYP1A2, the substrate was EOMCC and the positive control inhibitor naphthoflavone; for CYP2D6, the substrate was EOMCC and the positive control inhibitor quinidine. The assays were performed using the excitation and emission wavelengths recommended by the manufacturer. To run the assay, 50 μL of Master Pre-Mix was added with 40 μL of THC, curcumin and calebin-A, at 0.01, 0.1, 1.0, 10.0, 50.0 and 100.0 μM dissolved in DMSO. The plate was incubated for 10 min at room temperature (25 ± 1 °C) on a plate shaker. Then, 10 μL of Vivid® Substrate was added to each well to start the reaction. Less than 2 min after the reaction had started, the measurement of fluorescence was performed using the Synergy HT multi-well plate reader and Gen5 data analysis software (Biotek Instruments Inc., Winooski, VT, USA). The assay was done in triplicate. The reading was performed at 1 min intervals for 60 min. Inhibition was calculated as $(1 - (X - B/A - B)) \times 100\%$, where X was the average of compound fluorescence, A was the average of solvent control and B was the average of inhibition in the presence of positive inhibitor control. The percent inhibition was calculated relative to a fixed concentration of the positive control. For more information of assay protocols, please refer to the instructions for the kits (Vivid® CYP2C9 Green Screening Kit—Cat. no. P2860; Vivid® CYP3A4 Green Screening Kit—Cat. No. P2857; Vivid® CYP1A2 Blue Screening Kit—Cat. No. P2863 and Vivid® CYP2D6 Blue Screening Kit—Cat. No. P2972 from Life Technologies).

2.8. Antioxidant Capacity Determination

Total antioxidant capacity of THC, curcumin and calebin-A was measured using the antioxidant assay kit (Cayman Chemical, Ann Arbor, MI, USA) following the standard protocol from the manufacturer. The assay measures the inhibition of oxidation of 2,2′-azino-bis(3-ethylbenzothiazoline-6-sulphonic acid) (ABTS) by metmyoglobin. THC, curcumin and calebin-A were prepared in DMSO for concentrations of 1, 5, 10, 50 and 100 μg/mL. The antioxidant capacity of each curcuminoid was expressed as Trolox equivalents. The assay was performed in triplicate and absorbance at 750 nm was measured using the Synergy HT plate reader (Biotek Instruments Inc., Winooski, VT, USA). For more information regarding the assay protocol, please refer to the instructions for the kit (Antioxidant Assay kit from Cayman Chemical—Cat. No. 709091).

2.9. Cyclooxygenase Inhibition Determination

Cyclooxygenase is a bifunctional enzyme exhibiting both COX and peroxidase activities. This assay was used to measure the inhibition of COX-1 and -2 of THC, curcumin and calebin-A. Concentrations of 1, 10 and 250 μg/mL of THC, curcumin and calebin-A were prepared using DMSO. The assay was performed in quadruplet using a COX Inhibitor Screening Assay Kit from Cayman

Chemical (Cat. No. 560131) according to the manufacturer's instructions. The measurement of absorbance was performed at 415 nm within 10 min at room temperature using the Synergy HT multi-well plate reader and Gen5 data analysis software (Biotek Instruments Inc., Winooski, VT, USA).

2.10. *Lipoxygenase Inhibition*

We detected the lipoxygenase activity of the curcuminoids using a Lipoxygenase Inhibitor Screening Assay Kit from Cayman Chemical (Ann Arbor, MI, USA, Cat. No. 760700a) using linoleic acid as the substrate according to the manufacturer's recommended instructions. Briefly, concentrations of 1, 10 and 250 μg/mL of THC, curcumin and calebin-A were prepared in DMSO and 10 μL of each were combined with 90 μL of 15-lipoxygenase derived from soybean. 10 μL of linoleic acid was added to start the reaction. The plate was covered and placed on a shaker for 5 min. Then, 100 μL of chromogen was added. The plate was covered and placed on a shaker for 5 min again. The assay was performed in triplicate. The absorbance was measured at 500 nm using the Synergy HT multi-well plate reader and Gen5 data analysis software (Biotek Instruments Inc., Winooski, VT, USA). For additional information of assay protocol, please refer to the instructions for the kit.

2.11. *Cellular Growth Inhibition Assay (MTS)*

The CellTiter 96® AQueous One Solution Cell Proliferation Assay (MTS, Promega, Madison, WI, USA) was used to measure proliferation inhibition of cultured cells. Briefly, Sup-T1 cells were cultured in RPMI 1640 supplemented with 10% FBS and 1% penicillin/streptomycin at 37 °C and 5% CO_2. 2×10^5 cells/mL were seeded in each well and THC, curcumin and calebin-A, at 0.1, 0.5, 1.0, 5.0, 10.0, 50.0 and 100.0 μM dissolved in DMSO, were added to their respective wells and incubated for 24, 48 and 72 h. The MTS reagent was added and incubated for 4 h. Absorbance was recorded at 490 nm in Synergy HT multi-well plate reader and Gen5 data analysis software (Biotek Instruments Inc., Winooski, VT, USA). Sup-T1 cells were used in this study because curcuminoids are thought in part to work via an HDAC inhibitor mechanism and as some HDACs are approved for some T-cell lymphomas, we used Sup-T1 cells because they are a T-cell lymphoma cell line that is established. To the best of our knowledge no other study has measured the effects of THC on Sup-T1 cells.

2.12. *Cellular Inflammatory Cytokine Release Assay (TNF-α)*

Sup-T1 cells were prepared and seeded as above and separately treated with THC, curcumin and calebin-A at 5, 10, 50 and 100 μM. Cell culture supernatant was collected and used to determine released TNF-α using the Human TNF-alpha DuoSet ELISA kit (DY210, R & D systems, Minneapolis, MN, USA) following the standard manufacturer's protocol, optimized using recombinant TNF-α. The optical density was determined in Synergy HT multi-well plate reader and Gen5 data analysis software (Biotek Instruments Inc., Winooski, VT, USA). The data were analyzed using SigmaPlot 12.2 (Systat Software Inc., San Jose, CA, USA).

2.13. *HDAC1 and PCAF Inhibition Assays*

Curcuminoids were tested for direct HDAC1 and PCAF inhibitory activity using the fluorescent-based HDAC1 or PCAF inhibitor screening assay kit ((HDAC1) 10011564, (PCAF) 10006515, Cayman, Ann Arbor, MI, USA) according to manufacturer's instructions. THC, curcumin and calebin-A, at 0.1, 1.0, 10.0, 50.0, 100.0 and 250.0 μg/mL dissolved in DMSO, were prepared and screened. Fluorescence was measured for both assays using excitation/emission wavelengths of 340/460 nm using Synergy HT multi-well plate reader and Gen5 data analysis software (Biotek Instruments Inc., Winooski, VT, USA).

Data for the PCAF and HDAC1 inhibition and viability assays were used to derive percent changes based on no treatment controls. Each of three data sets were then fit to a 4-parameter logistic regression using SigmaPlot 12.2 to derive IC_{50} values, which were then used to determine the mean and SD.

3. Results

3.1. Chromatography

The central 3,5-dione structure of THC and curcumin allows for keto–enol tautomerism. We optimized chromatographic conditions for both tautomers of THC to be resolved easily as the keto and enol forms that had a retention time of 1.4 min and 2.7 min, respectively. Similarly, the keto and enol tautomers of curcumin were easily resolved, having retention times of 1.2 min and 3.2 min, respectively (Figure 2). The enol and keto forms of each compound have the same molecular weight and fragmentation spectra, so the mass spectrometer on its own is incapable of differentiating the two tautomers of each analyte. We reconciled the retention times of each tautomer based on the previous studies which showed that curcumin is primarily in the enol form in solutions of ~50% acetonitrile, which is very similar to the conditions we used [17]. Corroborating this, other similar studies have shown that in aqueous solutions with increasing amounts of alcohol the enol tautomer predominates [18]. We defined the larger peak with the longer retention time to be the enol tautomer for curcumin, as has been observed by others under similar conditions [17], and used the same relative retention to identify the tautomers of THC (Figure 2). For THC, we found that the two tautomers were in roughly equal proportion under these chromatographic conditions, while curcumin appeared to favour the enol tautomer by a 5:1 ratio. The sum of the peak areas for both tautomers was used to calculate the concentrations in the samples. Blank plasma samples showed that there were no interfering peaks that co-eluted with THC and curcumin (data not shown).

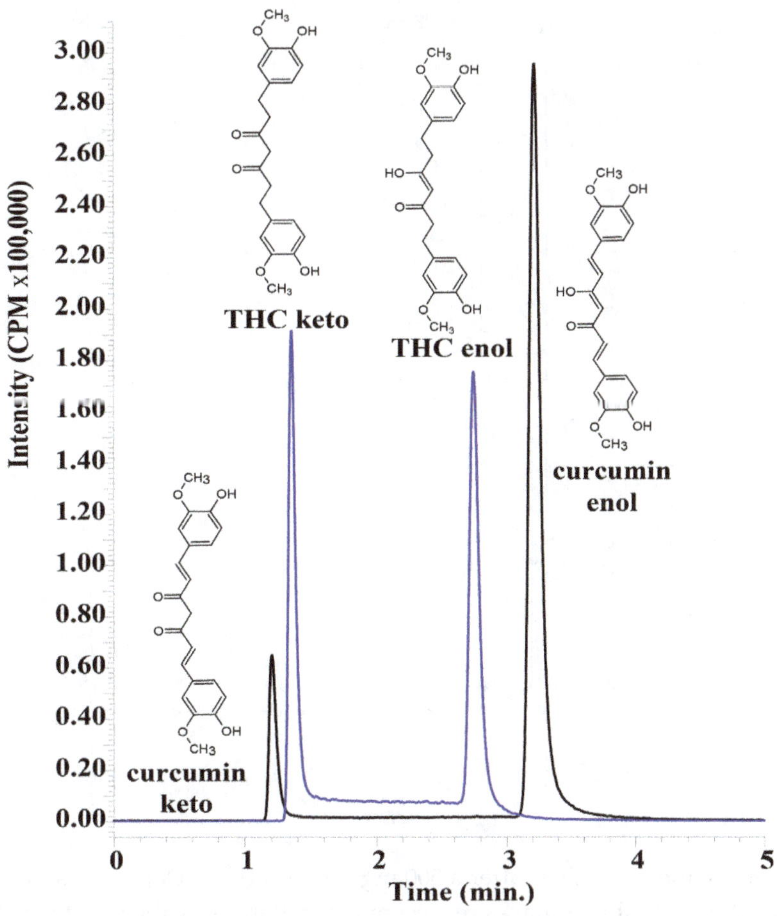

Figure 2. A representative chromatogram of curcumin and tetrahydrocurcumin (THC) Shown are the enol and keto forms of curcumin and THC using the LC–MS/MS assay. Both compounds are at a concentration of 1 µg/mL dissolved in acetonitrile.

3.2. Pharmacokinetics

The serum THC concentration versus time curve shows that more than one absorption and distribution phase was present. Initially, a rapid absorption phase with an average T_{max} of 6.8 μg/mL at 1 h was observed, followed by a short elimination phase. This was followed by two redistributions with two smaller THC maxima at 6 and 24 h (Figure 3A). Both redistribution phases had similar maxima of about 1 μg/mL (Figure 3A). The total amount of THC excreted unchanged in urine was up to 8 μg at 24 h (Figure 3B). Coinciding with the first short elimination phase, the rate of urinary excretion reached a maximum of just under 3 μg/h at 2 h. In addition, an increase in excretion rate can be observed at 12 after the second distribution. Finally, a second excretion rate maximum coincided with the final distribution phase at 24 h.

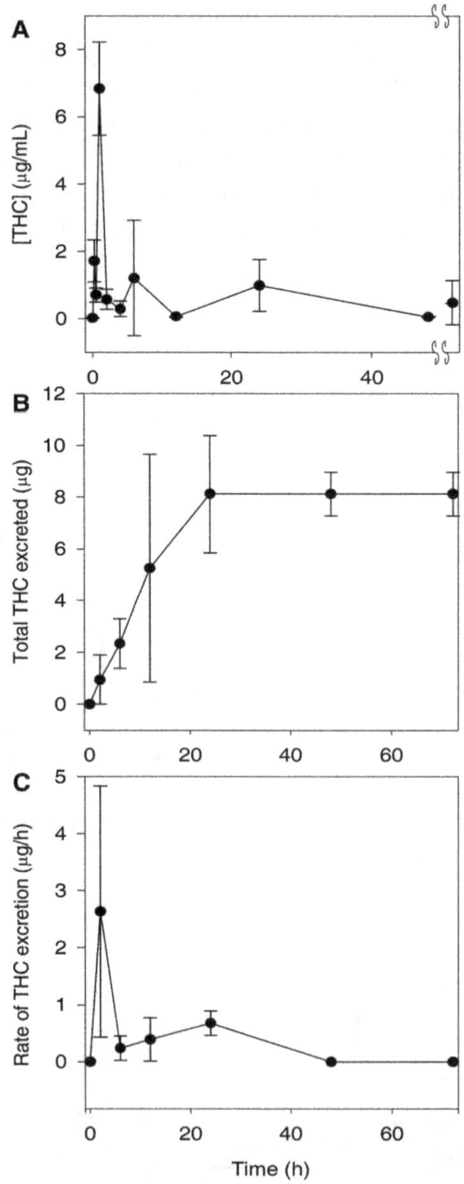

Figure 3. The pharmacokinetics of THC after a 500 mg/kg oral dose. Depicted is the serum disposition of THC in μg/mL (**A**) (the double S-marks represent a break in the Time axis from 49 to 71 h and the final time point is 72 h); the total amount of THC excreted in the urine in μg after oral administration (**B**); and the rate of urinary excretion of THC in μg/mL (**C**). All values represent a mean of 3 with standard deviation.

3.3. Cytochrome P450 Inhibition

The three curcuminoids were tested for their ability to inhibit CYP 2C9, 3A4, 1A2 and 2D6. THC, curcumin and calebin-A yielded dose-dependent inhibition of CYP2C9, and to a lesser extent, CYP3A4. All three exhibited maximum inhibition of CYP2C9 (Figure 4A) and CYP3A4 (Figure 4B) at 50 to 100 μM, compared to the positive controls sulphaphenazole and ketoconazole. Curcumin, calebin-A and THC did not show a consistent dose-response inhibition of CYP1A2 (Figure 4C) or CYP2D6 (Figure 4D) over the range of concentrations tested. In some cases, the percent inhibition exceeded 100%; this may be because percent inhibition is calculated relative to a fixed concentration of a positive control inhibitor. In those cases where percent inhibition exceeds 100%, it may be because the curcuminoid being studied is a more effective inhibitor of the CYP in question than the positive control. For Figure 4D, in some cases, curcumin appears to produce negative inhibition or increased activity, but the error associated with these values makes it difficult to determine if this is the case.

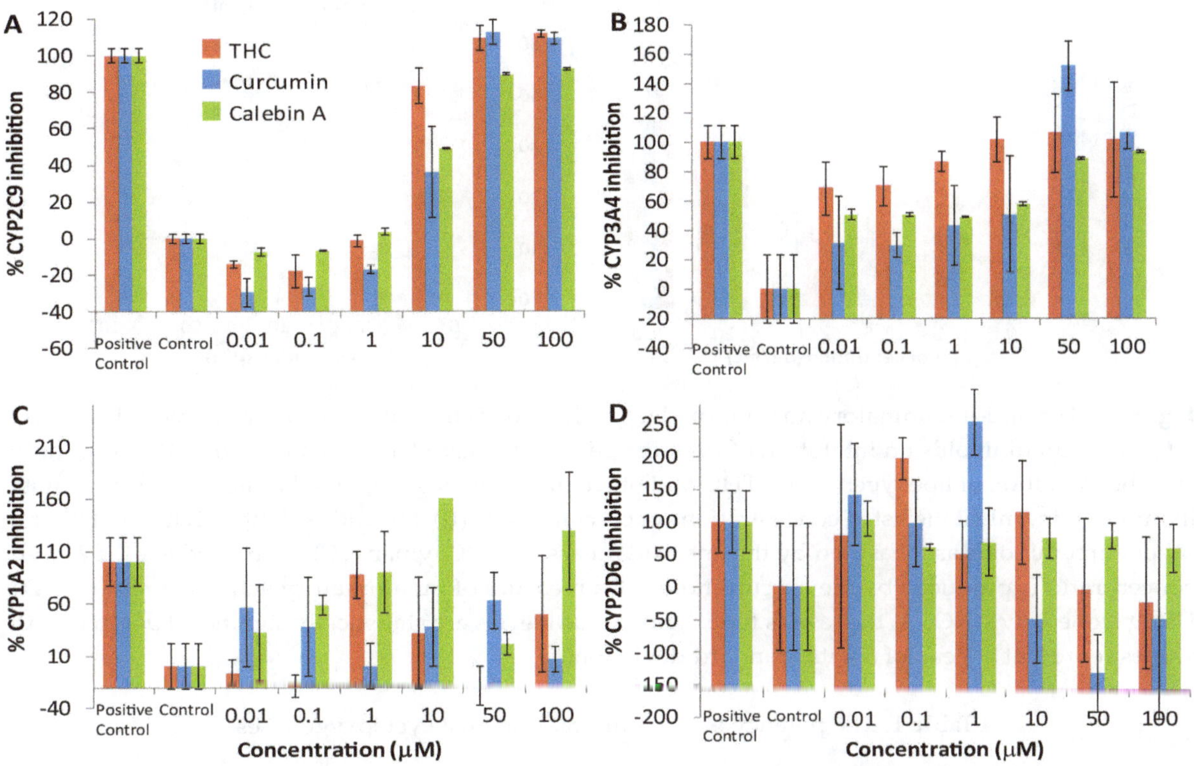

Figure 4. The inhibition of selected common drug-metabolizing enzymes by curcuminoids. Displayed are graphs showing the inhibition of CYP 2C9 (**A**); CYP3A4 (**B**); CYP1A2 (**C**); and CYP 2D6 (**D**) by THC, curcumin and calebin-A with solvent and positive controls using commercial assay kits.

3.4. Anti-Inflammatory Activity

The potential anti-inflammatory activity of HAT inhibitors, like curcumin and other curcuminoids, is thought to involve inhibition of expression of pro-inflammatory genes such as the *NF-κB* family and *COX-2*, however, it is still unclear if there is any direct inhibitory activity for curcuminoids against these pro-inflammatory proteins. Therefore, the inhibition of cyclooxygenase and lipoxygenase by THC, curcumin and calebin-A was measured using assay kits described in the methods. For the cyclooxygenase inhibition assay, we measured COX-2 and COX-1 IC_{50} and reported their COX-2/COX-1 ratios. Calebin-A and THC have similar ratios around 1, demonstrating approximately equal propensity to directly inhibit COX-2 and COX-1. Curcumin appears to show higher COX-2 inhibition with a COX-2/COX-1 ratio of 0.19 (Figure 5A). None of the curcuminoids were particularly effective inhibitors of either COX-1 or -2, with curcumin being the most effective against COX-2 with an IC_{50} of ~600 µM (Table 1). We evaluated the potential lipoxygenase inhibitory activity because we found marginal COX inhibition. Calebin-A did not show any activity, but both curcumin and THC inhibited lipoxygenase as low as 1 µM (Figure 5B).

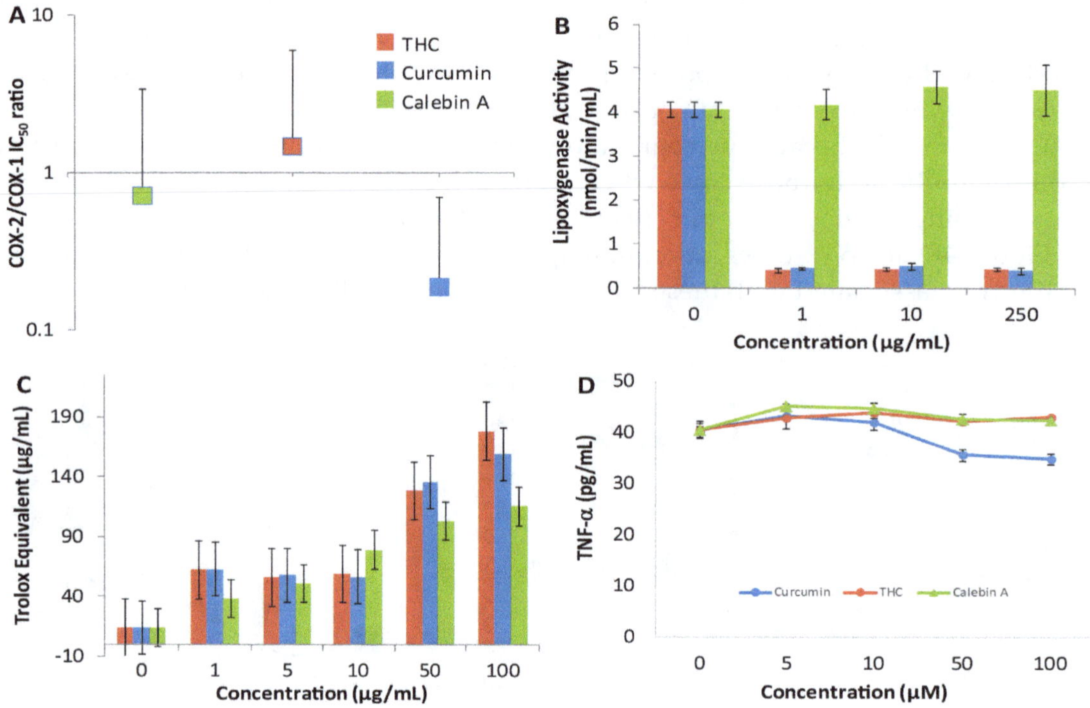

Figure 5. The anti-inflammatory and antioxidant activity of THC and other curcuminoids. The direct effects of curcuminoids on inhibition of cyclooxygenase displayed as the COX-2 to COX-1 IC_{50} ratio (**A**); the inhibition of lipoxygenase by THC and other curcuminoids displayed as lipoxygenase activity in mmol/min/mL at the listed concentrations of curcuminoids (**B**); the antioxidant activity of THC and other curcuminoids as measured by the antioxidant assay kit (Cayman) (**C**); displayed are the TNF-α concentrations produced by the curcuminoids as a measure of inflammatory activity in pg/mL (**D**). Using a one-way ANOVA, the results for 50 and 100 µM levels are statistically significant $p < 0.001$. All values represent a mean of 3 with standard deviation.

Table 1. The potency of curcuminoids against cyclooxygenases.

Curcuminoid	COX-1 IC_{50} (µM)	COX-2 IC_{50} (µM)
THC	918 ± 1300	1348 ± 3641
Curcumin	3392 ± 8982	635 ± 367
Calebin-A	1069 ± 490	784 ± 2200

The total antioxidant activity of THC, curcumin and calebin-A was calculated with respect to Trolox as a measure of antioxidant capacity. Both THC and curcumin (and to a lesser extent calebin-A) showed their greatest antioxidant effect at 100 µM (Figure 5C).

In order to fully evaluate the anti-inflammatory activity of the curcuminoids, the concentrations of the pro-inflammatory mediators TNF-α, IFN-γ, MIG and IP-10 were measured using an ELISA assay in Sup-T1 cells treated with increasing concentrations of THC, curcumin and calebin-A. The measurements for IFN-γ, MIG and IP-10 were below detection levels for all curcuminoids. There also appeared to be no dose-response change in the concentration of TNF-α in Sup-T1 cells treated with THC and calebin-A. However, a slight decrease in TNF-α compared to no-treatment control appears to be present at the 50 and 100 µM levels for curcumin (Figure 5D).

3.5. Cell Viability

One potential therapeutic use of curcumin and THC is for the treatment of cancer [3]. It has been shown that curcumin and potentially other curcuminoids are inhibitors of HDAC and HAT. Such compounds that inhibit histone lysine acetylation and deacetylation are already being explored for their cancer treatment potential [9]. The effect of THC, curcumin and calebin-A on cancer cell viability was measured. Sup-T1 cells, T-cell lymphoblastic lymphoma cells, were treated with the curcuminoids to determine their ability to induce growth inhibition using an MTS assay, and the corresponding IC_{50} values were in the mid-to-high micromolar range (Table 2). Curcumin and calebin-A were the most potent, but THC was more than 4-fold less potent than curcumin, and at the most, resulted in a 40% growth inhibition (Figure 6A).

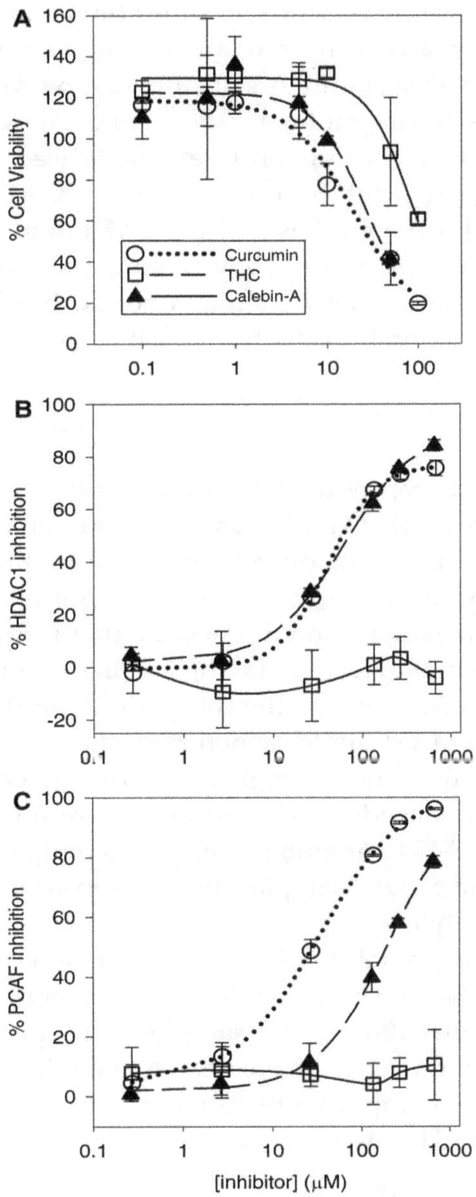

Figure 6. Cell viability and HDAC and HAT inhibition. The viability of Sup-T1 cells with increasing concentrations of the curcuminoids (**A**); the direct inhibition of the HAT PCAF by the curcuminoids as measured by an ELISA assay (**B**); the direct inhibition of the HDAC HDAC1 by the curcuminoids as measured by an ELISA assay (**C**). For each graph the points are the means of three values with an SD.

Table 2. The potency of curcuminoids on Sup-T1 growth inhibition and HDAC1/PCAF inhibition.

Curcuminoid	Viability IC_{50} (μM)	HDAC1 IC_{50} (μM)	PCAF IC_{50} (μM)
THC	82 ± 116	NA	NA
Curcumin	19.0 ± 11	39.8 ± 3.2	33.1 ± 2.8
Calebin-A	26.2 ± 17	61.3 ± 11	200.0 ± 31

3.6. HDAC1 and HAT Inhibition

Having established the antioxidant, anti-inflammatory and cancer cell growth inhibitory properties of these curcuminoids, their activity against histone acetyltransferases (HAT) and histone deacetylases (HDAC) was evaluated, since it has been previously reported that this may be one of the many possible mechanisms for their anticancer and anti-inflammatory activities. HAT inhibitors are currently being explored as a new class of cancer treatments and have been shown to reduce expression of pro-inflammatory mediators. HDAC inhibitors are already in use alone or in combination to treat various cancers such as cutaneous T-cell lymphoma. We therefore tested the ability of the curcuminoids to inhibit HDAC1 and the HAT PCAF, using a fluorescence-based assay described in the methods. Here, we show curcumin is a potent inhibitor of the HAT PCAF (Figure 6B), an effect that has not been reported previously [4]. Calebin-A is also a PCAF inhibitor but is 6-fold less potent than curcumin (Table 2). Interestingly, THC shows no above-control inhibition of PCAF at any concentration (Figure 6C). Also as expected, curcumin and calebin-A both exhibit HDAC inhibition [5], but with similar potency, and THC shows no inhibitory activity against PCAF or HDAC1 at any concentration (Figure 6 and Table 2).

4. Discussion

A sensitive, accurate and reproducible assay was developed for the detection of tetrahydrocurcumin using UHPLC–MS/MS. It was possible to obtain baseline separation between keto and enol forms of THC and curcumin, despite the obvious similarities between the tautomers (Figure 2). Both tautomeric forms of THC and curcumin are present because of the 45% acetonitrile in the mobile phase, and they interconvert on a timescale that results in two peaks on the UHPLC chromatogram that are easily separable [17,18]. Having an alkaline mobile phase would result in only the enol form that would form an enolate, and the two peaks would converge. However, this would necessitate detection in negative MRM mode, which results in a decrease in sensitivity. The acidic mobile phase was important in obtaining the highly sensitive detection of THC and curcumin, but resulted in two separate peaks that needed to be summed in order to calculate total THC and total curcumin. We used UHPLC–MS/MS to unambiguously differentiate curcumin and THC from other serum peaks, and as expected, the plasma samples did not appear to have any other peaks that were erroneously detected as either analyte.

The choice of curcumin as an internal standard is rational in the sense that its chemical properties and structure are similar to THC. However, as mentioned above, curcumin can be metabolized to THC in the liver, and it is still possible that after plasma samples were spiked with curcumin as the internal standard, a small amount of curcumin could have been metabolized in the plasma. To mitigate this, plasma proteins in the samples were rapidly precipitated with ice-cold acetonitrile, and this would also remove any possible plasma reductases.

4.1. Disposition, Metabolism and Elimination of THC

Preliminary pharmacokinetic studies indicate that un-optimized formulations of THC have poor oral bioavailability, and it appears to only be detectable in serum and urine as glucuronides [19]. In order to detect curcumin and THC by the UHPLC–MS/MS assay, samples were treated with β-glucuronidase in order to proceed with the analysis in serum and urine. Its presence in urine indicates that THC was orally absorbed and was eliminated at least in part through the renal route.

However, it has already been long established that curcumin is excreted primarily in the bile as a glucuronide conjugate of THC [20]. More recent evidence suggests that curcumin is excreted into the bile via the active transport ABCC2 drug efflux pump [21]. Therefore, the most likely route of elimination of THC is in the bile as a glucuronide conjugate. This, together with the poor bioavailability of THC, explains why we found low concentrations of THC in the urine (Figure 3B).

4.2. *THC, Curcumin and Calebin-A Inhibit CYP2C9 and CYP3A4*

Curcuminoids have demonstrated inhibition of many human drug-metabolizing enzymes, especially the Phase I CYP family of oxidases in vitro [22]. We showed that THC, calebin-A and curcumin produced a consistent inhibitory dose-response relationship with CYP2C9 and 3A4, but no such dose-response relationship could be detected with CYP 1A2 and 2D6. These results suggest that THC, curcumin and calebin-A are inhibitors of CYP 2C9 and 3A4. It is not immediately obvious how these curcuminoids inhibit CYP enzymes. Curcuminoids are unlikely to be important as substrates for CYPs, as previous studies have shown that curcumin is reduced to THC by reductases and primarily converted into a THC glucuronide [19,20]. Despite this, a small proportion of each of the curcuminoids may undergo *O*-dealkylation by demethylation of the aromatic methoxy groups, and the occupancy of the enzyme may result in inhibition that is competitive. As has been observed, some curcuminoids have the potential to alkylate enzymes through the α,β-unsaturated carbonyl (Michael acceptor) [9]. This has been the mechanism proposed for curcumin and its activity against p300, however, this cannot be the mechanism of action of CYP inhibition because THC does not have such a Michael acceptor group and yet exhibits CYP inhibition. An alternative mechanism of inhibition may be nucleophilic addition at the enolic carbon (Michael donor) shared between THC and curcumin.

4.3. *Curcuminoids Inhibit Some Pro-Inflammatory Mediators*

None of the curcuminoids were particularly effective inhibitors of either COX-1 or -2, with curcumin being the most effective, yielding a modest IC_{50} of ~600 μM (Table 1). Nevertheless, curcumin showed a slight inhibitory preference for COX-2, suggesting it may have an effect on the activity of COX during acute inflammation. The COX ratios of calebin-A and THC were sufficiently close to 1 and the errors large enough to make it difficult to suggest that either curcuminoid exhibited a preference for either COX enzyme. Furthermore, treatment with THC and calebin-A did not reduce TNF-α release in Sup-T1 cells, and curcumin only had a moderate effect at higher doses. None of the curcuminoids tested altered the concentrations of the cytokines, IFN-γ, MIG and IP-10 in SupT1 cells. Another important group of pro-inflammatory mediators are the leukotrienes, produced by lipoxygenase. Both THC and curcumin inhibited soybean 1,5-lipoxygenase at all doses tested in comparison to a control, while calebin-A showed no such inhibitory activity. As with CYP inhibition, the inhibition of lipoxygenase activity is unclear and cannot be caused by direct Michael addition reaction because THC does not possess a Michael acceptor group, however, both THC and curcumin are very similar in structure, suggesting that this structure may be important for binding to lipoxygenase. Previous studies have used molecular docking approaches to propose potential binding sites for THC on lipoxygenase. These studies suggest that THC scavenges peroxides acting as a redox inhibitor of lipoxygenase, showing mixed inhibition [23]. Other studies confirm that curcumin and THC potently inhibit human lipoxygenase, showing that the inhibition may be clinically significant [24]. The inhibition of lipoxygenase presents the possibility that THC and curcumin may be used as a treatment for inflammatory conditions such as asthma. Lipoxygenase inhibitors such as zileuton are currently in use for treatment of asthma in children where glucocorticoids are less desirable or contraindicated.

Our data showed that THC does not inhibit HDAC or HAT; therefore, its narrower spectrum may make it a superior choice as a lipoxygenase inhibitor anti-inflammatory, because in this case, HDAC and HAT inhibitory activities would represent off-target effects. This is especially significant because we found that THC has a peak concentration of greater than 6 μg/mL (Figure 3A), with concentrations of greater than 1 μg/mL being found up to 20 h later. As we found that THC has potent lipoxygenase inhibition at 1 μg/mL (Figure 5B), this suggests that despite its poor bioavailability, THC reaches concentrations in vivo that can inhibit lipoxygenase. As far as we know, no other group has measured these activities and parameters together and made the suggestion that THC may be used as a lipoxygenase inhibitor to treat asthma and that it may be superior to curcumin. However, we acknowledge that the formulation of THC would need to be dramatically improved or an alternate route of administration chosen. In this particular case, the poor bioavailability of THC may warrant formulation into an intrapulmonary delivery system such as a metered-dose inhaler.

4.4. Curcuminoids Are Potent Antioxidants

All curcuminoids tested exhibited antioxidant capacity equivalent to the vitamin E analog antioxidant Trolox in a dose-dependent manner as measured by their free-radical-scavenging activity (ABTS) in the antioxidant assay [16]. All curcuminoids appear to be more potent than Trolox at the 50 and 100 μg/mL levels. However, the data does not suggest there is any difference in antioxidant potency among the curcuminoids. These results suggest that the curcuminoids tested have potential as potent antioxidants if their poor bioavailability can be overcome.

4.5. Curcumin and Calebin-A Potently Inhibit Sup-T1 Growth

Consistent with the previously discovered anticancer activity, curcumin induced reductions in the T-cell lymphoblastic lymphoma Sup-T1 cell line. Calebin-A also reduced viability with a similar potency to curcumin (Table 2). However, THC was at least 4-fold less cytotoxic to SupT1 cells compared to curcumin and calebin-A. This difference is likely larger as we were unable to reduce the viability of the Sup-T1 cells below the 50% level over the concentration range used. Therefore, our estimation of the IC_{50} for THC is likely higher than it would be if we were able to reduce the viability below 50%. The Sup-T1 cell line only represents one particular cell line of one type of cancer, and the different curcuminoids may have varying efficacy against different cell and cancer types. For example, THC has been shown to potently inhibit the growth of colorectal cancer cells such as SW480 and HT-29 cells, either alone or in combination [25,26]. In fact, THC has been shown to be more effective than curcumin in colon and other cancers [27,28]. Moreover, the measure of potency for reducing cell viability may not be an accurate reflection of the clinical usefulness of any drug for cancer treatment, as animal cancer models (though outside of the scope for this work) are usually more informative.

4.6. Curcumin and Calebin-A Inhibit PCAF and HDAC1

Consistent with previous findings, curcumin inhibits HDAC and HAT activity. Although previous studies have shown that curcumin binds to and inhibits the HAT activity of p300/CBP [4], as far as we know, this is the first study to show that curcumin and calebin-A inhibit PCAF. These results are not unexpected, as PCAF binds to p300/CBP and all three proteins have HAT activity, albeit with slightly different substrate specificities [29]. The suggested mechanism for inhibition of HAT activity by curcumin is alkylation of the HAT via the Michael acceptor on curcumin. This is thought to happen through HAT active-site cysteine residues [9]. Given this, it is not surprising that calebin-A also inhibits HAT, because it has a similar Michael acceptor group (Figure 1). Previous groups have identified calebin-A as having anticancer activity against a multidrug-resistant human gastric cancer line through its activity in modulating the expression of the MAP kinase family, but the mechanism of this activity was not determined directly [1]. This was recently corroborated by the finding that calebin-A inhibits phosphorylation by suppressing NF-κB signaling activation associated with osteoporosis [30]. This result is important because NF-κB is modulated through the acetylation activity of p300/CBP [31]. Here, for the first time, we can justify the activities against MAPK/NF-κB and the resulting anticancer effects of calebin-A through its direct effect inhibiting PCAF. Furthermore, calebin-A shows similar potency inhibiting HDAC1 compared to curcumin (Figure 6B), which may contribute to their anticancer activities and may be attributed to the presence of the Michael acceptor moiety on each compound. Therefore, the lack of both HDAC1 and PCAF inhibition by THC may be attributed to its lack of double bonds, which form the Michael acceptor groups present in curcumin and calebin-A (Figure 1). The observed absence of HDAC/PCAF inhibition by THC is not entirely surprising as it has long been suspected to have a different anticancer mechanism than curcumin [3]. Several studies have shown that THC is a potent antioxidant, and this study is in agreement with these findings [32–34]. Moreover, the finding that THC reduces lipoxygenase activity adds a potential anti-inflammatory mechanism that, in conjunction with its antioxidant activity, may explain the anticancer activity of THC.

Our results show that curcumin is 6-fold more potent with respect to PCAF inhibition than calebin-A, but both curcuminoids have similar IC_{50} values for inhibition of HDAC1. It is not clear why this might be the case, as both compounds are very similar. It is unlikely that enzymatic or non-enzymatic hydrolysis of the ester of calebin-A might affect its potency, as both compounds have similar potency against HDAC1 under similar conditions to the HAT assay. However, this ester is almost certainly a route of metabolism for calebin-A—that is not present in curcumin or THC—that may affect its in-vivo activity.

Acknowledgments: The authors acknowledge support from the Paul H.T. Thorlakson Foundation Fund, The Manitoba Medical Services Foundation [8-2014-03 2014], University of Manitoba Research Grants Program [UM Project # 43887, 2015], the Natural Sciences and Engineering Research Council (NSERC) Canada [RGPIN-2015-06543, 2015-2020] (to Ted M. Lakowski), the Leslie F. Buggey Graduate Scholarship, 2014 and the Research Manitoba Fellowship (to Ryan Lillico), a Canada, Brazil Science without Borders Summer Studentship (to Julia T. Novaes), and a graduate scholarship from Kuwait University, Kuwait (to Samaa Al-Rushaid). This work was also partially funded by the Sabinsa Corporation (to Neal M. Davies).

Author Contributions: Stephanie E. Martinez, Casey L. Sayre, Neal M. Davies, Kalyanam Nagabhushanam, Muhammed Majeed, Yufei Chen and Ryan Lillico conceived and designed the experiments; Julia T. Novaes, Anna P. Oliveira, Stephanie E. Martinez, Ryan Lillico, Samaa Alrushaid, performed the experiments; Julia T. Novaes, Stephanie E. Martinez, Neal M. Davies, Kalyanam Nagabhushanam, Muhammed Majeed, Ted M. Lakowski and Ryan Lillico analyzed the data; Ted M. Lakowski, Emmanuel Ho, Kalyanam Nagabhushanam, Muhammed Majeed and Neal M Davies contributed reagents/materials/analysis tools; Julia T. Novase, Ted M. Lakowski, Neal M. Davies, and Ryan Lillico wrote the paper..

References

1. Li, Y.; Li, S.; Han, Y.; Liu, J.; Zhang, J.; Li, F.; Wang, Y.; Liu, X.; Yao, L. Calebin-A induces apoptosis and modulates MAPK family activity in drug resistant human gastric cancer cells. *Eur. J. Pharmacol.* **2008**, *591*, 252–258. [CrossRef] [PubMed]
2. Oliveira, A.L.; Martinez, S.E.; Nagabushnam, K.; Majeed, M.; Alrushaid, S.; Sayre, C.L.; Davies, N.M. Calebin A: Analytical Development for Pharmacokinetics Study, Elucidation of Pharmacological Activities and Content Analysis of Natural Health Products. *J. Pharm. Pharm. Sci.* **2015**, *18*, 494–514. [CrossRef] [PubMed]
3. Aggarwal, B.B.; Deb, L.; Prasad, S. Curcumin differs from tetrahydrocurcumin for molecular targets, signaling pathways and cellular responses. *Molecules* **2015**, *20*, 185–205. [CrossRef] [PubMed]
4. Balasubramanyam, K.; Varier, R.A.; Altaf, M.; Swaminathan, V.; Siddappa, N.B.; Ranga, U.; Kundu, T.K. Curcumin, a novel p300/CREB-binding protein-specific inhibitor of acetyltransferase, represses the acetylation of histone/nonhistone proteins and histone acetyltransferase-dependent chromatin transcription. *J. Biol. Chem.* **2004**, *279*, 51163–51171. [CrossRef] [PubMed]
5. Reuter, S.; Gupta, S.C.; Park, B.; Goel, A.; Aggarwal, B.B. Epigenetic changes induced by curcumin and other natural compounds. *Genes Nutr.* **2011**, *6*, 93–108. [CrossRef] [PubMed]
6. Wang, S.H.; Lin, P.Y.; Chiu, Y.C.; Huang, J.S.; Kuo, Y.T.; Wu, J.C.; Chen, C.C. Curcumin-Mediated HDAC Inhibition Suppresses the DNA Damage Response and Contributes to Increased DNA Damage Sensitivity. *PLoS ONE* **2015**, *10*, e0134110. [CrossRef] [PubMed]
7. Lee, S.J.; Krauthauser, C.; Maduskuie, V.; Fawcett, P.T.; Olson, J.M.; Rajasekaran, S.A. Curcumin-induced HDAC inhibition and attenuation of medulloblastoma growth in vitro and in vivo. *BMC Cancer* **2011**, *11*, 144. [CrossRef] [PubMed]
8. Farria, A.; Li, W.; Dent, S.Y. KATs in cancer: Functions and therapies. *Oncogene* **2015**, *34*, 4901–4913. [CrossRef] [PubMed]

9. Lillico, R.; Stesco, N.; Amhad, T.K.; Cortes, C.; Namaka, M.P.; Lakowski, T.M. Inhibitors of enzymes catalyzing modifications to histone lysine residues: Structure, function and activity. *Future Med. Chem.* **2016**, *8*, 879–897. [CrossRef] [PubMed]
10. Dekker, F.J.; van den Bosch, T.; Martin, N.I. Small molecule inhibitors of histone acetyltransferases and deacetylases are potential drugs for inflammatory diseases. *Drug Discov. Today* **2014**, *19*, 654–660. [CrossRef] [PubMed]
11. Van den Bosch, T.; Boichenko, A.; Leus, N.G.; Ourailidou, M.E.; Wapenaar, H.; Rotili, D.; Mai, A.; Imhof, A.; Bischoff, R.; Haisma, H.J.; et al. The histone acetyltransferase p300 inhibitor C646 reduces pro-inflammatory gene expression and inhibits histone deacetylases. *Biochem. Pharmacol.* **2016**, *102*, 130–140. [CrossRef] [PubMed]
12. Zhu, X.Y.; Huang, C.S.; Li, Q.; Chang, R.M.; Song, Z.B.; Zou, W.Y.; Guo, Q.L. p300 exerts an epigenetic role in chronic neuropathic pain through its acetyltransferase activity in rats following chronic constriction injury (CCI). *Mol. Pain* **2012**, *8*, 84. [CrossRef] [PubMed]
13. Gerich, J. Pathogenesis and management of postprandial hyperglycemia: Role of incretin-based therapies. *Int. J. Gen. Med.* **2013**, *6*, 877–895. [CrossRef] [PubMed]
14. Pari, L.; Amali, D.R. Protective role of tetrahydrocurcumin (THC) an active principle of turmeric on chloroquine induced hepatotoxicity in rats. *J. Pharm. Pharm. Sci.* **2005**, *8*, 115–123. [PubMed]
15. Limtrakul, P.; Chearwae, W.; Shukla, S.; Phisalphong, C.; Ambudkar, S.V. Modulation of function of three ABC drug transporters, P-glycoprotein (ABCB1), mitoxantrone resistance protein (ABCG2) and multidrug resistance protein 1 (ABCC1) by tetrahydrocurcumin, a major metabolite of curcumin. *Mol. Cell. Biochem.* **2007**, *296*, 85–95. [CrossRef] [PubMed]
16. Esatbeyoglu, T.; Huebbe, P.; Ernst, I.M.; Chin, D.; Wagner, A.E.; Rimbach, G. Curcumin—From molecule to biological function. *Angew. Chem. Int. Ed. Engl.* **2012**, *51*, 5308–5332. [CrossRef] [PubMed]
17. Kawano, S.; Inohana, Y.; Hashi, Y.; Lin, J. Analysis of keto-enol tautomers of curcumin by liquid chromatography/mass spectrometry. *Chin. Chem. Lett.* **2013**, *24*, 685–687. [CrossRef]
18. Manolova, Y.; Deneva, V.; Antonov, L.; Drakalska, E.; Momekova, D.; Lambov, N. The effect of the water on the curcumin tautomerism: A quantitative approach. *Spectrochim. Acta Part A Mol. Biomol. Spectrosc.* **2014**, *132*, 815–820. [CrossRef] [PubMed]
19. Zhongfa, L.; Chiu, M.; Wang, J.; Chen, W.; Yen, W.; Fan-Havard, P.; Yee, L.D.; Chan, K.K. Enhancement of curcumin oral absorption and pharmacokinetics of curcuminoids and curcumin metabolites in mice. *Cancer Chemother. Pharmacol.* **2012**, *69*, 679–689. [CrossRef] [PubMed]
20. Holder, G.M.; Plummer, J.L.; Ryan, A.J. The metabolism and excretion of curcumin (1,7-bis-(4-hydroxy-3-methoxyphenyl)-1,6-heptadiene-3,5-dione) in the rat. *Xenobiotica* **1978**, *8*, 761–768. [CrossRef] [PubMed]
21. Lee, J.H.; Oh, J.H.; Lee, Y.J. Biliary excretion of curcumin is mediated by multidrug resistance-associated protein 2. *Biol. Pharm. Bull.* **2012**, *35*, 777–780. [CrossRef] [PubMed]
22. Volak, L.P.; Ghirmai, S.; Cashman, J.R.; Court, M.H. Curcuminoids inhibit multiple human cytochromes P450, UDP-glucuronosyltransferase, and sulfotransferase enzymes, whereas piperine is a relatively selective CYP3A4 inhibitor. *Drug Metab. Dispos.* **2008**, *36*, 1594–1605. [CrossRef] [PubMed]
23. Sneharani, A.H.; Singh, S.A.; Srinivas, P.; Rao, A.G.A. Inhibition of lipoxygenase-1 by tetrahydrocurcumin. *Eur. Food Res. Technol.* **2011**, *233*, 561. [CrossRef]
24. Hong, J.; Bose, M.; Ju, J.; Ryu, J.H.; Chen, X.; Sang, S.; Lee, M.J.; Yang, C.S. Modulation of arachidonic acid metabolism by curcumin and related beta-diketone derivatives: Effects on cytosolic phospholipase A(2), cyclooxygenases and 5-lipoxygenase. *Carcinogenesis* **2004**, *25*, 1671–1679. [CrossRef] [PubMed]
25. Chen, C.Y.; Yang, W.L.; Kuo, S.Y. Cytotoxic activity and cell cycle analysis of hexahydrocurcumin on SW 480 human colorectal cancer cells. *Nat. Prod. Commun.* **2011**, *6*, 1671–1672. [CrossRef] [PubMed]
26. Srimuangwong, K.; Tocharus, C.; Chintana, P.Y.; Suksamrarn, A.; Tocharus, J. Hexahydrocurcumin enhances inhibitory effect of 5-fluorouracil on HT-29 human colon cancer cells. *World J. Gastroenterol.* **2012**, *18*, 2383–2389. [CrossRef] [PubMed]
27. Lai, C.S.; Wu, J.C.; Yu, S.F.; Badmaev, V.; Nagabhushanam, K.; Ho, C.T.; Pan, M.H. Tetrahydrocurcumin is more effective than curcumin in preventing azoxymethane-induced colon carcinogenesis. *Mol. Nutr. Food Res.* **2011**, *55*, 1819–1828. [CrossRef] [PubMed]

28. Wu, J.C.; Tsai, M.L.; Lai, C.S.; Wang, Y.J.; Ho, C.T.; Pan, M.H. Chemopreventative effects of tetrahydrocurcumin on human diseases. *Food Funct.* **2014**, *5*, 12–17. [CrossRef] [PubMed]
29. Henry, R.A.; Kuo, Y.M.; Andrews, A.J. Differences in specificity and selectivity between CBP and p300 acetylation of histone H3 and H3/H4. *Biochemistry* **2013**, *52*, 5746–5759. [CrossRef] [PubMed]
30. Tyagi, A.K.; Prasad, S.; Majeed, M.; Aggarwal, B.B. Calebin A downregulates osteoclastogenesis through suppression of RANKL signalling. *Arch. Biochem. Biophys.* **2016**, *593*, 80–89. [CrossRef] [PubMed]
31. Greene, W.C.; Chen, L.F. Regulation of NF-kappaB action by reversible acetylation. *Novartis Found. Symp.* **2004**, *259*, 208–217. [PubMed]
32. Naito, M.; Wu, X.; Nomura, H.; Kodama, M.; Kato, Y.; Osawa, T. The protective effects of tetrahydrocurcumin on oxidative stress in cholesterol-fed rabbits. *J. Atheroscler. Thromb.* **2002**, *9*, 243–250. [CrossRef] [PubMed]
33. Somparn, P.; Phisalaphong, C.; Nakornchai, S.; Unchern, S.; Morales, N.P. Comparative antioxidant activities of curcumin and its demethoxy and hydrogenated derivatives. *Biol. Pharm. Bull.* **2007**, *30*, 74–78. [CrossRef] [PubMed]
34. Sugiyama, Y.; Kawakishi, S.; Osawa, T. Involvement of the beta-diketone moiety in the antioxidative mechanism of tetrahydrocurcumin. *Biochem. Pharmacol.* **1996**, *52*, 519–525. [CrossRef]

A Simple and Sensitive Liquid Chromatography with Tandem Mass Spectrometric Method for the Simultaneous Determination of Anthraquinone Glycosides and their Aglycones in Rat Plasma: Application to a Pharmacokinetic Study of *Rumex acetosa* Extract

Hossain Mohammad Arif Ullah †, Junhyeong Kim †, Naveed Ur Rehman, Hye-Jin Kim, Mi-Jeong Ahn * and Hye Jin Chung *

College of Pharmacy and Research Institute of Pharmaceutical Sciences, Gyeongsang National University, Jinju 52828, Korea; arifpha@ymail.com (H.M.A.U.); jhk6914@naver.com (J.K.); naveed.rehman50@gmail.com (N.U.R.); black200203@gmail.com (H.-J.K.)

* Correspondence: amj5812@gnu.ac.kr (M.-J.A.); hchung@gnu.ac.kr (H.J.C.)

† These authors contributed equally to this work.

Abstract: *Rumex acetosa* (*R. acetosa*) has been used in folk remedies for gastrointestinal disorders and cutaneous diseases. *Rumex* species, in particular, contain abundant anthraquinones. Anthraquinone glycosides and aglycones show different bioactive effects. However, information on the pharmacokinetics of anthraquinone glycosides is limited, and methods to quantify anthraquinone glycosides in plasma are rarely available. A simple and sensitive liquid chromatography-tandem mass spectrometric bioanalytical method for the simultaneous determination of both anthraquinone glycosides and their aglycones, including emodin, emodin-8-*O*-β-D-glucoside, chrysophanol, chrysophanol-8-*O*-β-D-glucoside, physcion, and physcion-8-*O*-β-D-glucoside , in a low volume of rat plasma (20 μL) was established. A simple and rapid sample preparation was employed using methanol as a precipitating agent with appropriate sensitivity. Chromatographic separation was performed on HPLC by using a biphenyl column with a gradient elution using 2 mM ammonium formate (pH 6) in water and 2 mM ammonium formate (pH 6) in methanol within a run time of 13 min. The anthraquinones were detected on triple-quadrupole mass spectrometer in negative ionization mode using multiple-reaction monitoring. The method was validated in terms of selectivity, linearity, accuracy, precision, recovery, and stability. The values of the lower limit of quantitation of anthraquinones were 1–20 ng/mL. The intra-batch and inter-batch accuracies were 96.7–111.9% and the precision was within the acceptable limits. The method was applied to a pharmacokinetic study after oral administration of *R. acetosa* 70% ethanol extract to rats at a dose of 2 g/kg.

Keywords: anthraquinone; glycoside; aglycone; LC-MS/MS; plasma; protein precipitation

---

1. Introduction

Rumex acetosa L. (*R. acetosa*), belonging to the Polygonaceae family, is a perennial herb that is listed in the Korean Food Code (Korea Food and Drug Administration) as a food material and has been used in folk remedies for gastrointestinal disorders and cutaneous diseases [1]. Extracts of *R. acetosa* have been reported to have various biological activities, including anti-ulcerogenic, anti-inflammatory, anti-proliferative, and anti-viral effects [2–4]. They contain a number of bioactive compounds, including anthraquinones, flavonoids, and polysaccharides [5]. In particular, *Rumex* species contain abundant anthraquinones, including emodin, chrysophanol, and physcion in all parts of the plant, in free and glycoside forms [6]. A difference in anthraquinone physiological activity between these forms has been described [7]. Previous studies reported a number of quantitative methods of anthraquinones in plasma [8–10]. However, we found that most of these studies focused on determining aglycones (free anthraquinones). Methods to quantify anthraquinone glycosides in plasma are rarely available.

As interest in natural drugs has increased in the pharmaceutical industry, research is underway to develop potential applications of *R. acetosa*, which has already proven its efficacy. Therefore, a simple and sensitive analytical method to examine bioactive anthraquinones in biological samples is needed to evaluate the potential of new treatments.

The aim of this study is to establish a simple, rapid, and sensitive liquid chromatography-tandem mass spectrometry (LC-MS/MS) method to simultaneously quantify emodin (E), emodin-8-*O*-β-D-glucoside (EG), chrysophanol (C), chrysophanol-8-*O*-β-D-glucoside (CG), physcion (P), and physcion-8-*O*-β-D-glucoside (PG) in rat plasma within one chromatographic run. The method was applied to determine pharmacokinetic parameters after oral administration of *R. acetosa* 70% ethanol extract in rat. The results of this study might be helpful in the development of a new type of medicine using *R. acetosa*.

2. Materials and Methods

2.1. Materials

The plant of *R. acetosa* L. (Polygonaceae) was collected from the Sancheong province of Korea in April 2014 and identified by Mi-Jeong Ahn of the College of Pharmacy, Gyeongsang National University (Jinju, Korea). The voucher specimen (APG-1403) was deposited in the Herbarium of the College of Pharmacy, Gyeongsang National University. The standards of the six anthraquinones (E, EG, C, CG, P, and PG) were isolated from the whole part of *R. acetosa* and their structures (Figure 1) were elucidated using spectroscopy such as MS and nuclear magnetic resonance spectroscopy (data not shown) [11]. The purity of anthraquinone compounds isolated from *R. acetosa* was confirmed to be more than 95% by NMR and HPLC-UV. Diclofenac used as an internal standard (IS) was purchased from Sigma Aldrich (St. Louis, MO, USA). HPLC-grade acetonitrile, methanol, and water were products of Fisher Scientific Korea Ltd. (Seoul, Korea). All reagents were analytical grade.

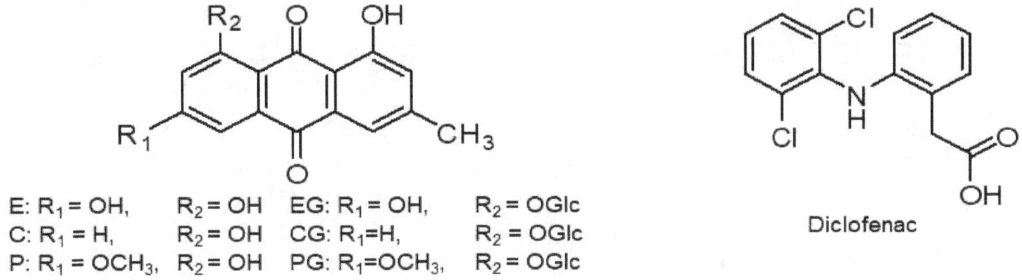

Figure 1. The chemical structures of six anthraquinones and diclofenac (internal standard). E, emodin; EG, emodin-8-*O*-β-D-glucoside; C, chrysophanol; CG, chrysophanol-8-*O*-β-D-glucoside; P, physcion; PG, physcion-8-*O*-β-D-glucoside.

2.2. Chromatographic Condition

The analysis was performed on an Agilent 1260 series (Agilent Technologies, Waldbronn, Germany) HPLC system. Chromatographic separation of the samples was carried out on a Kinetex Biphenyl column (100 × 3.0 mm, 2.6 μm, 110 Å, Phenomenex, Torrance, CA, USA). The mobile phase consisted of 2 mM ammonium formate (pH 6) in water (A) and 2 mM ammonium formate (pH 6) in methanol (B). The gradient program was used at a flow rate of 0.3 mL/min while maintaining the column temperature at 40 °C. The mobile phase initial composition of 25% B was maintained for 2 min. It was then increased linearly from 25% to 95% B for 0.5 min and held for 7 min. The gradient was then changed back to the initial condition for 0.5 min and kept at the initial condition for 3 min. The total analysis time was 13 min for each sample. The injection volume was 15 μL.

2.3. Mass Spectrometric Condition

The mass spectrometric detection was performed on an Agilent 6460 triple-quadruple mass spectrometer (Agilent Technologies, Singapore) with an electrospray ionization source. It was operated in the negative ion detection mode because of its higher sensitivity than that in the positive ionization mode on multiple reaction monitoring (MRM). The data were acquired and processed using Mass Hunter Workstation B.06.00 software (Agilent Technologies, Singapore). The mass spectrometric parameters of each compound are summarized in Table 1 [12]. The MS spectra of the six anthraquinones are shown in Figure 2. The source parameters were also optimized as follows: a drying gas flow and temperature at 6 L/min and 350 °C were used, respectively; the sheath gas flow and temperature were maintained at 12 L/min and 350 °C, respectively; the nebulizing gas (N_2) pressure was set at 25 psi; and the capillary and nozzle voltages were set at 3500 V and 500 V, respectively.

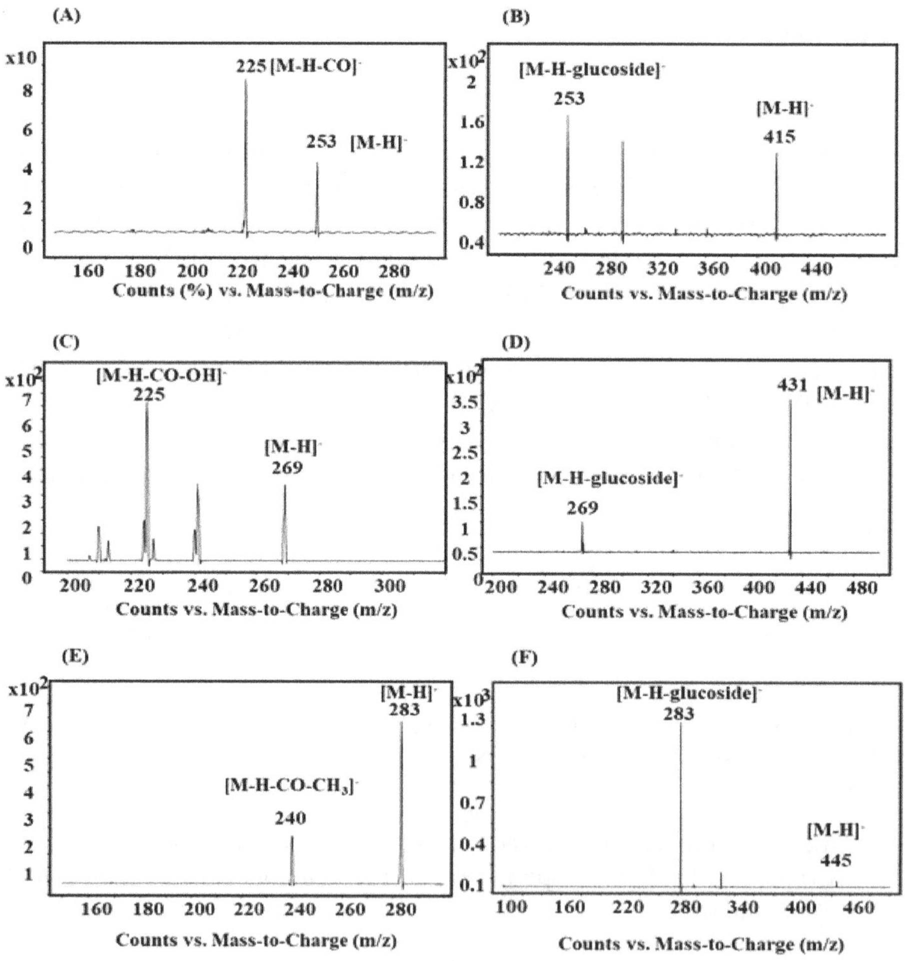

Figure 2. MS/MS scan spectra of six anthraquinones. (**A**) chrysophanol; (**B**) chrysophanol-8-*O*-β-D-glucoside; (**C**) emodin; (**D**) emodin-8-*O*-β-D-glucoside; (**E**) physcion; (**F**) physcion-8-*O*-β-D-glucoside.

Table 1. Summary of the MS/MS parameters.

Compounds	MRM Transition (m/z) [a] Precursor Ion → Product Ion	Fragmentor (V)	Collision Energy (V)
E	269 → 225	145	20
EG	431 → 269	150	24
C	253 → 225	175	22
CG	415 → 253	89	13
P	283 → 240	157	16
PG	445 → 283	95	5
IS (Diclofenac)	294 → 250	65	1

[a] MRM transitions refer to the reference [12]. MRM, multiple reaction monitoring; E, emodin; EG, emodin-8-*O*-β-D-glucoside; C, chrysophanol; CG, chrysophanol-8-*O*-β-D-glucoside; P, physcion; PG, physcion-8-*O*-β-D-glucoside; IS, internal standard.

2.4. Preparation of *R. acetosa* Extract

The dried plant material (100 g) was ground and extracted with 70% ethanol. The extract was filtered using filter papers (Whatman No. 40) and concentrated through a rotary evaporator. The concentrate was lyophilized and stored at −80 °C. The exact amount was weighed and used as the samples for the animal studies. The contents of E, EG, C, CG, P, and PG in *R. acetosa* extract were 0.94 ± 0.15%, 1.29 ± 0.06%, 0.68 ± 0.09%, 0.77 ± 0.12%, 0.17 ± 0.02%, and 0.41 ± 0.05% (w/w), respectively. The values were expressed as mean ± standard deviation.

2.5. Preparation of the Calibration Standard and Quality Control (QC) Samples

The primary stock solutions of E, EG, C, CG, P, PG, and IS were prepared in dimethyl sulfoxide at a concentration of 1 mg/mL and stored at −80 °C. The mixture stock solutions to obtain the standard solutions were serially diluted in methanol. The IS stock solution of 5 ng/mL was prepared in methanol. The calibration standards were prepared by spiking 10 µL of above standard solutions into 90 µL of blank rat plasma to yield concentration ranges of 1–300 ng/mL for E, 20–300 ng/mL for P and C, 1–150 ng/mL for EG, 10–150 ng/mL for CG and PG. Twenty microliters of aliquots were prepared and stored at −80 °C until analysis.

The QC samples were prepared in the same way as the calibration samples for E, EG, C, CG, P, and PG in rat plasma at low, middle, and high concentrations. All the solutions were kept at −80 °C.

2.6. Sample Preparation

To 20 µL aliquot of the rat plasma samples, 60 µL of 5 ng/mL IS in methanol was added. The mixture was vortexed for 30 s and kept at 4 °C for 30 min. The mixture was centrifuged at 10,000× *g* for 10 min. The supernatant was transferred to an HPLC vial, and 15 µL of the processed sample was injected onto the LC-MS/MS system.

2.7. Method Validation

The method validation was performed according to the United States Food and Drug Administration's guidance on bioanalytical method validation [13].

2.7.1. Selectivity

The selectivity study was performed by comparing the chromatograms of the six different rat plasma samples to investigate the interference near the retention time of the analytes and the IS.

2.7.2. Calibration Curves and Sensitivity

The linearity of each calibration curve was determined by plotting the peak area ratio of the analyte to IS versus the plasma concentrations. The least-square method was used to achieve a linear regression equation. Sensitivity was defined by calculating the lower limit of detection and the lower limit of quantification (LLOQ) based on a signal-to-noise ratio of greater than 3 and 10, respectively. Besides signal-to-noise ratio, LLOQ values with acceptable precision and accuracy values were chosen. The criteria of precision and accuracy at LLOQ are within 20% relative standard deviation (RSD) for precision and between 80–120% for accuracy.

2.7.3. Precision and Accuracy

Precision and accuracy were investigated by analyzing six replicates of four QC levels on the same batch (intra-batch) and five different batches (inter-batch) of four QC levels (LLOQ, low QC, middle QC, and high QC). The intra- and inter-batch precision was expressed by RSD (%), and accuracy was evaluated by expressing it as a percentage of the theoretical value (the mean calculated concentration/nominal concentration) × 100%. The acceptance criteria are within 15% RSD except 20% at LLOQ for precision and ±15% of nominal concentrations except ±20% at LLOQ for accuracy.

2.7.4. Extraction Recovery and Matrix Effect

The extraction recovery was evaluated by comparing the peak area of the extracted sample with that of the post-extracted sample at three replicates of three QC levels. The matrix effect of the analytes was investigated by comparing the peak area of the post-extracted sample with the peak area obtained by the corresponding standard solutions in pH 7.4 buffer at three QC levels. Matrix effects were determined using the equation below.

$$\left(\frac{\text{peak area of the analytes for the sample spiked with the target compounds after extraction}}{\text{peak area of the analytes for the standard solutions}}\right) \times 100\%$$

2.7.5. Stability

The stability of the analytes in rat plasma was evaluated by analyzing triplicates of three QC levels at room temperature for 4 h (short-term stability), −80 °C for one month (long-term stability), three freeze-thaw cycles from −80 °C to room temperature (freeze and thaw stability), and 4 °C for 24 h (processed sample stability). The stability of analytes in stock solution was also evaluated. The peak areas obtained from freshly prepared stock solutions were compared with stock solutions stored for 4 h at room temperature.

2.8. Pharmacokinetic Study

Male Sprague-Dawley rats (8-week-old, weighing 250 ± 10 g) were obtained from Koatech (Pyeongtaek, Korea). They were housed and acclimated in the Animal Laboratory, Gyeongsang National University, under controlled temperature and humidity and regular 12 h light cycle, freely accessible to food and water for 7 days before the experiment. The rats were cannulated into the carotid artery and allowed to recover for one day. Before the pharmacokinetic study, all rats were fasted for 12 h with free access to water. *R. acetosa* extract suspended in a solution (ethanol:polysorbate 80:water = 1:2:7, *v*/*v*/*v*) was orally administered to the three rats at a dose of 2 g/kg. The calculated doses of compounds based on the contents in the extract were 18.8, 25.8, 13.6, 15.4, 3.4, and 8.2 mg/kg for E, EG, C, CG, P, and PG, respectively. Blood samples (100 μL) were collected via the cannulated carotid vessel at 0, 15, 30, 45 min, 1, 2, 3, 4, 6, 8, 12, and 24 h after oral administration. To collect plasma, the blood samples were immediately centrifuged at 10,000× *g* for 5 min. All plasma samples were stored at −80 °C until analysis. All experimental procedures of the animal study were approved (GNU-130618-R0038) by the Animal Care and Use Committee of Gyeongsang National University, Korea.

3. Results

3.1. Method Validation

3.1.1. Specificity and Selectivity

The representative MRM chromatograms of blank rat plasma and that spiked with six anthraquinones and IS are shown in Figure 3. No interference from endogenous substances near the retention time of the analytes or the IS was observed.

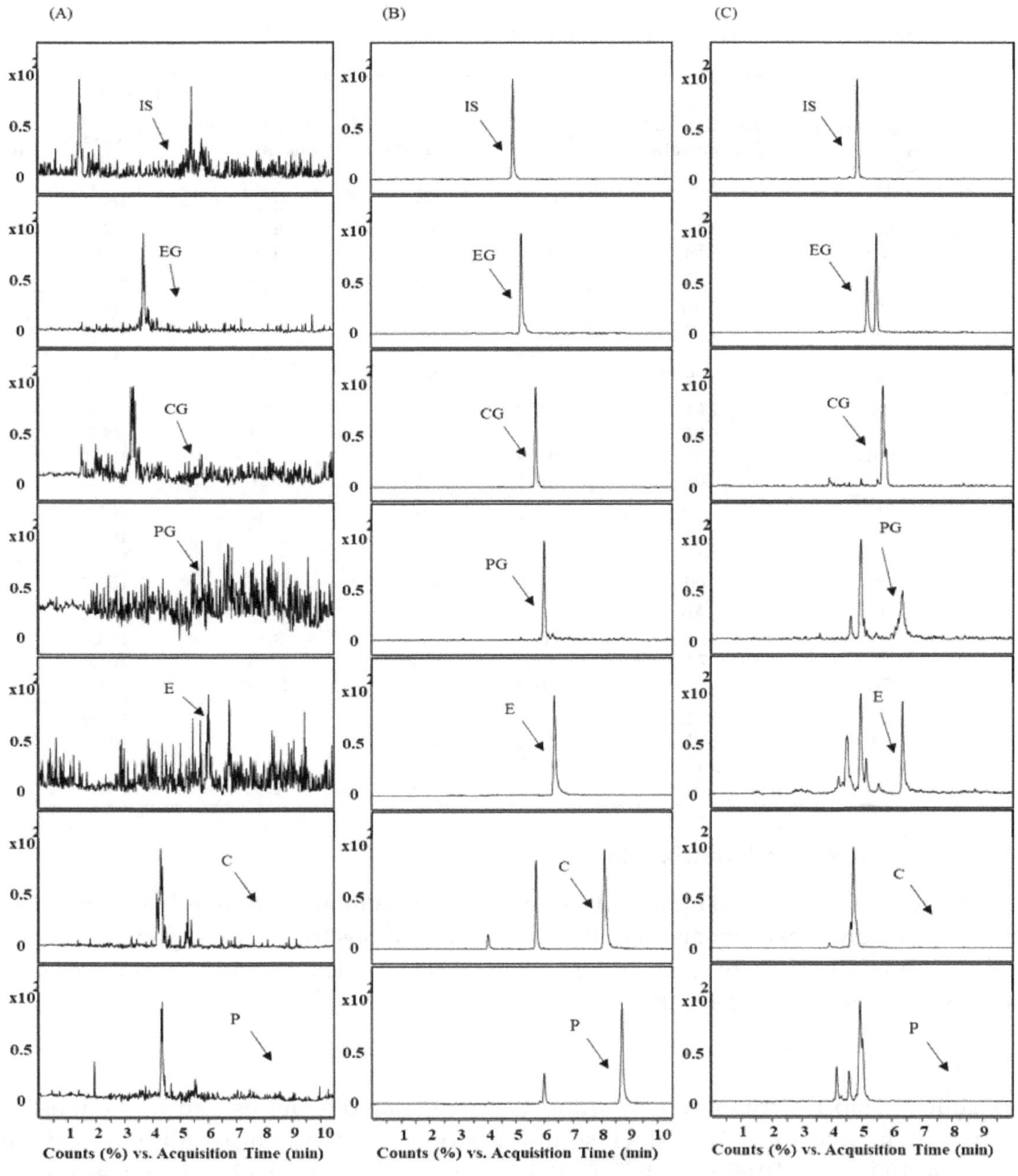

Figure 3. Representative MRM chromatograms of IS, EG, CG, PG, E, C, and P in rat plasma. (**A**) blank plasma; (**B**) blank plasma spiked with six anthraquinones (250 ng/mL for aglycones and 125 ng/mL for glycosides) and IS; (**C**) plasma sample obtained from rats 45 min after oral administration of *R. acetosa* extract (2 g/kg).

3.1.2. Linearity and Sensitivity

The calibration curves showed good linearity over their corresponding ranges for the analytes ($R^2 > 0.9934$).

3.1.3. Precision and Accuracy

The intra- and inter-batch precision and accuracies are presented in Table 2. The RSD values for the intra- and inter-batch were below 13.5%, except for EG at LLOQ (18.9%). The accuracies were between 85% and 115%. All results showed acceptable accuracy and precision.

Table 2. Accuracy and precision of anthraquinones in rat plasma ($n = 6$). RSD: relative standard deviation.

Analyte	Nominal Concentration (ng/mL)	Intra-Batch			Inter-Batch		
		Mean Calculated Concentration (ng/mL)	Accuracy (%)	RSD (%)	Mean Calculated Concentration (ng/mL)	Accuracy (%)	RSD (%)
P	20	20.5	102.5	8.83	21.3	106.4	11.2
	60	58.0	96.7	4.69	63.4	105.6	7.72
	150	156	104.2	3.98	158	105.3	5.90
	300	308	102.6	2.80	312	104.1	5.54
E	1	1.10	110.1	13.5	1.05	104.6	11.1
	3	3.31	110.3	6.87	3.12	103.9	6.87
	150	155	103.4	2.32	154	102.8	2.66
	300	309	103.0	3.45	299	99.8	2.28
C	20	21.8	109.2	9.23	19.8	98.9	2.98
	60	64.1	106.9	7.79	59.3	98.9	5.75
	150	153	101.9	4.91	155	103.1	6.85
	300	303	101.1	3.94	321	107.0	4.20
PG	10	10.2	102.1	10.7	10.2	102.3	12.1
	30	32.1	107.1	6.83	31.7	105.7	5.72
	75	80.3	107.1	5.38	80.5	107.3	4.95
	150	160	106.5	4.13	159	106.2	4.89
EG	1	1.10	110.1	18.9	1.05	105.2	9.10
	3	3.35	111.8	5.49	3.27	108.9	12.9
	75	77.3	103.0	1.59	78.5	104.6	3.85
	150	156	104.1	1.24	153.9	102.6	4.34
CG	10	11.2	111.9	8.34	11.0	109.9	8.00
	30	31.5	105.0	4.13	31.6	105.4	5.79
	75	76.3	101.7	2.72	76.5	102.0	3.16
	150	154	102.9	3.87	157	104.5	2.12

3.1.4. Extraction Recovery and Matrix Effect

The extraction recoveries and matrix effects of the anthraquinone compounds are shown in Table 3. The matrix effects were consistent among different concentrations for each compound. The recoveries ranged from 96.0% to 112.7% for the analytes at the QC levels. The matrix effects were constant for each analyte with different concentrations.

3.1.5. Stability

The stability of stock solution was determined. As compared with fresh stock solutions, the mean concentration of analytes ($n = 3$) in stock solutions stored at room temperature for 4 h were 99.2, 94.8, 95.9, 102.4, 100.4, and 101.7% for P, E, C, PG, EG, and CG, respectively. There was no detectable degradation of compounds in dimethyl sulfoxide and methanol stored at room temperature for 3 months based on HPLC-UV chromatogram. The stability results of the analytes in rat plasma under different conditions are shown in Table 4.

Table 3. Extraction recovery and matrix effect of anthraquinones in rat plasma (n = 3).

Analyte	Nominal Concentration (ng/mL)	Extraction Recovery (%)		Matrix Effect (%)	
		Mean	RSD	Mean	RSD
P	60	106.5	4.85	185.6	2.29
	150	106.4	1.23	185.1	3.13
	300	98.6	1.49	183.9	3.92
E	3	101.3	2.74	70.1	6.65
	150	105.6	0.82	87.0	1.46
	300	100.4	1.90	92.3	2.77
C	60	112.7	8.71	143.0	1.04
	150	102.1	1.07	144.3	1.62
	300	96.6	1.04	144.6	4.11
PG	30	106.4	13.0	42.5	8.41
	75	107.4	5.60	44.3	6.07
	150	96.6	3.14	51.4	2.33
EG	3	97.6	3.48	286.5	4.29
	75	100.5	0.77	277.6	3.60
	150	97.6	1.25	277.8	2.84
CG	30	96.0	1.36	113.8	6.64
	75	96.6	6.01	121.9	3.24
	150	96.5	6.89	126.7	2.02

Table 4. Stability of anthraquinones in rat plasma (n = 3).

Analyte	Conc. (ng/mL)	Short Term Stability (%)		Long Term Stability (%)		Freeze and Thaw Stability (%)		Processed Sample Stability (%)	
		Accuracy	RSD	Accuracy	RSD	Accuracy	RSD	Accuracy	RSD
P	60	104.9	2.05	107.3	5.31	103.6	8.18	102.2	9.10
	150	98.9	5.64	100.1	2.34	103.9	4.48	101.6	2.87
	300	103.8	2.39	98.0	2.00	104.2	3.21	102.7	5.76
E	3	103.2	3.46	106.8	4.25	107.5	2.38	108.2	5.26
	150	100.7	2.55	107.8	1.87	104.5	4.32	108.0	5.96
	300	101.8	2.44	107.7	0.93	102.0	3.47	104.6	3.60
C	60	103.5	6.23	104.3	8.67	89.7	0.76	101.5	9.60
	150	98.6	1.07	97.9	7.67	91.8	3.94	103.7	5.43
	300	101.2	2.97	102.6	2.98	92.4	8.25	102.3	6.47
PG	30	98.9	9.48	97.7	5.64	101.5	9.06	98.8	6.33
	75	91.8	6.60	98.5	5.36	94.3	6.57	92.7	4.64
	150	96.7	1.62	97.1	2.85	93.6	2.16	96.8	1.19
EG	3	99.8	5.11	102.9	4.02	100.4	6.39	91.5	3.11
	75	108.5	2.79	107.9	1.54	112.3	3.60	107.9	2.88
	150	98.9	1.81	102.8	2.14	100.9	1.69	100.3	4.14
CG	30	97.6	9.29	97.5	4.04	98.3	4.81	91.1	2.45
	75	96.9	0.56	100.6	1.38	101.0	2.23	100.2	7.38
	150	101.8	5.27	101.5	2.52	97.0	5.66	96.7	5.93

3.2. Pharmacokinetics Study

The validated LC-MS/MS method was applied to the pharmacokinetic study after oral administration of *R. acetosa* extract at a dose of 2 g/kg to the rats. The concentrations of EG and P were not high enough to determine the pharmacokinetic parameters. The concentrations of C and PG were below the LLOQ from 6 h after administration of extract, CG and E could be detected until 8 and 24 h, respectively. The mean plasma concentration–time profiles of the analytes are presented in Figure 4. The major pharmacokinetic parameters of C, E, CG, and PG calculated by non-compartmental analysis are listed in Table 5. The data were expressed as mean ± standard deviation. The concentrations of emodin fluctuated and were insufficient to calculate the half-life of elimination ($t_{1/2}$). Meanwhile, rapid absorption of aglycones was observed because of the higher lipophilic character with T_{max} of 0.25 (0.25–0.5) h and 0.25 (0.25–0.75) h, compared with that of glycosides.

Table 5. The pharmacokinetic parameters of anthraquinones after oral administration of *R. acetosa* extract to rats at a dose of 2 g/kg (n = 3).

Analyte	$AUC_{0\text{–}last}$ [a] (ng h/mL)	C_{max} (ng/mL)	T_{max} [b] (h)	MRT (h)	$t_{1/2}$ (h)
C	265.6 ± 70.9	155.6 ± 86.0	0.25 (0.25–0.5)	2.4 ± 0.2	3.9 ± 0.6
E	1165 ± 336.1	123.5 ± 41.7	0.25 (0.25–0.75)	7.7 ± 3.0	NA
CG	158.0 ± 12.3	28.7 ± 4.7	2 (0.75–2)	2.4 ± 0.08	4.8 ± 0.5
PG	82.8 ± 13.8	20.5 ± 1.4	0.75 (0.5–2)	2.7 ± 0.6	6.2 ± 3.9

The values were expressed as mean ± standard deviation except T_{max}. [a] The last measured time points for C, E, CG, and PG were 6, 24, 8, and 6 h. [b] Median (range). $AUC_{0\text{–}last}$, total area under the plasma concentration–time curve from time zero to last measured time; C_{max}, maximum plasma concentration; T_{max}, time to reach C_{max}; MRT, mean residence time; $t_{1/2}$, half-life; NA, not available.

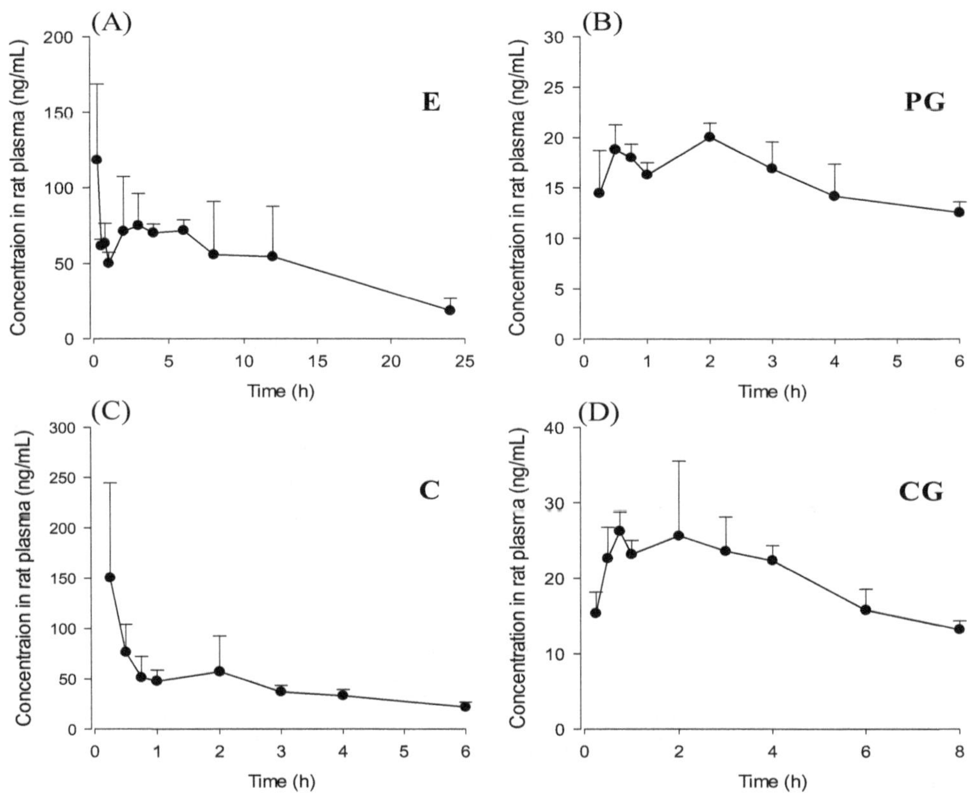

Figure 4. Mean plasma concentration–time profiles after oral (n = 3) administration of *R. acetosa* extract (2 g/kg) to SD male rats. Bars represent standard deviation. (**A**) emodin; (**B**) physcion-8-*O*-β-D-glucoside; (**C**) chrysophanol; (**D**) chrysophanol-8-*O*-β-D-glucoside.

4. Discussion

The objective of this study was to develop a bioanalytical method that simultaneously quantified the bioactive glycosides and aglycones of anthraquinones. The developed LC-MS/MS method could quantify six anthraquinones simultaneously in rat plasma in an accurate, reproducible, and simple way. Reported bioanalytical methods which simultaneously determine both aglycones and glycosides of anthraquinones are rarely available. In this study, simultaneous determination achieved by using biphenyl column. The column could prolong retention time of hydrophilic glycosides compare to C18 column at the same mobile phase composition.

There was no interfering peak when the compound mixture was spiked to blank rat plasma. However, there were small peaks appeared near CG and PG peaks after oral administration of plant extract. It is suggested that those peaks came from the extract or the metabolites of components in the extract. It is known that emodin is extensively glucuronized after absorption [14] and the molecular weight of emodin glucuronide is same as PG. There is some possibility that emodin glucuronide could interfere PG. However, the MS/MS fragment pattern of emodin glucuronide is different from PG. Emodin glucuronide might cause little interference. We could quantify CG and PG by adjusting the baselines because the interfering peaks were small.

A simple and rapid sample preparation was utilized on a low volume of rat plasma sample (20 μL) by using methanol as a precipitating agent with appropriate sensitivity compare to the reported methods [8,12,15]. The comparison with reported analytical methods for aglycones and glycosides of anthraquinones was shown in Table 6.

Table 6. Comparison with reported analytical methods for aglycones and glycosides of anthraquinone.

Analytical Condition		Our Method	Lin et al. [8]	Wang et al. [12]	Ma et al. [15]
Sample volume		20 μL	25 μL	25 μL	100 μL
Sample preparation		Protein precipitation	Solid phase extraction	Liquid-liquid extraction	Liquid-liquid extraction
Target compounds		E, C, P, EG, CG, PG	EG, E	E, C, P, EG, CG, PG	EG, E
LLOQ (ng/mL)	E	1	1	2	9.6
	C	20	-	50	-
	P	20	-	50	-
	EG	1	1	2	33.7
	CG	10	-	2	-
	PG	10	-	1	-

The method was acceptably validated and used to perform a pharmacokinetic study of anthraquinones after oral administration of *R. acetosa* in rats. As shown in Figure 4, C, E, CG, and PG could be detected in every rat from the first sampling time, 15 min. All of the studied anthraquinones were absorbed rapidly from rat gastrointestinal tract. Median T_{max} value of C and E was 15 min (Table 5). This result was consistent with reported values [8,10]. Emodin could be detected for the longest time among four compounds even though the concentrations fluctuated. The fluctuated concentration was also reported in other pharmacokinetic studies of emodin in rats [9,15]. This was possibly due to enterohepatic circulation [16]. In some other works [17], emodin rapidly and extensively metabolized to form its glucuronide and the parent form was almost undetectable after administration of emodin even the doses were similar (40 mg/kg) to our study (18.8 mg/kg for E and 25.8 mg/kg for EG). Free emodin could be measured until 24 h after oral administration because of the low LLOQ level of emodin using the method developed in this work.

Generally, plant glycosides have been considered to be hydrolyzed to aglycones by microflora in the gastrointestinal tract before absorption [18]. Glycosides have large molecular weights and low lipophilicity, so they might be difficult to be absorbed. However, recent studies show that emodin glycoside can be absorbed in an intact form after oral administration of plant extract [8]. The absorption of the glycosides of anthraquinones in an intact form was confirmed by studying in vivo absorption in rats in this study. Pharmacokinetics of anthraquinone aglycones and their glycosides after oral administration of *R. acetosa* was first evaluated. CG and PG were detected in rat plasma after oral administration of *R. acetosa* extract. Interestingly, the T_{max} of C and that of CG were different after oral administration of the extract. It might be due to different lipophilicity. Glycosides and aglycones have been proposed to have different degrees of absorption and metabolic patterns. Note that second peaks in the plasma concentrations of aglycones were observed. This could be due to delayed absorption of aglycones hydrolyzed from glycosides by microflora in the gastrointestinal tract and enterohepatic circulation of anthraquinones [16]. A number of published studies have reported pharmacokinetics of anthraquinones. However, we found that most of these studies focused on determining aglycones. Pharmacokinetics of anthraquinone glycosides is rarely available. Wang et al. [12] recently reported the pharmacokinetics of anthraquinone aglycones and their glycosides in hyperlipidemic hamsters after administration of rhubarb. The plasma concentration-time profile patterns of anthraquinones were similar to our study even though the composition (dose ratio of compounds) of rhubarb extract might be quite different from *R. acetosa* extract and physiological differences between rats and hamsters probably exist. T_{max} values of glycosides were slightly longer than aglycones. Similar to our results, emodin glucoside was not detected even though emodin could be detected until 36 h. It is suggested that emodin glycoside probably rapidly hydrolyzed to emodin and was poorly absorbed as an intact form in the gastrointestinal tract.

Our pharmacokinetic study has some limitations. The number of animals ($n = 3$) is not enough to achieve statistically significant pharmacokinetic parameters after administration of an herbal product. The pharmacokinetic parameters obtained in this study might b not sufficient to represent the animal population. Nevertheless, this study showed the possibility that our bioanalytical method could be used in pharmacokinetic studies of *R. acetosa* extract. Another issue to consider is that *R. acetosa* extract contained a number of other compounds besides anthraquinones. Further studies with a large sample size and studies of the effects of other compounds on the pharmacokinetics of anthraquinones are needed for better understanding of the pharmacokinetics of anthraquinones.

5. Conclusions

A simple and sensitive LC-MS/MS method for the determination of the glycosides and aglycones of anthraquinones in rat plasma was developed. The method was acceptably validated and applied to a pharmacokinetic study of anthraquinones after oral administration of *R. acetosa* extract in rats. The absorption of the glycosides of anthraquinones in an intact form was confirmed in the pharmacokinetic study. The results of this study could be relevant to a better understanding of the pharmacokinetics and pharmacodynamics of anthraquinone glycosides and aglycones.

Author Contributions: Conceptualization, M.-J.A. and H.J.C.; Formal analysis, J.K.; Funding acquisition, M.-J.A. and H.J.C.; Investigation, H.M.A.U., J.K., N.U.R., and H.-J.K; Methodology, H.J.C.; Project administration, H.J.C.; Writing—original draft, H.M.A.U.; Writing—review and editing, J.K., M.-J.A. and H.J.C.

Abbreviations

LC-MS/MS	liquid chromatography-tandem mass spectrometry
MRM	multiple reaction monitoring
E	emodin
EG	emodin-8-*O*-β-D-glucoside
C	chrysophanol
CG	chrysophanol-8-*O*-β-D-glucoside
P	physcion
PG	physcion-8-*O*-β-D-glucoside

References

1. Lee, N.-J.; Choi, J.-H.; Koo, B.-S.; Ryu, S.-Y.; Han, Y.-H.; Lee, S.-I.; Lee, D.-U. Antimutagenicity and cytotoxicity of the constituents from the aerial parts of *Rumex acetosa*. *Biol. Pharm. Bull.* **2005**, *28*, 2158–2161. [CrossRef] [PubMed]
2. Kucekova, Z.; Mlcek, J.; Humpolicek, P.; Rop, O.; Valasek, P.; Saha, P. Phenolic compounds from *Allium schoenoprasum*, *Tragopogon pratensis* and *Rumex acetosa* and their antiproliferative effects. *Molecules* **2011**, *16*, 9207–9217. [CrossRef] [PubMed]

3. Gescher, K.; Hensel, A.; Hafezi, W.; Derksen, A.; Kühn, J. Oligomeric proanthocyanidins from *Rumex acetosa* L. inhibit the attachment of herpes simplex virus type-1. *Antivir. Res.* **2011**, *89*, 9–18. [CrossRef] [PubMed]
4. Bae, J.-Y.; Lee, Y.S.; Han, S.Y.; Jeong, E.J.; Lee, M.K.; Kong, J.Y.; Lee, D.H.; Cho, K.J.; Lee, H.-S.; Ahn, M.-J. A comparison between water and ethanol extracts of *Rumex acetosa* for protective effects on gastric ulcers in mice. *Biomol. Ther.* **2012**, *20*, 425–430. [CrossRef] [PubMed]
5. Bicker, J.; Petereit, F.; Hensel, A. Proanthocyanidins and a phloroglucinol derivative from *Rumex acetosa* L. *Fitoterapia* **2009**, *80*, 483–495. [CrossRef] [PubMed]
6. Fairbairn, J.W.; Reigal, E. Chemotaxonomy of anthraquinones in *Rumex*. *Phytochemistry* **1972**, *11*, 263–268. [CrossRef]
7. Uddin, Z.; Song, Y.H.; Curtis-Long, M.J.; Kim, J.Y.; Yuk, H.J.; Park, K.H. Potent bacterial neuraminidase inhibitors, anthraquinone glucosides from *Polygonum cuspidatum* and their inhibitory mechanism. *J. Ethnopharmacol.* **2016**, *193*, 283–292. [CrossRef] [PubMed]
8. Lin, L.; Ni, B.; Lin, H.; Cao, S.; Yang, C.; Zhao, Y.; Xue, D.; Ni, J. Simultaneous determination and pharmacokinetic study of P-hydroxybenzaldehyde, 2,3,5,4′-tetrahydroxystilbene-2-*O*-β-glucoside, emodin-8-*O*-β-D-glucopyranoside, and emodin in rat plasma by liquid chromatography tandem mass spectrometry after oral administration of *Polygonum multiflorum*. *Anal. Methods* **2015**, *7*, 244–252. [CrossRef]
9. Wu, W.; Yan, R.; Yao, M.; Zhan, Y.; Wang, Y. Pharmacokinetics of anthraquinones in rat plasma after oral administration of a rhubarb extract. *Biomed. Chromatogr.* **2014**, *28*, 564–572. [CrossRef] [PubMed]
10. Yan, D.; Ma, Y. Simultaneous quantification of five anthraquinones in rat plasma by high-performance liquid chromatography with fluorescence detection. *Biomed. Chromatogr.* **2007**, *21*, 502–507. [CrossRef] [PubMed]
11. Vasas, A.; Orbán-Gyapai, O.; Hohmann, J. The genus rumex: Review of traditional uses, phytochemistry and pharmacology. *J. Ethnopharmacol.* **2015**, *175*, 198–228. [CrossRef] [PubMed]
12. Wang, M.; Hu, G.; Tian, Y.; Zhang, Z.; Song, R. Influence of wine-processing on the pharmacokinetics of anthraquinone aglycones and glycosides from rhubarb in hyperlipidemic hamsters. *RSC Adv.* **2016**, *6*, 24871–24879. [CrossRef]
13. US Food and Drug Administration. *Guidance for Industry: Bioanalytical Method Validation, Draft Guidance*; US Food and Drug Administration: Silver Spring, MD, USA, 2013.
14. Dong, X.; Fu, J.; Yin, X.; Cao, S.; Li, X.; Lin, L.; Huyiligeqi; Ni, J. Emodin: A review of its pharmacology, toxicity and pharmacokinetics. *Phytother. Res.* **2016**, *30*, 1207–1218. [CrossRef] [PubMed]
15. Ma, J.; Zheng, L.; He, Y.S.; Li, H.J. Hepatotoxic assessment of *Polygoni multiflori* radix extract and toxicokinetic study of stilbene glucoside and anthraquinones in rats. *J. Ethnopharmacol.* **2015**, *162*, 61–68. [CrossRef] [PubMed]
16. Shia, C.S.; Tsai, S.Y.; Lin, J.C.; Li, M.L.; Ko, M.H.; Chao, P.-D.L.; Huang, Y.C.; Hou, Y.C. Steady-state pharmacokinetics and tissue distribution of anthraquinones of Rhei rhizoma in rats. *J. Ethnopharmacol.* **2011**, *137*, 1388–1394. [CrossRef] [PubMed]
17. Shia, C.S.; Hou, Y.C.; Tsai, S.Y.; Huieh, P.H.; Leu, Y.L.; Chao, P.D. Differences in pharmacokinetics and ex vivo antioxidant activity following intravenous and oral administrations of emodin to rats. *J. Pharm. Sci.* **2010**, *99*, 2185–2195. [CrossRef] [PubMed]
18. Moreau, J.P.; Moreau, S.; Skinner, S. Comparative physiological disposition of some anthraquinone glycosides and aglycones. *Biopharm. Drug Dispos.* **1985**, *6*, 325–334. [CrossRef] [PubMed]

13

A High-Performance Liquid Chromatography Assay Method for the Determination of Lidocaine in Human Serum

Hamdah M. Al Nebaihi [1], Matthew Primrose [2], James S. Green [2] and Dion R. Brocks [1,*]

[1] Faculty of Pharmacy and Pharmaceutical Sciences, University of Alberta, Edmonton, AB T6G 2E1, Canada; alnebaih@ualberta.ca

[2] Department of Anesthesiology and Pain Medicine, Faculty of Medicine and Dentistry, University of Alberta, Edmonton, AB T6G 2B7, Canada; mprimros@ualberta.ca (M.P.); jgreen2@ualberta.ca (J.S.G.)

* Correspondence: dbrocks@ualberta.ca

Abstract: Here we report on the development of a selective and sensitive high-performance liquid chromatographic method for the determination of lidocaine in human serum. The extraction of lidocaine and procainamide (internal standard) from serum (0.25 mL) was achieved using diethyl ether under alkaline conditions. After liquid–liquid extraction, the separation of analytes was accomplished using reverse phase extraction. The mobile phase, a combination of acetonitrile and monobasic potassium phosphate, was pumped isocratically through a C18 analytical column. The ultraviolet (UV) wavelength was at 277 nm for the internal standard, and subsequently changed to 210 for lidocaine. The assay exhibited excellent linearity ($r^2 > 0.999$) in peak response over the concentration ranges of 50–5000 ng/mL lidocaine HCl in human serum. The mean absolute recoveries for 50 and 1000 ng/mL lidocaine HCl in serum using the present extraction procedure were 93.9 and 80.42%, respectively. The intra- and inter-day coefficients of variation in the serum were <15% at the lowest, and <12% at other concentrations, and the percent error values were less than 9%. The method displayed a high caliber of sensitivity and selectivity for monitoring therapeutic concentrations of lidocaine in human serum.

Keywords: lidocaine; pharmacokinetics; ultraviolet detection

1. Introduction

Lidocaine [also known as 2-(diethylamino)-*N*-(2,6-dimethylphenyl) acetamide] is commonly used as a local anesthetic and antiarrhythmic drug [1]. It can also be used for the management of extensive pain via either central or peripheral administration [2]. For these reasons, lidocaine is considered an essential medication for a wide array of clinical conditions [3]. Lidocaine is not a new medication, and hence many methods are available for its quantitation in biological specimens. The available methods are wide ranging, as is evident from the summary provided in Table 1. The most commonly used approach is to use reverse phase high performance liquid chromatography for separation, and ultraviolet (UV) absorbance as the detection method. This is not surprising considering that lidocaine by itself has poor fluorescence properties, and UV detectors are commonly available in laboratories.

Recently, our involvement in a clinical study necessitated that we measure lidocaine from human serum. Most of the previously available methods were based on volumes of 0.5 to 1 mL of specimen. In order to ensure that we could assay all of the samples available, we sought to develop a method that would use only 0.25 mL of specimen. Here we report on an alternative analytical method for lidocaine that was sufficiently sensitive to measure the drug in the serum using a volume of 0.25 mL.

Table 1. Comparisons of some published methods for assaying lidocaine in human matrices.

Volume of Specimen (mL)	Validated LLQ (ng/mL)	Type of Human Matrix	Sample Preparation Method	Analytical Column	Detection Method	References
0.2	50	Plasma	SPE	DB-1	GC–MS	[4]
0.5	200	Serum	LLE	C8	UV	[5]
0.1	680	Plasma	Protein ppt	C18	UV	[6]
0.5	200	Plasma	LLE	C18	UV	[7]
1	10	Serum	LLE	C18	UV	[8]
0.5	50	Plasma	LLE	C18	UV	[9]
0.1	400	Plasma	Protein ppt	C18	UV	[10]
0.5	100	Plasma	LLE	Phenyl	UV	[11]
0.5–1	25	Plasma	LLE	C18	Fluorescence of derivative	[12]
0.25	NS	Plasma	NS	C18	UV	[13]
1	1000	Plasma	LLE	C18	UV	[14]
0.01	200	Plasma	Protein ppt	C18	LC-MS/MS	[15]
1	0.2	Plasma	LLE	C18	LC-MS/MS	[16]
1	20	Serum	None	C18	UV	[17]
0.25	43	Serum	LLE	C18	UV	Current method

2. Materials and Methods

Lidocaine HCl (0.4% in 5% dextrose for injection) USP (Baxter Healthcare Corporation, Deerfield, IL, USA) was utilized as a source of lidocaine (Figure 1). Procainamide HCl was obtained from Sigma-Aldrich (St. Louis, MO, USA) (Figure 1). Ethyl ether, acetonitrile, water (all HPLC grade), triethylamine, potassium phosphate (monobasic) and sulfuric acid were purchased from Caledon Laboratories Ltd. (Georgetown, ON, Canada).

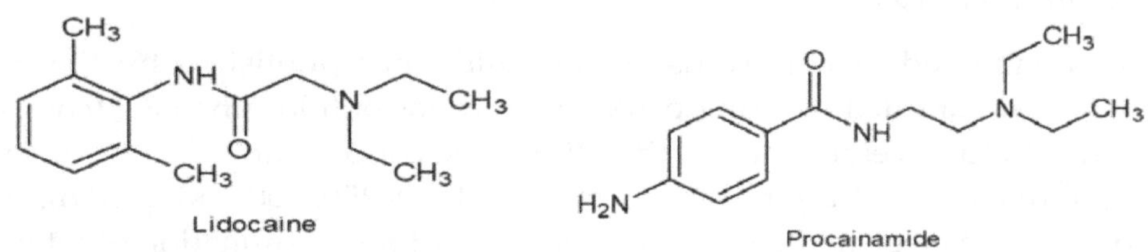

Figure 1. Chemical structure of lidocaine and procainamide, the internal standard.

2.1. Instrumentation and Chromatographic Conditions

The chromatographic system consisted of a Waters (Milford, MA, USA) 600 E multi-solvent delivery system pump, an autosampler with a variable injection valve (Waters 717), and a UV–visible tunable absorbance detector (Waters 486). The chromatograms were recorded using EZStart software (Scientific Software, Pleasanton, CA, USA) in a Windows-based computer system for data collection and processing. The chromatographic separation of lidocaine and procainamide (internal standard) were achieved using a 150 × 4.6 mm i.d., 3.5 μm particle size Alltima C18-column (Alltech, Deerfield, IL, USA) attached to a pre-guard column (Grace Alltech All-Guard™ Guard Cartridges, 7.5 mm 5 μm, Deerfield, IL, USA). The mobile phase consisted of a mixture of acetonitrile and phosphate solution (25 mM KH_2PO_4-3 mM sulfuric acid-3.6 mM triethylamine) in a ratio of 12:88 (v/v). The mobile phase was degassed prior to use by filtering it under vacuum pressure through a 0.45 μm pore size nylon filter, then pumped at a flow rate of 0.9 mL/min at room temperature.

Immediately after injection, the UV detection wavelength was set at 277 nm (the UV_{max} for procainamide). At 4 min post-injection, the UV detector was programmed to switch to a wavelength of 210 nm (the UV_{max} for lidocaine). The total analytical run time was <13 min.

2.2. Standard and Stock Solutions

The stock drug solution was 0.4% lidocaine HCl in 5% dextrose for injection. The working standard solutions were prepared daily from the stock solution by serial dilution with HPLC grade water to provide final concentrations of 40, 4 and 0.4 μg/mL lidocaine. The internal standard (IS) stock solution was prepared by dissolving 17 mg of procainamide HCl in 100 mL of water. All stock solutions were refrigerated between use. For the construction of a standard curve, samples of (0.25 mL) were prepared by adding lidocaine HCl equivalent to 50, 125, 250, 500, 1000, 2000, 2500 and 5000 ng/mL.

2.3. Extraction Procedure

A one-step liquid–liquid extraction step was used to extract lidocaine from human serum. After adding 50 μL volume of the IS stock solution and 200 μL of 1 M NaOH to 0.25 mL of human serum, 3 mL of diethyl ether was added. This was followed by vortex mixing of tubes for 30 s and centrifugation at 3000 *g* for 3 min. The organic solvent layer was pipetted to new tubes, then evaporated to dryness in vacuo. The dried residues were reconstituted using 150 μL of HPLC grade water with up to 75 μL being injected into the chromatographic system.

2.4. Recovery

Recovery was determined with lidocaine HCl concentrations of 50 and 1000 ng/mL and with an IS concentration of 0.17 mg/mL in human serum. The extraction efficiency was determined using five replicates of each concentration and comparing the extracted peak heights of analyte in the extracted samples to the peak heights of the same amounts of analyte directly injected into the HPLC without extraction.

2.5. Calibration, Accuracy and Validation

The assay was validated, generally using the guidelines published by the EMA [18]. The calibration curves were quantified by using peak height ratios of lidocaine HCl (concentration range from 50 to 5000 ng/mL) to IS versus the nominal lidocaine concentration. Intra-day validation was assessed at four different concentrations of lidocaine HCl (50, 250, 500 and 2000 ng/mL) per day in five replicates. This step was repeated on three separate days for determination of inter-day validation. For each daily run, an independent set of calibration curves samples was prepared. Accuracy and precision were assessed using the mean intra- and inter-day percentage error and percent coefficient of variation (CV%), respectively. Calibration curves were weighted by a factor of concentration^{-2} due to the wide range of concentrations (50–5000) used in the calibration curves.

Intraday, accuracy and precision of the assay were determined using a range of concentrations of lidocaine HCl. The selected concentrations were 50, 250, 500 and 2000 ng/mL of lidocaine HCl in human serum. Each concentration had five replicates. To permit the assessment of interday accuracy and precision in human serum, the assay was repeated on three separate days. For each daily run, a set of calibration samples separate from the validation samples were prepared to permit the quantification of the peak height ratios of lidocaine to IS. Precision was assessed by percentage coefficient of variation (CV%), while accuracy was represented by determining the mean intra- or inter-day percentage error.

2.6. Applicability

For the standard curve and validation samples, the serum was obtained from two healthy individuals on two separate occasions. For two of the samplings, each individual was asked to refrain from ingesting any caffeine-laden foods or drinks for 24 h before sampling.

The method was employed to determine the lidocaine concentration in human serum from one surgical patient after the injection of lidocaine as a reservoir within the rectus sheath (200 mg single dose). The patient provided written consent, and the study was approved by the University of Alberta Health Research Ethics Board. After the injection of the dose, blood samples were drawn serially into serum collection tubes until 24 h from the time of dosing. The blood samples were left for 30 min to clot, then centrifuged for 10 min. The serum was then separated and frozen at −20 °C until assayed.

3. Results

The chromatographic retention times were ~10 min for lidocaine and 2.5 min for IS (Figure 2). The chromatography displayed symmetrical peak shapes and high specificity, with a baseline resolution of IS and lidocaine. For both analytes, there was an absence of interference from endogenous components in serum (Figure 2). It was of note that the chromatograms from the serum of the healthy volunteers used in the assay development had a significant peak present that eluted at about 6.4 min, which was not seen in the patient serum sample obtained at 10 min. However, this did not interfere with the analysis of lidocaine, nor the internal standard.

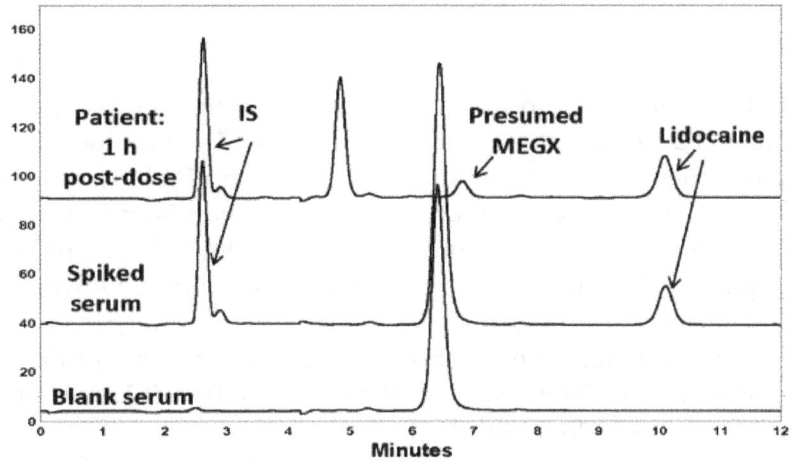

Figure 2. HPLC-UV chromatograms of blank (drug-free) serum from a healthy volunteer, volunteer serum spiked with 1000 ng/mL of lidocaine, and serum obtained 1 h after a 200 mg injection of lidocaine. The peak in the patient sample appearing at 6.8 min in the patient sample was presumed to be the lidocaine metabolite, monoethylglycinexylidide (MEGX). The peak at ~6.4 min was presumed to be from food components ingested by the volunteers who were not fasted.

The average recoveries were 97.7 ± 21% and 81.0 ± 2.4% for 50 and 1000 ng/mL lidocaine HCl in serum, respectively. The average extraction recoveries for IS at the concentration used in the assay was 55.4 ± 4.1%. There were excellent linear relationships (>0.9995) noted between the peak height ratios and lidocaine HCl concentrations over ranges of 50–5000 ng/mL serum.

From regression analysis of the concentration vs. peak height ratios of lidocaine to IS, the observed average slopes and intercepts were 0.00024 and 0.0011, respectively. The mean correlation coefficient of regression (r^2) for the serum standard curves were 0.9995. The CV of intra-and inter-day assessments were less than 15% (Table 2). The mean inter-day error in human serum was less than 9% (Table 2).

The validation assessments revealed that the assay was precise and possessed low bias. Overall, all intraday measures for mean error and CV% of the lowest concentration were less than 15%, and for the other concentrations only one fell above 10% (day three of the 216 ng/mL concentration). Except for the lowest concentration, all of the interday measures of CV% were less than 10%. All interday measures for mean error were less than 10%.

When tested for applicability in the patient samples, lidocaine serum concentrations could be measured for the full 24 h period following administration of the lidocaine dose. The observed maximal concentration was 1644 ng/mL, which occurred at 0.5 h post-dose.

The assay was reproducible and relatively fast in terms of preparation. To assay 30 samples, from the time of adding components to serum to completion of the evaporation of extracted solvent, took less than 40 min.

Table 2. Validation data for the assay of lidocaine in human serum, $n = 5$.

Nominal Concentration of Lidocaine *, ng/mL	Intraday			Interday		
	Mean ± SD ng/mL (CV%)			Mean ± SD ng/mL	CV%	Error%
43.3	45.9 ± 4.54 (9.90)	38.5 ± 5.37 (14.0)	40.8 ± 6.05 (14.8)	41.7 ± 5.32	12.9	−3.57
216	2158 ± 11.5 (5.35)	220 ± 9.60 (4.35)	226 ± 26.6 (11.8)	221 ± 15.9	7.16	1.99
433	379 ± 28.7 (7.56)	395 ± 25.6 (6.46)	407 ± 38.5 (9.47)	394 ± 30.9	7.83	−8.97
1731	1489 ± 60.5 (4.06)	1704 ± 43.3 (2.53)	1635 ± 47.1 (2.87)	1609 ± 50.3	3.16	−7.02

* To convert to lidocaine HCl salt, divide by 0.865.

4. Discussion

The HPLC method described here represents an accurate and precise avenue to determine the concentration of lidocaine in 0.25 mL volumes of human serum. The volumes of serum required are at the lower end of those volumes used by other analytical methods (Table 1). Additionally, the reported validated lower limits of quantitation are frequently greater than 50 ng/mL (Table 1). The lowest validated quantifiable concentration was found in the literature to be 10 ng/mL, though a serum volume of 1 mL was required [8]. Sintov et al. reported that the validated lower limit of quantification by using fluorescence detector was 25 ng/mL, which also required larger volumes of specimen up to 1 mL and derivatization following the extraction process [12], thereby adding elements of expense and time into sample preparation. The lower limit of quantitation (LLQ) in the current method is comparable to 50 ng/m by the GC-MS method [4].

Alkaline conditions were used to force lidocaine into its free base form, which promotes its extraction into a suitable organic solvent [12]. For the extraction of lidocaine from biological matrices, different solvents have been used in HPLC methods. These include an ethyl acetate/hexane/methanol mixture [14], dichloromethane [5], ethyl acetate [7,11], and a mixture of diethyl ether/dichloromethane [8]. Qin et al. had previously used diethyl ether as an extraction solvent for local anesthetics in human plasma, including procaine, ropivacaine, tetracaine, bupivacaine, including lidocaine [9]. The extraction of lidocaine from plasma in their hands was virtually complete, similar to what we had found. For this reason, we adopted the extraction method of Qin for use in the currently described assay method. Qin et al. had used carbamazepine as their internal standard. Due to its late elution time compared to procainamide [9], we chose to use procainamide instead. Although its recovery was less than that of lidocaine, it nevertheless extracted very consistently and provided excellent standard curves and validation indices. Procainamide would be an unlikely interfering substance in a patient as while it is chemically similar to lidocaine, it is not a popular antiarrhythmic currently, nor is it used as an anesthetic agent. The disadvantage of procainamide is that it requires that the UV detector possess the ability to program a change in wavelength after the elution of the internal standard.

In terms of mobile phase composition, acetonitrile and phosphate solution are the most common components in most of the reported studies (Table 1). Only Tam et al. and Qin et al. supplemented the mobile phase with 0.15% and 0.16% of triethylamine (TEA), respectively [7,9], while Chen et al. supplied the mobile phase with 1% diethylamine [6]. In the current method, 0.15% of triethylamine was added as it improved the peak symmetries and reduced the peak tailing of the compounds of interest, as has been noted for other compounds [19,20]. From the literature, the retention time for the compound of interest ranged from 3.6 to less than 13 min (Table 1).

The measured serum concentrations in the patient were in accordance with measures of plasma concentrations observed previously in patients administered the same dose of lidocaine HCl as depot parenteral injections [21]. The presence of a peak at 6.4 min was noticed in HPLC-UV chromatograms of blank (drug-free) human serum. Unfortunately, the appearance of this peak in the blank serum (with or without a caffeine-free period) virtually coincided with the elution of monoethylglycylxylidide (MEGX), a major metabolite of lidocaine [22]. In the first sample taken from the patient 10 min after the dose, although lidocaine was present, there was no peak observed eluting between 6 and 7 min. In later timed samples, such as 1 h after dosing (Figure 3) a peak virtually coinciding with MEGX was apparent. However, because in the volunteer serum, a large, mostly interfering peak was present, it was not possible to quantify the MEGX concentrations in the serum of the patient using the chromatographic conditions optimal for lidocaine elution. The patient differed from those subjects contributing volunteer serum in that the patients were required to fast before the surgery. Hence, it is possible that the peak in the healthy serum was from a food component, as none of the healthy volunteers had consumed any medications before contributing the blood for serum. The assay of metabolite was not a primary aim of this study, so we did not further pursue assay work as it would have meant a longer analytical run time for lidocaine, our primary analyte of interest. We did check for the elution of caffeine, and indeed it eluted at the same time as the large interfering peak in the serum of the volunteers who drank caffeine, but it was still present even after a 24 h caffeine fast. Therefore, it most likely derived from some other component of food. The patient also received other medications during surgery, and we believe that one of these may have been represented by the peak at 5.8 min (Figure 3), as it was not also seen in the volunteer serum, none of whom ingested any other drugs orally.

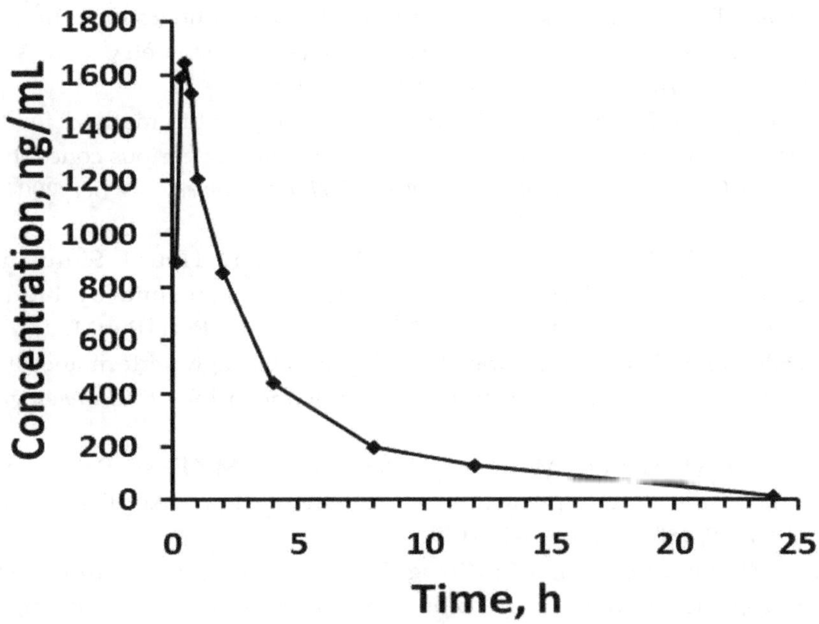

Figure 3. Serum lidocaine concentration vs. time profiles after rectus sheath injection of 200 mg lidocaine HCl to the patient volunteer.

5. Conclusions

The method demonstrated high calibers of sensitivity and selectivity for monitoring concentrations of lidocaine in human serum. The method was uncomplicated in terms of sample preparation and extraction. It was precise and accurate and was shown to have utility as a means to measure lidocaine concentration as part of a pharmacokinetic study.

Acknowledgments: Hamdah M. Al Nebaihi is the recipient of Government of Saudi Arabia scholarship.

Author Contributions: Hamdah M. Al Nebaihi performed most of the analytical method work including assay of samples and validation, and was extensively involved in data analysis and writing of the paper. Matthew Primrose and James S. Green contributed towards the concept and clinical aspect of the work. Dion R. Brocks was involved in concept, initial method workup and writing of the paper.

Abbreviations

CV%	Coefficient of variation expressed as percent
LLQ	Lower limit of quantitation
SPE	Solid phase extraction
GC-MS	Gas chromatography-mass spectrometry
ppt	Precipitation
IS	Internal standard
LLE	Liquid-liquid extraction
UV	Ultraviolet detection
NS	Not specified or unclear

References

1. Benowitz, N.L.; Meister, W. Clinical pharmacokinetics of lignocaine. *Clin. Pharmacokinet.* **1978**, *3*, 177–201. [CrossRef] [PubMed]
2. Tremont-Lukats, I.; Teixeira, G.; Backonja, M. Systemic administration of local anesthetic agents to relieve neuropathic pain. *Anesth. Analg.* **2005**, *101*, 1736–1737.
3. World Health Organization. WHO Model List of Essential Medicines: 20th List, March 2017. Available online: http://www.who.int/medicines/publications/essentialmedicines/20th_EML2017_FINAL_amendedAug2017.png?ua=1 (accessed on 15 November 2017).
4. Ohshima, T.; Takayasu, T. Simultaneous determination of local anesthetics including ester-type anesthetics in human plasma and urine by gas chromatography-mass spectrometry with solid-phase extraction. *J. Chromatogr. B Biomed. Sci. Appl.* **1999**, *726*, 185–194. [CrossRef]
5. Piwowarska, J.; Kuczynska, J.; Pachecka, J. Liquid chromatographic method for the determination of lidocaine and monoethylglycine xylidide in human serum containing various concentrations of bilirubin for the assessment of liver function. *J. Chromatogr. B Anal. Technol. Biomed. Life Sci.* **2004**, *805*, 1–5. [CrossRef] [PubMed]
6. Chen, L.; Liao, L.; Zuo, Z.; Yan, Y.; Yang, L.; Fu, Q.; Chen, Y.; Hou, J. Simultaneous determination of nikethamide and lidocaine in human blood and cerebrospinal fluid by high performance liquid chromatography. *J. Pharm. Biomed. Anal.* **2007**, *43*, 1757–1762. [CrossRef] [PubMed]
7. Tam, Y.K.; Tawfik, S.R.; Ke, J.; Coutts, R.T.; Gray, M.R.; Wyse, D.G. High-performance liquid chromatography of lidocaine and nine of its metabolites in human plasma and urine. *J. Chromatogr.* **1987**, *423*, 199–206. [CrossRef]
8. Lotfi, H.; Debord, J.; Dreyfuss, M.F.; Marquet, P.; Ben Rhaiem, M.; Feiss, P.; Lachâtre, G. Simultaneous determination of lidocaine and bupivacaine in human plasma: Application to pharmacokinetics. *Ther. Drug Monit.* **1997**, *19*, 160 164. [CrossRef] [PubMed]
9. Qin, W.W.; Jiao, Z.; Zhong, M.K.; Shi, X.J.; Zhang, J.; Li, Z.D.; Cui, X.Y. Simultaneous determination of procaine, lidocaine, ropivacaine, tetracaine and bupivacaine in human plasma by high-performance liquid chromatography. *J. Chromatogr. B Anal. Technol. Biomed. Life Sci.* **2010**, *878*, 1185–1189. [CrossRef] [PubMed]
10. Bhusal, P.; Sharma, M.; Harrison, J.; Procter, G.; Andrews, G.; Jones, D.S.; Hill, A.G.; Svirskis, D. Development, validation and application of a stability indicating HPLC method to quantify lidocaine from polyethylene-co-vinyl acetate (EVA) matrices and biological fluids. *J. Chromatogr. Sci.* **2017**, *55*, 832–838. [CrossRef] [PubMed]
11. Nation, R.L.; Peng, G.W.; Chiou, W.L. High-performance liquid chromatographic method for the simultaneous determination of lidocaine and its N-dealkylated metabolites in plasma. *J. Chromatogr.* **1979**, *162*, 466–473. [CrossRef]
12. Sintov, A.; Siden, R.; Levy, R.J. Sensitive high-performance liquid chromatographic assay using 9-fluorenylmethylchloroformate for monitoring controlled-release lidocaine in plasma. *J. Chromatogr.* **1989**, *496*, 335–344. [CrossRef]
13. Kihara, S.; Miyabe, M.; Kakiuchi, Y.; Takahashi, S.; Fukuda, T.; Kohda, Y.; Toyooka, H. Plasma concentrations of lidocaine and its principal metabolites during continuous epidural infusion of lidocaine with or without epinephrine. *Reg. Anesth. Pain Med.* **1999**, *24*, 529–533. [CrossRef] [PubMed]

14. Dusci, L.J.; Hackett, L.P. Simultaneous determination of lidocaine, mexiletine, disopyramide, and quinidine in plasma by high performance liquid chromatography. *J. Anal. Toxicol.* **1985**, *9*, 67–70. [CrossRef] [PubMed]
15. Ter Weijden, E.; Van den Broek, M.; Ververs, F. Easy and fast LC–MS/MS determination of lidocaine and MEGX in plasma for therapeutic drug monitoring in neonates with seizures. *J. Chromatogr. B* **2012**, *881*, 111–114. [CrossRef] [PubMed]
16. Bo, L.D.; Mazzucchelli, P.; Marzo, A. Highly sensitive bioassay of lidocaine in human plasma by high-performance liquid chromatography-tandem mass spectrometry. *J. Chromatogr. A* **1999**, *854*, 3–11. [PubMed]
17. Ochoa-Aranda, E.; Esteve-Romero, J.; Rambla-Alegre, M.; Martinavarro-Domnguez, A.; Marcos-Toms, J.V.; Bose, D. Monitoring disopyramide, lidocaine, and quinidine by micellar liquid chromatography. *J. AOAC Int.* **2011**, *94*, 537–542. [PubMed]
18. Guideline on Bioanalytical Method Validation. Available online: http://www.ema.europa.eu/docs/en_GB/document_library/Scientific_guideline/2011/08/WC500109686.png (accessed on 15 November 2017).
19. Roos, R.W.; Lau-Cam, C.A. General reversed-phase high-performance liquid chromatographic method for the separation of drugs using triethylamine as a competing base. *J. Chromatogr.* **1986**, *370*, 403–418. [CrossRef]
20. Ruiz-Angel, M.; Torres-Lapasió, J.; Carda-Broch, S.; García-Alvarez-Coque, M. Improvement of peak shape and separation performance of β-blockers in conventional reversed-phase columns using solvent modifiers. *J. Chromatogr. Sci.* **2003**, *41*, 350–358. [CrossRef] [PubMed]
21. Chen, L.; Wang, Q.; Shi, K.; Liu, F.; Liu, L.; Ni, J.; Fang, X.; Xu, X. The Effects of Lidocaine Used in Sciatic Nerve on the Pharmacodynamics and Pharmacokinetics of Ropivacaine in Sciatic Nerve Combined with Lumbar Plexus Blockade: A Double-Blind, Randomized Study. *Basic Clin. Pharmacol. Toxicol.* **2013**, *112*, 203–208. [CrossRef] [PubMed]
22. Bargetzi, M.J.; Aoyama, T.; Gonzalez, F.J.; Meyer, U.A. Lidocaine metabolism in human liver microsomes by cytochrome P450IIIA4. *Clin. Pharmacol. Ther.* **1989**, *46*, 521–527. [CrossRef] [PubMed]

14

Pharmacokinetic Interaction between Metformin and Verapamil in Rats: Inhibition of the OCT2-Mediated Renal Excretion of Metformin by Verapamil

Seung Yon Han and Young Hee Choi *

College of Pharmacy and Integrated Research Institute for Drug Development, Dongguk University_Seoul, 32 Dongguk-lo, Ilsandong-gu, Goyang-si 10326, Korea; hsyglory@gmail.com
* Correspondence: choiyh@dongguk.edu

Abstract: The incidence of hypertension in diabetic patients has been increasing and contributing to the high mortality of diabetic patients. Recently, verapamil use was found to lower fasting blood glucose levels in diabetic patients, which led to a new indication of verapamil as combination treatment with anti-diabetic agents such as metformin. As pharmacokinetic (PK) interaction can affect drug efficacy and safety in drug combination, their PK-based interaction is recommended to be evaluated in preclinical levels as well as clinical levels. In case of metformin and verapamil, organic cation transporter (OCT) 1 and 2 primarily mediate metformin distribution to the liver and its elimination into urine, whereas cytochrome P450 is responsible for the hepatic metabolism of verapamil. Verapamil is also known as a potential OCT2 inhibitor. Thus, PK interaction between metformin (30 mg/kg) and verapamil (20 mg/kg) were investigated after their simultaneous administration to rats. In our results, verapamil inhibited the OCT2-mediated renal excretion of metformin, subsequently leading to increase of the systemic exposure of metformin. In contrast, metformin did not influence the pharmacokinetic pattern of verapamil. Although the further clinical investigation is required, our finding suggests a possibility of OCT2-mediated interaction of metformin and verapamil.

Keywords: metformin; verapamil; drug interaction; organic cation transporter 2; renal excretion

---

1. Introduction

The incidences of diabetic mellitus and hypertension are rapidly growing worldwide, and hypertension is an important cardiovascular risk factor in patients with type 2 diabetes mellitus (T2DM) [1–3]. The dramatically increased (two- to four-fold) risk of cardiovascular diseases in T2DM patients is their leading cause of mortality [4–6]. Insulin resistance and compensatory hyperinsulinemia are also frequent findings in hypertensive patients [7,8]. Since blood pressure-lowering treatment is important to reduce the risk of developing cardiovascular complications in T2DM patients, a combination of anti-diabetic and anti-hypertension drugs is needed and increasingly used [9].

Metformin, an oral biguanide antihyperglycemic agent, increases hepatic and skeletal muscle insulin sensitivity and decreases hepatic glucose production without causing hypoglycemia [10–12]. Metformin also reduces cardiovascular disease complications such as high blood pressure in patients with type 2 diabetic mellitus (T2DM) [3,13,14]. Metformin pharmacokinetics (PK) and pharmacodynamics (PD) rely on the organic cation transporter (OCT) 1 in the sinusoidal membrane of hepatocytes to transport metformin into the liver, its pharmacological target site. The metformin concentration in the liver determines the metformin's effect on inhibiting glucose production [15–17]. OCT2 in the basolateral membrane of the renal proximal tubules mediates the renal excretion of metformin as ~70% of the metformin dose [16,18]. Reduced renal excretion of metformin via renal

OCT2 inhibition causes an increase of systemic exposure (i.e., plasma concentration of metformin), which can result in lactic acidosis [19]. Previous reports that metformin suppresses P-glycoprotein (P-gp) and pregnane X receptor (PXR)-regulated transactivation of the cytochrome P450 (CYP) 3A4 gene [20,21] suggest that the potential for a PK-based drug-drug interaction (DDI) occurrence between metformin and verapamil.

Verapamil, as a calcium channel blocker, is recently emerged as a combination drug in DM patients with hypertension, because verapamil lowers fasting blood glucose levels and enhances insulin secretion in T2DM patients [22,23]. In particular, it is an important issue to regulate insulin secretion as a compensatory mechanism of hyperinsulinemia in hypertensive patients [7,8]. Verapamil has been popularly used for treatment of hypertension and supraventricular tachyarrhythmias [22–27]. Orally administered verapamil is rapidly and well-absorbed, and then it is eliminated via extensive cytochrome P450 (CYP)-mediated hepatic metabolism [25–29]. An *N*-methylated metabolite, norverapamil, has been shown to have a vasodilator effect in vitro [13]. Verapamil also has an inhibitory effect on P-gp and OCT2 in in vitro and clinical studies [16,30,31]. Although it was reported that verapamil reduced the maximum blood glucose concentration and area under the blood glucose concentration-time curve in healthy adults orally administered with metformin and verapamil together [32], there was no direct measurement of metformin concentration in liver, which may be a substantial evidence on its glucose tolerance activity. Moreover, there has been no report to explain whether transporter and/or metabolic enzyme-mediated PK changes of metformin and verapamil in their combination. In the meantime, new findings regarding positive effect of verapamil for the treatment of hypertension in DM patients have been introduced [22,23], there is a need to investigate how the plasma and tissue concentrations of metformin and verapamil change in DDI events, especially at preclinical levels [33,34]. Since changes in plasma and tissue concentrations of these drugs in combination are associated with their efficacy and toxicity [35,36], the PK interactions of metformin and verapamil were evaluated in rats based on their plasma and tissue concentration changes.

2. Materials and Methods

2.1. Chemicals

Metformin hydrochloride was donated from Daelim Pharmaceutical Company (Seoul, Korea). Verapamil hydrochloride, norverapamil, ipriflavone (internal standard (IS) for the high-performance liquid chromatography (HPLC) analysis of metformin) and propranolol (IS for the HPLC analysis of verapamil and norverapamil), the reduced form of β-nicotinamide adenine dinucleotide phosphate, tris(hydroxymethyl)-aminomethane (Tris) buffer and ethylenediamine tetraacetic acid were purchased from Sigma–Aldrich Corporation (St. Louis, MO, USA). HEK-293 cells overexpressing OCT1 (SLC22A1) and OCT2 (SLC22A2) were purchased from Corning Life Sciences (Corning, NY, USA). Other chemicals were of reagent or HPLC grade.

2.2. Animals

The protocol for the animal studieswas approved by the Animal Care and Use Committee of the College of Pharmacy, Dongguk University-Seoul, Korea (approval no. IACUC-2013-006, 15 December 2013). Male Sprague–Dawley rats (5–7 weeks old, weighing 190–260 g) were purchased from Taconic Farms Inc. (Samtako Bio Korea, O-San, Korea). The rats were housed and handled similarly based on the reported methods [17,33,34].

2.3. Pharmacokinetic Studies of Metformin, Verapamil and Both Drugs in Rats

Early in the morning, the carotid artery (for blood sampling in the intravenous and oral studies) and the jugular vein (for intravenous drug administration only in the intravenous study) of the rats were cannulated, similar to previously reported methods [17,33,34]. The rats were not restrained during the experimental period.

For the intravenous study, 30 mg (2 mL)/kg of metformin (as metformin hydrochloride dissolved in 0.9% NaCl-injectable solution; $n = 6$), 20 mg (2 mL)/kg of verapamil (as verapamil hydrochloride dissolved in 0.9% NaCl-injectable solution; $n = 6$) and both drugs together ($n = 6$) were administered to the rats. Blood samples (approximately 0.12 or 0.22 mL for each drug alone or both drugs together, respectively) were collected via the carotid artery at 0, 1, 5, 15, 30, 60, 90, 120, 180, 240, 300 or 360 min after the start of the drug administration. After each blood sampling, 0.3 mL of 0.9% NaCl-injectable solution containing heparin (20 U/mL) was immediately flushed into each cannula to prevent blood clotting. The blood samples were immediately centrifuged and a 50 μL (or two 50 μL for both drugs) of plasma sample was stored at −80 °C (Revco ULT 1490 D-N-S; Western Mednics, Asheville, NC, USA). The 24-h urine sample ($Ae_{0\text{–}24\,h}$) and the gastrointestinal tract (including its contents and feces) sample at 24 h ($GI_{24\,h}$) were prepared following previously reported methods [17,33,34], and the samples were also stored at −80 °C.

For the oral study, after overnight fasting with free access to water, the same doses of metformin ($n = 5$), verapamil ($n = 5$) and both drugs together ($n = 5$) were orally administered (total oral volume of 6 mL/kg) to the rats using a gastric gavage tube. Blood samples were collected via the carotid artery at 0, 5, 15, 30, 60, 90, 120, 180, 240, 360, 480 or 600 min after the drug administration. Other procedures were similar to those for the intravenous study.

2.4. *Effect of Verapamil on Metformin Uptake in HEK-293 Cells Overexpressing OCT1 or OCT2*

To investigate whether OCT1 and OCT2, as the main transporters affecting metformin pharmacokinetics, were changed by verapamil, the effect of verapamil on OCT1- or OCT2-mediated metformin uptake was investigated in HEK-293 cells overexpressing OCT1 or OCT2 following previously published procedures [33,34]. Briefly, a density of 4.0×10^5 cells/well of HEK-293 cells overexpressing either OCT1 or OCT2 were seeded into 24-well plates coated with poly-D-lysine (Corning Incorporated, Corning, NY, USA) and incubated with Dulbecco's Modified Eagle Medium supplemented with 10% fetal bovine serum for 24 h. After washing twice with pre-warmed Hank's Balanced Salt Solution with Ca^{2+} and Mg^{2+} (Hank's buffer) and pre-incubating the cells with Hank's buffer for 10 min, Hank's buffer was replaced to Hank's buffer containing 10 μM metformin with verapamil added as an inhibitor (0–100 μM). The concentrations of metformin and verapamil were chosen in the ranges of concentrations used in HEK-293 cells overexpressing OCT1 or OCT2 in the previous reports [33,34] and a protocol of in vitro screening method for human SLC uptake transporter inhibition (OCT1 and OCT2) by Cyprotex. Metformin uptake was initiated at this time and the cells were incubated at 37 °C for 10 min. At 10 min after starting metformin uptake, Hank's buffer was removed and the cells were immediately washing twice with ice-cold Hank's buffer to stop metformin uptake. The cells were lysed with distilled water and harvested by scraping them off in 200 μL distilled water followed by ultra-sonification at 4 °C for 10 s. After centrifuging the cells at 15,000× *g* for 10 min at 4 °C, the supernatant was determined by LC/MS/MS analysis of metformin [33,34]. The half-maximal inhibitory constant (IC_{50}) values of verapamil for the inhibition of OCT1 or OCT2-mediated metformin uptake are expressed as % of metformin uptake without verapamil (exposed to vehicle instead of verapamil) in HEK-293 cells overexpressing OCT1 or OCT2, arbitrarily set at 100% ($n = 2$ for each dose). From percentages of metformin uptake versus inhibitor concentrations, a sigmoid shaped curve was fitted to the data and IC_{50} was calculated by fitting Hill equation to the data using GraphPad Prism 5 (GraphPad Software Inc., San Diego, CA, USA).

2.5. *Effect of Verapamil on Metformin Concentration in the Liver and Kidneys*

To investigate whether verapamil changes the metformin concentration in the liver and kidneys, a tissue distribution study of metformin with and without verapamil was conducted following a previously reported method [17,33,34]. At 0.5, 1, 3 and 6 h after intravenous or oral administration of metformin with and without verapamil at the same doses as in the pharmacokinetic study, as much blood as possible was collected and each rat was then sacrificed by lethal blood loss. The liver and kidneys were excised, weighed and homogenized in a 4-fold volume of 0.9% NaCl-injectable solution ($n = 4$ for each organ). After centrifuging each homogenate at 15,000× g for 10 min at 4 °C, the supernatant was collected and stored at −80 °C.

2.6. Effect of Metformin on Verapamil Metabolism in Rat Hepatic and Intestinal Microsomes

To investigate the effect of metformin on verapamil metabolism, the measurement of kinetic constants, such as V_{max} (maximum velocity) and K_m (apparent Michaelis–Menten constant; the concentration at which the rate is one half of the V_{max}) for verapamil metabolism, with and without metformin, in hepatic and intestinal microsomes were conducted. Hepatic and intestinal microsomes were prepared by the previously reported method as followings [17,37,38]: freshly excised livers were cut in pieces, washed extensively with ice-cold solution (KCl 0.15 M) to remove remaining blood and were homogenized with Tris-HCl buffer (pH 7.5) containing 0.15 M KCl + 50 mM Tris, 1 mM EDTA in a Potter-Elvehjem glass homogenizer for 30 s. The homogenate was centrifuged for 10 min at 10,000× g and 4 °C and then followed by ultracentrifugation of the remaining supernatant for 1 h at 100,000× g and 4 °C. Microsomal pellets were then re-suspended in the same buffer with a hand homogenizer and re-centrifuged for 1 h at 100,000× g and 4 °C. The supernatant was discarded, and the microsomal pellets were carefully overlaid with 0.15 mol KCl buffer and stored at −80 °C. Intestinal microsomes were prepared using freshly excised proximal and middle sections of the small intestine. This part of intestine was excised, rinsed with ice-cold 0.01 M potassium phosphate buffer with 1.15% KCl (pH 7.4), filled with solution A (1.5 mM KCl + 96 mM NaCl + 27 mM sodium citrate + 8 mM KH_2PO_4 + 5.6 mM Na_2HPO_4 + 40 µg/mL PMSF). The intestine filled with solution A was incubated in a 37 °C water bath for 15 min. After discarding solution A, the intestine was filled with ice-cold solution B (phosphate-buffered saline + 1.5 mM EDTA + 0.5 mM dithiothreitol + 40 µg/mL PMSF), wound around a middle finger and tapped against the finger three times. The upper villus cells were released into solution B during this process, and the collected cells were pooled. The pooled solution was centrifuged at 10× g and 4 °C for 5 min. After discarding the supernatant, approximately 15 mL of ice-cold solution C (5 mM histidine + 0.25 M sucrose + 0.5 mM EDTA + 40 µg/mL PMSF) was added into each centrifuge tube, which was inverted twice. Following the discard of the supernatant, the cells were resuspended in fresh ice-cold solution C, homogenized with a Pyrex glass Potter-Elvehjem homogenize and centrifuged at 10,000× g and 4 °C for 20 min. The supernatant was then centrifuged at 100,000× g and 4 °C for 65 min. The pellet of intestinal microsome was resuspended in 0.2 mM EDTA/20% glycerol/80% 0.1 M phosphate buffer (pH 7.4), homogenized and stored at −80 °C. Protein contents in hepatic and intestinal microsomes were measured by the reported method [39].

In hepatic microsomes (equivalent to 1 mg protein), 2.5 µL of 0.9% NaCl-injectable solution containing 2.5, 5, 10, 20 or 50 µM verapamil (the substrate) as final concentrations, 2.5 µL of 0.9% NaCl-injectable solution containing 10 µM metformin (the inhibitor) as a final concentration and 50 µL of 1 mM of NADPH dissolved in 0.1 M phosphate buffer of pH 7.4 were added. The total volume, 0.5 mL, was adjusted by adding 0.1 M phosphate buffer (pH 7.4), and then the components were incubated at 37 °C using a thermomixer at 500 opm. In intestinal microsomes, verapamil (as the substrate) concentrations of 5, 10, 20, 50 or 200 µM were used and the other conditions were the same as in the hepatic microsome study. After incubation for 15 or 30 min of the hepatic and intestinal microsomes, respectively, 1 mL of diethylether containing 1 µg/mL of propranolol, as an IS, was added to terminate the reaction. The verapamil concentration in each sample was determined by HPLC analysis [29].

The K_m and V_{max} for the verapamil metabolism were calculated using a non-linear regression method [40]. The unweighted kinetic data from the hepatic and intestinal microsomes were fitted using a single-site Michaelis–Menten equation; $V = V_{max} \times [S]/(K_m + [S])$, in which [S] was the substrate concentration. The intrinsic clearance (CL_{int}) was calculated by dividing the V_{max} by the K_m.

2.7. Rat Plasma Protein Binding of Metformin and Verapamil Using Equilibrium Dialysis

Protein binding values of metformin and verapamil with and without each other were measured in the fresh plasma of control rats using equilibrium dialysis ($n = 4$ for each; [17]). A 1 mL aliquot of the plasma was dialyzed against 1 mL of isotonic Sørensen phosphate buffer (pH 7.4) containing 3% dextran (*w/v*) in a dialysis cell (Spectrum Medical Industries, Laguna Hills, CA, USA) using a Spectra/Por 4 membrane (mol. wt. cutoff 12–14 KDa; Spectrum Medical Industries, USA). After 24 h incubation, two 50 μL aliquots were collected from each compartment, and the samples were stored at −80 °C.

2.8. Analytical Methods for Metformin, Verapamil and Norverapamil

In the HPL-UV system, the metformin concentration in the sample was determined using the analytical method developed by Choi et al. [17]. The quantitation limits of metformin in rat plasma, urine and GI samples were 0.05, 0.1 and 0.1 μg/mL, respectively. The inter- and intra-day coefficients of variation were below 8.94%. Additionally, the metformin concentration in the sample from the metformin uptake study was determined by LC-MS/MS analysis [33,34]. The quantitation limits of metformin in rat plasma, urine and GI samples were 0.01, 0.02 and 0.02 μg/mL, respectively. The inter- and intra-day coefficients of variation were below 9.53%. Verapamil and norverapamil concentrations in the sample were also determined by the HPLC-UV analytical method of Hong et al. [29]. The quantitation limits of verapamil in rat plasma, urine and GI samples were 0.01, 0.05 and 0.05 μg/mL, respectively. The corresponding values of norverapamil in all biological samples was 0.02 μg/mL; the inter- and intra-day coefficients of variation were below 12.9%.

2.9. Pharmacokinetic Analysis

Standard methods [41] were used to calculate the following pharmacokinetic parameters using non-compartmental analysis (WinNonlin; Pharsight Corporation, Mountain View, CA, USA): the total area under the plasma concentration–time curve from time zero to infinity (AUC), terminal half-life, time-averaged total body, renal, and non-renal clearances (CL, CL_R and CL_{NR}, respectively), and apparent volume of distribution at a steady state (V_{ss}). The peak plasma concentration (C_{max}) and time to reach C_{max} (T_{max}) were directly read from the experimental data.

2.10. Statistical Analysis

A p-value < 0.05 was deemed to be statistically significant using a Student's t-test between the two means for the unpaired data. All results are expressed as mean ± standard deviation (S.D.) except the medians (ranges) for T_{max}.

3. Results

3.1. Effect of Verapamil on Metformin Pharmacokinetics

The mean arterial plasma concentration–time profiles and relevant pharmacokinetic parameters of metformin after its intravenous administration with and without verapamil are shown in Figure 1 and Table 1, respectively. After intravenous administration of metformin with verapamil, the AUC was significantly greater (by 66.7%); CL and CL_R were significantly slower (by 50.8 and 70.7%, respectively); and $Ae_{0–24\,h}$ was significantly smaller (by 43.0%) than those without verapamil.

After oral administration of metformin with verapamil, the AUC was significantly greater (by 73.5%), C_{max} was significantly higher (by 60.5%), CL_R was significantly slower (by 68.4%) and $Ae_{0–24\,h}$ was significantly smaller (by 46.0%) than those without verapamil.

Table 1. Mean (± S.D.) pharmacokinetic parameters of metformin after its intravenous and oral administration with and without verapamil to rats. Doses of metformin and verapamil were 30 and 20 mg/kg, respectively.

Parameter	Intravenous (n = 6 for Each)		Parameter	Oral (n = 5 for Each)	
	Without Verapamil	With Verapamil		Without Verapamil	With Verapamil
Body weight (g)	203 ± 8.80	209 ± 6.65	Body weight (g)	228 ± 19.2	217 ± 13.0
AUC (μg min/mL)	1590 ± 613	2650 ± 449 [a]	AUC (μg min/mL)	472 ± 40.2	819 ± 82.3 [b]
Terminal half-life (min)	92.4 ± 26.4	80.5 ± 34.6	Terminal half-life (min)	137 ± 44.4	101 ± 48.0
MRT (min)	21.4 ± 5.28	18.4 ± 7.69	C_{max} (μg/mL)	2.00 ± 0.328	3.21 ± 1.04 [c]
V_{SS} (mL/kg)	349 ± 128	286 ± 92.4	T_{max} (min)	60 (60–120)	60 (60-120)
CL (mL/min/kg)	24.2 ± 3.02	11.9 ± 2.00 [b]	CL_R (mL/min/kg)	45.6 ± 5.66	14.4 ± 5.45 [b]
CL_{NR} (mL/min/kg)	8.12 ± 3.03	7.13 ± 0.932	$Ae_{0–24\ h}$ (% of dose)	71.3 ± 5.86	38.5 ±9.96 [b]
CL_R (mL/min/kg)	16.1 ± 3.18	4.72 ± 2.52 [b]	$GI_{24\ h}$ (% of dose)	3.57 ± 2.84	1.53 ± 1.57
$Ae_{0–24\ h}$ (% of dose)	66.5 ± 11.3	37.9 ± 14.9 [a]	F (%)	29.7	30.9
$GI_{24\ h}$ (% of dose)	0.471 ± 0.782	0.831 ± 0.787			

AUC, total area under the plasma concentration–time curve from time zero to infinity; MRT, mean residence time; V_{ss}, apparent volume of distribution at steady state; CL, time-averaged total body clearance; CL_{NR}, time-averaged non-renal clearance; CL_R, time-averaged renal clearance; $Ae_{0–24\ h}$, percentage of the dose excreted in the urine up to 24 h; $GI_{24\ h}$, percentage of the dose recovered from the gastrointestinal tract (including its contents and feces) at 24 h; C_{max}, peak plasma concentration of docetaxel; T_{max}, time to reach C_{max}; F, extent of absolute oral bioavailability. [a] Significantly different ($p < 0.01$) from with verapamil. [b] Significantly different ($p < 0.001$) from with verapamil. [c] Significantly different ($p < 0.05$) from with verapamil.

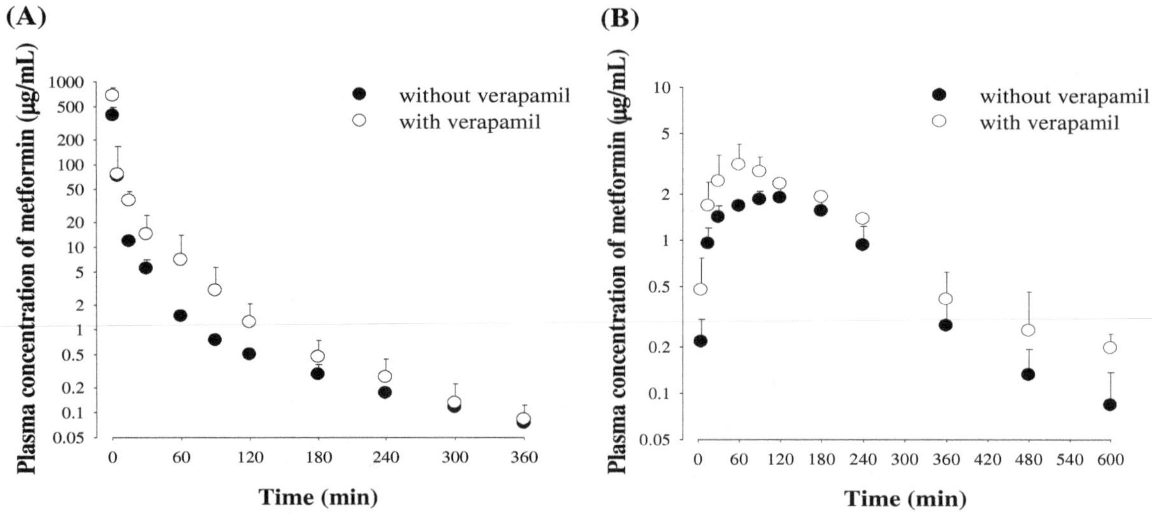

Figure 1. Mean (± S.D.) arterial plasma concentration–time profiles of metformin after intravenous (**A**; n = 6 for each) and oral (**B**; n = 5 for each) administration of metformin with (○) or without (•) verapamil to rats. Doses of metformin and verapamil were 30 and 20 mg/kg, respectively.

3.2. Effect of Verapamil on OCT1- or OCT2-Mediated Metformin Uptake in HEK-293 Cells Overexpressing OCT1 or OCT2

To examine the verapamil effect on OCT1 and OCT2 activities, the changes of metformin uptake with and without verapamil were compared in HEK-293 cells overexpressing OCT1 or OCT2. As shown in Figure 2, verapamil considerably inhibited metformin uptake in HEK-293 cells overexpressing either OCT1 or OCT2. The IC_{50} values of verapamil for inhibiting OCT1- and OCT2-mediated metformin uptake were 51.9 ± 1.09 and 19.3 ± 0.220 μM, respectively.

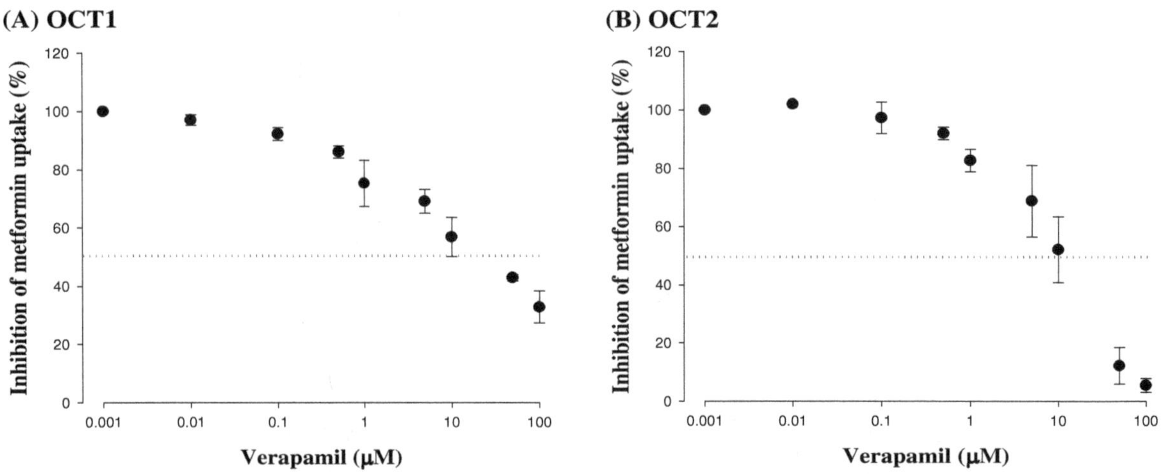

Figure 2. Mean (± S.D.) inhibitory effect of verapamil on metformin uptake in HEK293 cells overexpressing OCT1 (**A**, n = 2) or OCT2 (**B**, n = 2).

3.3. Effect of Verapamil on Metformin Concentrations in the Liver and Kidneys

After intravenous and oral administration of metformin with and without verapamil, metformin concentrations in the liver and kidneys are shown in Figure 3 and Table 2, respectively. After intravenous and oral administration of both drugs together, verapamil did not cause any change of the metformin concentration in the liver, but the metformin concentration in the kidneys was significantly decreased (by 38.6 and 48.7% at 1 and 3 h in the intravenous study and 42.9, 41.1 and 30.2% at 1, 3 and 6 h in the oral study, respectively) compared to metformin alone. Metformin concentrations in the plasma after intravenous and oral co-administration of metformin and verapamil were significantly lower than those after administration of metformin alone, showing similar patterns to the pharmacokinetic study.

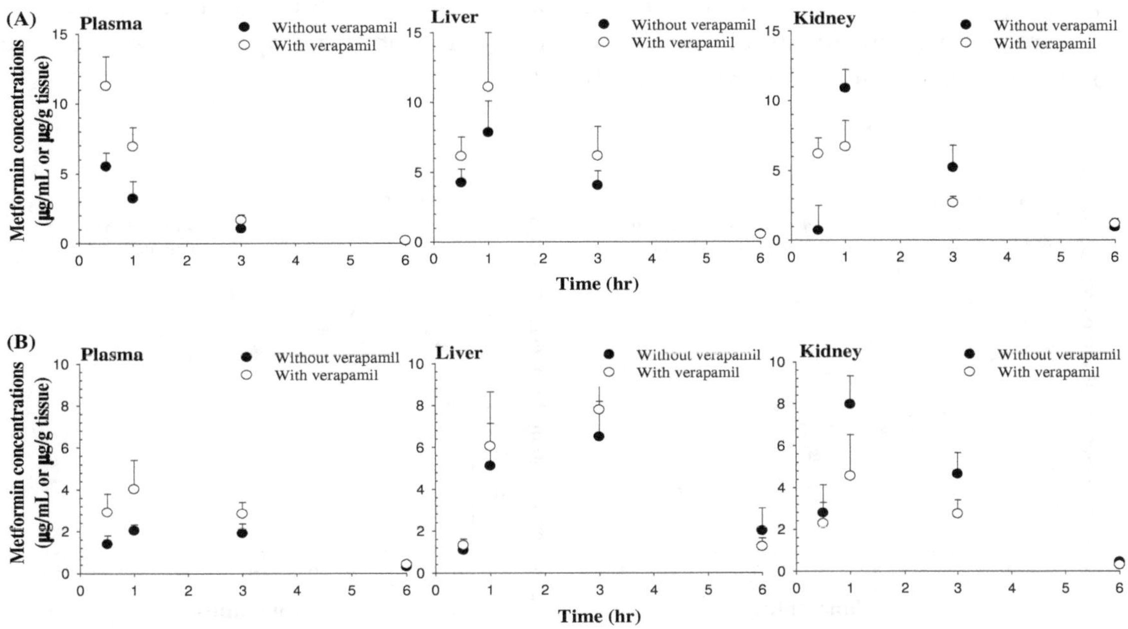

Figure 3. Mean (± S.D.) concentrations of metformin in the plasma, liver and kidneys after its intravenous (**A**, $n = 4$ for each) or oral (**B**, $n = 4$ for each) administration with (○) or without (•) verapamil. The dose of metformin and verapamil were 30 and 20 mg/kg, respectively.

Table 2. Mean (± S.D.) concentrations (μg/mL or μg/g tissue) of metformin in the plasma, liver and kidneys after intravenous or oral administration of metformin with and without verapamil.

	Intravenous (n = 4 for Each)		Oral (n = 4 for Each)	
Parameter	**Without Verapamil**	**With Verapamil**	**Without Verapamil**	**With Verapamil**
Plasma				
0.5	5.50 ± 0.988	11.3 ± 2.09 [a]	1.39 ± 0.415	2.91 ± 0.894 [b]
1	3.22 ± 1.22	6.94 ± 1.34 [a]	2.04 ± 0.281	4.03 ± 1.38 [b]
3	1.06 ± 0.214	1.68 ± 0.377 [b]	1.91 ± 0.455	2.84 ± 0.564 [b]
6	0.158 ± 0.0530	0.184 ± 0.0789	0.306 ± 0.0724	0.421 ± 0.0570 [b]
Liver				
0.5	4.25 ± 0.978	6.12 ± 1.39	1.09 ± 0.207	1.31 ± 0.300
1	7.84 ± 2.25	11.1 ± 3.84	5.11 ± 2.03	6.04 ± 2.60
3	4.04 ± 1.04	6.14 ± 2.10	6.49 ± 1.68	7.78 ± 1.11
6	0.553 ± 0.108	0.510 ± 0.222	1.99 ± 1.10	1.24 ± 0.407
Kidney				
0.5	0.706 ± 1.80	6.20 ± 1.12	2.78 ± 1.36	2.28 ± 1.01
1	10.9 ± 1.34	6.69 ± 1.87 [b]	7.97 ± 1.36	4.55 ± 1.98 [b]
3	5.22 ± 1.57	2.68 ± 0.471 [b]	4.65 ± 1.01	2.74 ± 0.675 [b]
6	0.935 ± 0.284	1.20 ± 0.342	0.443 ± 0.0640	0.309 ± 0.0767 [b]

[a] Significantly different ($p < 0.01$) from metformin. [b] Significantly different ($p < 0.05$) from metformin.

3.4. *Effect of Metformin on Verapamil Pharmacokinetics*

The mean arterial plasma concentration–time profiles and relevant pharmacokinetic parameters of verapamil and norverapamil after intravenous administration of verapamil with and without metformin are shown in Figure 4 and Table 3, respectively. After intravenous and oral administration of verapamil with metformin, all pharmacokinetic parameters of verapamil and norverapamil including the $AUC_{norverapamil}/AUC_{verapamil}$ ratio were comparable to those without metformin. The absorption of verapamil from the gastrointestinal tract and the formation of norverapamil were rapid based on the C_{max} of verapamil and norverapamil, respectively.

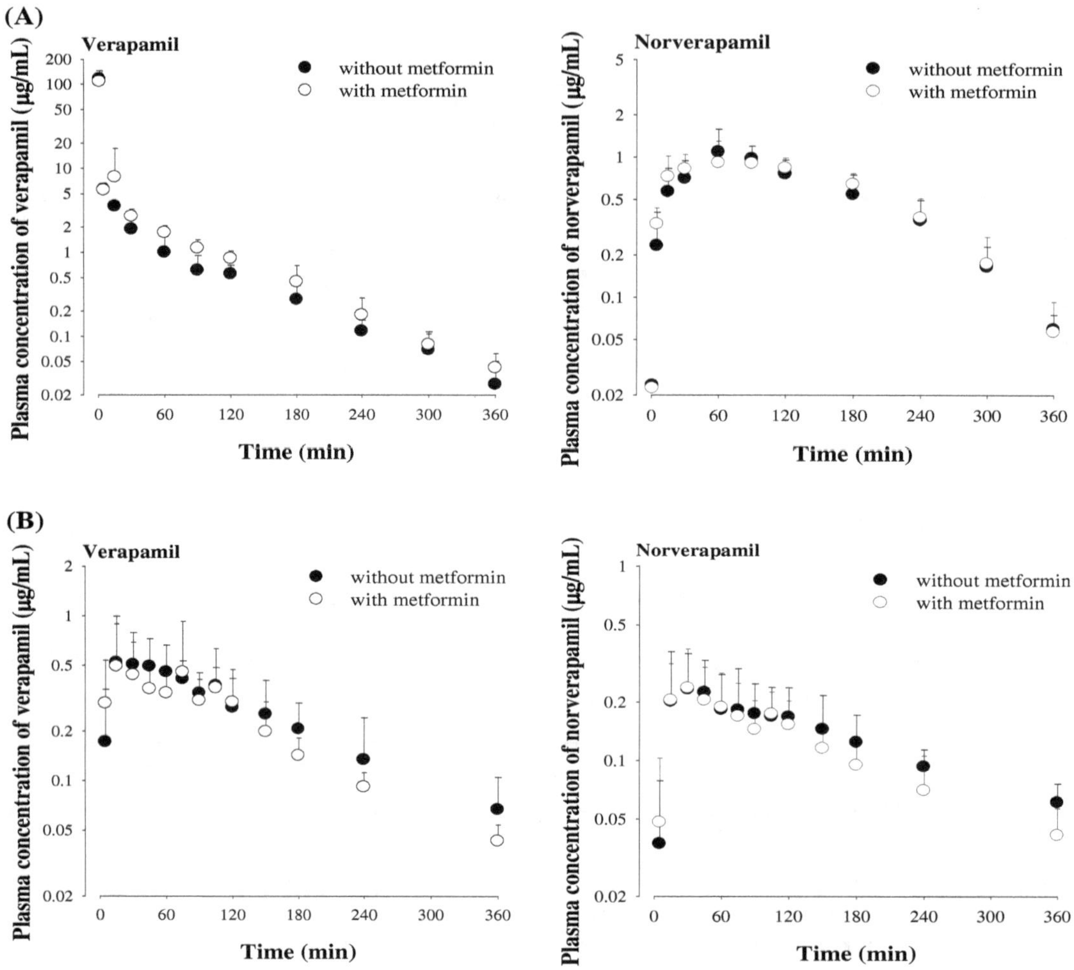

Figure 4. Mean (± S.D.) arterial plasma concentration–time profiles of verapamil and norverapamil after intravenous (**A**, $n = 6$ for each) or oral (**B**, $n = 5$ for each) administration of verapamil with (○) or without (•) metformin to rats. The doses of metformin and verapamil were 30 and 20 mg/kg, respectively.

Table 3. Mean (± S.D.) pharmacokinetic parameters of verapamil and norverapamil after intravenous or oral administration of verapamil without and with metformin to rats. The doses of metformin and verapamil were 30 and 20 mg/kg, respectively.

Parameter	Intravenous (n = 6 for Each)		Parameter	Oral (n = 5 for Each)	
	Without Metformin	With Metformin		Without Metformin	With Metformin
Verapamil			**Verapamil**		
Body weight (g)	205 ± 8.37	209 ± 6.65	Body weight (g)	214 ± 9.62	217 ± 13.0
AUC (μg min/mL)	441 ± 69.5	527 ± 134	AUC (μg min/mL)	103 ± 21.6	96.0 ± 30.6
Terminal half-life (min)	71.1 ± 19.0	79.1 ± 24.7	Terminal half-life (min)	128 ± 59.1	121 ± 57.5
MRT (min)	40.9 ± 7.75	42.4 ± 20.4	C_{max} (μg/mL)	0.678 ± 0.386	0.714 ± 0.452
V_{SS} (mL/kg)	1600 ± 861	1860 ± 535	T_{max} (min)	45 (15-105)	30 (15-75)
CL (mL/min/kg)	46.3 ± 7.14	40.0 ± 9.45	CL_R (mL/min/kg)	0.671 ± 0.748	0.489 ± 0.256
CL_{NR} (mL/min/kg)	46.1 ± 7.08	39.8 ± 9.40	$Ae_{0–24\ h}$ (% of dose)	0.308 ± 0.215	0.231 ± 0.102
CL_R (mL/min/kg)	0.147 ± 0.121	0.108 ± 0.0726	$GI_{24\ h}$ (% of dose)	0.291 ± 0.339	0.200 ± 0.135
$Ae_{0–24\ h}$ (% of dose)	0.306 ± 0.219	0.258 ± 0.125	F (%)	23.4	18.2
$GI_{24\ h}$ (% of dose)	0.148 ± 0.201	0.117 ± 0.0759			
Norverapamil			**Norverapamil**		
AUC (μg min/mL)	188 ± 34.7	199 ± 38.7	AUC (μg min/mL)	68.3 ± 38.6	53.9 ± 24.8
Terminal half-life (min)	50.8 ± 10.2	63.3 ± 15.2	Terminal half-life (min)	168 ± 73.2	117 ± 44.5
C_{max} (μg/mL)	1.24 ± 0.386	1.09 ± 0.308	C_{max} (μg/mL)	0.267 ± 0.141	0.273 ± 0.123
T_{max} (min)	60 (30–120)	60 (30–90)	T_{max} (min)	45 (15-120)	45 (15-105)
CL_R (mL/min/kg)	0.109 ± 0.102	0.0626 ± 0.0535	CL_R (mL/min/kg)	0.336 ± 0.107	0.562 ± 0.445
$Ae_{0–24\ h}$ (% of dose)	0.0872 ± 0.0691	0.0585 ± 0.0453	$Ae_{0–24\ h}$ (% of dose)	0.104 ± 0.0567	0.113 ± 0.0522
$GI_{24\ h}$ (% of dose)	0.146 ± 0.0841	0.126 ± 0.0927	$GI_{24\ h}$ (% of dose)	0.0870 ± 0.0665	0.0782 ± 0.0514
$AUC_{norverapamil}/AUC_{verapamil}$	43.0 ± 7.68	38.5 ± 11.6	$AUC_{norverapamil}/AUC_{verapamil}$	87.3 ± 26.7	89.7 ± 27.0

AUC, total area under the plasma concentration–time curve from time zero to infinity; MRT, mean residence time; V_{ss}, apparent volume of distribution at steady state; CL, time-averaged total body clearance; CL_{NR}, time-averaged non-renal clearance; CL_R, time-averaged renal clearance; $Ae_{0–24\ h}$, percentage of the dose excreted in the urine up to 24 h; $GI_{24\ h}$, percentage of the dose recovered from the gastrointestinal tract (including its contents and feces) at 24 h; C_{max}, peak plasma concentration of docetaxel; T_{max}, time to reach C_{max}; F, extent of absolute oral bioavailability.

3.5. *Effect of Metformin on Verapamil Metabolism in Rat Hepatic and Intestinal Microsomes*

The V_{max}, K_m and CL_{int} for the metabolism of verapamil with and without metformin in rat hepatic and intestinal microsomes are shown in Figure 5 and Table 4, respectively. There was no change of V_{max}, K_m or CL_{int} for verapamil metabolism in the presence of metformin, indicating that metformin did not affect verapamil metabolism in rat hepatic and intestinal microsomes under these conditions.

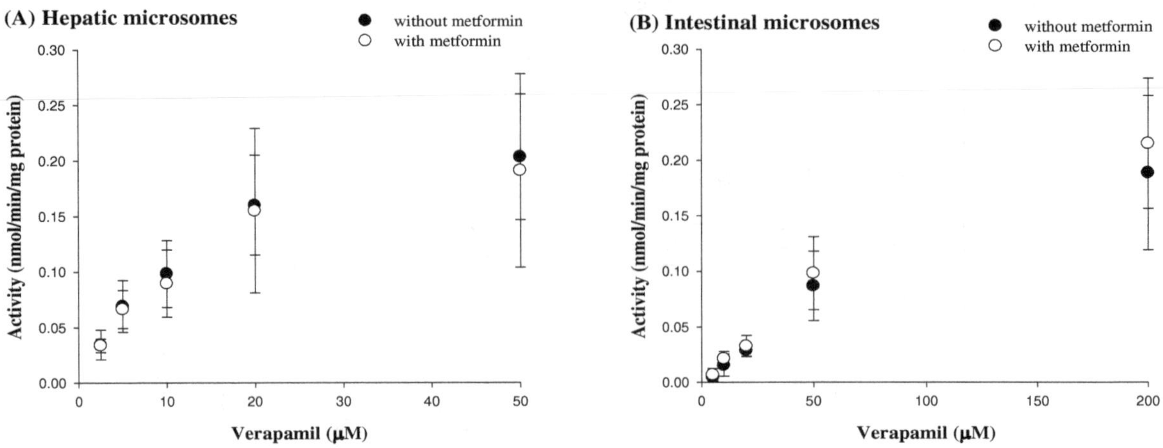

Figure 5. Nonlinear regression for mean values (± S.D.) of verapamil metabolism activity with (○) or without (•) metformin in rat hepatic (**A**, $n = 5$ for each) or intestinal (**B**, $n = 4$ for each) microsomes.

Table 4. Mean (± S.D.) K_m, V_{max} and CL_{int} for the metabolism of verapamil with and without metformin in hepatic and intestinal microsomes.

Parameter	Without Metformin	With Metformin
Hepatic	**$n = 5$ for Each**	
K_m (μM)	11.0 ± 3.11	13.8 ± 1.26
V_{max} (nmol/min/mg protein)	0.225 ± 0.0951	0.289 ± 0.151
CL_{int} (μL/min/mg protein)	0.0199 ± 0.00419	0.0205 ± 0.00911
Intestinal	**$n = 4$ for Each**	
K_m (μM)	148 ± 53.5	171 ± 11.4
V_{max} (nmol/min/mg protein)	0.332 ± 0.125	0.412 ± 0.0908
CL_{int} (μL/min/mg protein)	0.00181 ± 0.00150	0.00240 ± 0.000409

K_m, the concentration at which the rate is one-half of the V_{max}; V_{max}, maximum velocity; CL_{int}, intrinsic clearance.

3.6. *Rat Plasma Protein Binding of Verapamil and Metformin Using Equilibrium Dialysis*

The concentration of 5 g/mL of each drug was chosen based on previous reports [17,42]. Protein binding values of metformin with and without verapamil were 13.5% ± 5.39% and 11.6% ± 6.10%, respectively. The corresponding values for verapamil with and without metformin were 93.0% ± 38.9% and 85.1% ± 26.3%, respectively. Metformin and verapamil did not affect the rat plasma protein binding to each other.

4. Discussion

The ratio of AUC of a drug with an inhibitor (AUC_i)/ AUC of a drug without an inhibitor (AUC_0) of over 1.25 is classified as a relevant drug interaction by an inhibitor in U.S. FDA criteria [43]. In our study, the ratios of AUC_i/AUC of metformin with and without verapamil were 1.67 and 1.74 (i.e., relative bioavailability) after the intravenous and oral administration of both drugs (Table 1), indicating that verapamil might act as an inhibitor to cause a pharmacokinetic interaction with metformin.

In the intravenous study, the contribution of CL_R to CL, 66.5%, was a large portion of the metformin elimination pathway (Table 1), indicating that renal excretion is the main route of metformin elimination. The estimated CL_Rs of metformin considering the free fractions of metformin in the plasma ($CL_{R,fu}$s) were 4.08 and 14.2 mL/min/kg with and without verapamil, respectively. The $CL_{R,fu}$ of metformin without verapamil was faster than the reported glomerular filtration rate (GRF, represented by creatinine clearance), 5.24 mL/min/kg, in rats [44], indicating that active secretion of metformin as its renal excretion mechanism is changed by verapamil to glomerular filtration. Verapamil slowed the $CL_{R,fu}$ of metformin, 4.08 mL/min/kg, to the creatinine clearance level in rats, indicating that verapamil might cause metformin reabsorption in the renal tubules. The inhibited renal excretion pathway caused a dramatic increase in the systemic exposure (e.g., AUC) of metformin in this study similar as other references [18,45].

To investigate the inhibitory mechanism of verapamil on renal excretion of metformin, the IC_{50} of verapamil against metformin uptake in HEK-293 cells overexpressing OCT2 was conducted based on the known facts that metformin is an OCT2 substrate and verapamil inhibits OCT2 [15,16]. The inhibitory effect of verapamil on OCT2-mediated metformin uptake in HEK-293 cells overexpressing OCT2 (Figure 2) supported the reduced CL_R of metformin when co-administered with verapamil (Table 1). Verapamil significantly reduced the metformin concentration in the kidneys after intravenous and oral administration of metformin with verapamil (Table 2 and Figure 3), probably due to the inhibition of OCT2-mediated metformin uptake into the proximal renal tubules, as shown in the IC_{50} of verapamil in HEK-293 cells over-expressing OCT2 (Figure 2).

Considering that the metformin concentration in the liver is important to preserve the glucose-lowering effect of metformin [11,46,47], the metformin concentration in the liver was also measured after intravenous and oral administration of both drugs (Table 2 and Figure 3). However, the metformin concentration in the liver was not changed by verapamil, which might be due to verapamil not sufficiently inhibiting OCT1-mediated metformin uptake in the sinusoidal membrane of hepatocytes. Since OCT1 in the basolateral membrane uptakes metformin from the sinusoidal blood into hepatocytes, comparable metformin concentrations in the liver with and without verapamil could be supported by the relatively high IC_{50} of verapamil for inhibiting metformin uptake by HEK-293 cells over-expressing OCT1 (Figure 2). In other words, verapamil might have a stronger potential to inhibit OCT2 activity than OCT1 activity. Although verapamil inhibited OCT1 and OCT2-mediated metformin uptake in vitro (Figure 2), the inhibitory effect of verapamil on OCT1-mediated metformin uptake in hepatocytes might be almost negligible in in vivo studies (Table 2 and Figure 3). Therefore, verapamil is an OCT2 inhibitor in the renal proximal tubules, resulting in reduced renal excretion and increased systemic exposure of metformin.

On the other hand, the contribution of gastrointestinal (including biliary) excretion of unchanged metformin to its CL_{NR} was almost negligible; the $GI_{24\,h}$ was less than 0.471% of the intravenous dose (Table 1). Similarly, it has been reported that metformin is mainly eliminated via renal excretion, but the biliary excretion of metformin as a parent form into feces was negligible [11,17]. In the aspect of metformin and verapamil interactions, the unchanged CL_{NR} and $GI_{24\,h}$ of metformin by verapamil indicted that verapamil did not influence the non-renal elimination pathway (e.g., biliary excretion and metabolism) of metformin in rats.

After oral administration of metformin with and without verapamil, oral absorption of metformin was rapid and extensive regardless of co-administration of verapamil. For comparison, we estimated the mean 'true' unabsorbed fractions ('F_{unabs}') after oral metformin administration to rats with and without verapamil based on the following reported equation [48]:

$$\begin{aligned} 0.0357 &= \text{'}F_{unabs}\text{'} + (0.00471 \times 0.297) \qquad \text{without verapamil} \\ 0.0153 &= \text{'}F_{unabs}\text{'} + (0.00831 \times 0.309) \qquad \text{with verapamil} \end{aligned} \tag{1}$$

where 0.0357 (0.0153), 0.00471 (0.00831) and 0.297 (0.309) are the oral $GI_{24\,h}$, intravenous $GI_{24\,h}$ and F, respectively, of metformin without verapamil (with verapamil). The 'F_{unabs}' values thus estimated were 1.27% and 3.43% with and without verapamil, respectively, indicating that verapamil probably does not affect metformin absorption in the intestine (Table 1). Thus, the reduced AUC of metformin with verapamil could be due to the inhibition of renal excretion of metformin by verapamil, for the same reason as in the intravenous study.

In contrast, metformin did not change any pharmacokinetic profile of verapamil after intravenous and oral administration of metformin and verapamil together compared to verapamil alone. Metformin also did not affect the formation of norverapamil as an active metabolite of verapamil (Table 3). As hepatic metabolism via CYP3A is the main route of elimination of verapamil [28,49], and a suppressive effect of metformin on PXR-regulating CYP3A4 has been reported [21], the change of verapamil metabolism by metformin was evaluated with greater focus in this study. In parallel to the unchanged CL_{NR} of verapamil by metformin in the intravenous co-administration of metformin and verapamil (Table 3), metformin showed a negligible interaction with verapamil metabolism in in vitro hepatic and microsomal studies (Table 4). Considering that verapamil is a drug with a high (or intermediate) hepatic extraction ratio in rats [44], its hepatic clearance (metabolism) depends on the hepatic CL_{int} and free fraction (unbound to plasma proteins) of verapamil, and hepatic blood flow rate [50]. In our study, the unchanged CL_{NR}s of verapamil with and without metformin (Table 3) were supported by the comparable hepatic CL_{int}s and free unfound fractions of verapamil, and constant hepatic blood flow rate with and without metformin in rats. Metformin might not affect the hepatic blood flow rate based on studies in humans [51]. In other words, these findings indicated that metformin might inhibit the hepatic metabolism of verapamil including the formation of norverapamil (Table 3). Additionally, the unchanged K_ms and V_{max}s of verapamil with metformin compared to those without metformin in in vitro hepatic microsomal studies indicated that metformin did not affect the affinity between metabolic enzyme and verapamil and maximum rate of metabolism of verapamil.

Although the contribution of renal excretion of verapamil is minor in regards to its elimination, the renal excretion of verapamil with and without metformin was estimated as follows: the $CL_{R,fu}$s of verapamil with and without metformin adjusted by the free fraction of verapamil in the plasma were 0.00756 and 0.219 mL/min/kg, respectively. Both $CL_{R,fu}$s of verapamil were significantly slower than the reported GFR, indicating that glomerular filtration was a renal excretion mechanism of verapamil regardless of the presence of metformin and metformin did not inhibit its renal excretion in rats (Table 3).

After oral administration of both drugs, no effect of metformin on the pharmacokinetic profiles of verapamil and norverapamil was observed. The comparable AUCs of verapamil with and without metformin (Table 3) were likely due to the unchanged absorption of verapamil; the estimated 'F_{unabs}' values of verapamil were 0.00179 and 0.00256% for with and without metformin, respectively, from the equations [48]:

$$\begin{aligned} 0.00291 &= \text{'}F_{unabs}\text{'} + (0.00148 \times 0.234) \quad && \text{without metformin} \\ 0.00200 &= \text{'}F_{unabs}\text{'} + (0.00117 \times 0.182) \quad && \text{with metformin} \end{aligned} \tag{2}$$

where 0.00291 (0.00200), 0.00148 (0.00117) and 0.234 (0.182) are the oral $GI_{24\,h}$, intravenous $GI_{24\,h}$ and F of verapamil, respectively, without metformin (with metformin). Thus, metformin might not affect verapamil absorption in the intestine (Table 3). Orally administered metformin might also not inhibit verapamil metabolism in the liver and intestine, as supported by the unchanged verapamil metabolism by metformin in the in vitro hepatic and intestinal microsome studies (Table 4).

Although Cho et al. [32] reported the inhibitory effect of verapamil on the glucose tolerance activity of metformin without any change of metformin's AUC in healthy adults, verapamil has recently emerged as a new indication for the treatment of hypertension in DM patients [22,23]. Extrapolating the rat dose to human equivalent dose based on the equation by FDA [52], there is a slight difference: the estimated human equivalent doses of metformin and verapamil in our study are 340 mg/70 kg and 227 mg/70 kg, respectively, and the corresponding doses in Cho et al. [32] were 1000 mg and 180 mg per patient (average body weight of patients was 70.5 kg). This inconsistency of doses can be one reason for the result in the different PK interaction pattern in metformin and verapamil combination. In addition, the relatively lower doses were used to emphasize the potential for the occurrence of metformin and verapamil interaction, which can provide a clue to cause OCT mediated drug interaction as underlying mechanism for the further investigations using various dosage regimens in preclinical as well as clinical studies.

5. Conclusions

After intravenous and oral administration of both drugs, the significantly greater AUC of metformin could be due to the inhibition of OCT2-mediated renal excretion of metformin by verapamil, leading to increased systemic exposure of metformin. Interestingly, there was no interaction effect on the metformin concentration in the liver in spite of the inhibitory effect of verapamil on OCT1-mediated metformin uptake in vitro. In contrast, metformin did not influence the pharmacokinetic profile of verapamil. These results can provide essential knowledge about the drug interaction potential between metformin and verapamil for their clinical applications.

Author Contributions: Conceptualization, methodology and writing—original draft preparation, S.Y.H. and Y.H.C.; investigation, S.Y.H.; writing—review and editing, S.Y.H. and Y.H.C.; resources and supervision, Y.H.C. All authors have read and agreed to the published version of the manuscript.

References

1. De Boer, I.H.; Bangalore, S.; Benetos, A.; Davis, A.M.; Michos, E.D.; Muntner, P.; Rossing, P.; Zoungas, S.; Bakris, G. Diabetes and hypertension: A position statement by the American Diabetes Association. *Diabetes Care* **2017**, *40*, 1273–1284. [CrossRef]
2. Ferrannini, E.; Cushman, W.C. Diabetes and hypertension: The bad companions. *Lancet* **2012**, *380*, 601–610. [CrossRef]
3. Junior, V.C.; Fuchs, F.D.; Schaan, B.D.; Moreira, L.B.; Fuchs, S.C.; Gus, M. Effect of metformin on blood pressure in patients with hypertension: A randomized clinical trial. *Endocrine* **2019**, *63*, 252–258. [CrossRef] [PubMed]
4. Beckmman, J.A.; Creager, M.A.; Libby, P. Diabetes and antherosclerosis: Epidemiology, pathophysiology, and management. *JAMA* **2002**, *287*, 2570–2581. [CrossRef] [PubMed]
5. Hayward, R.A.; Reaven, P.D.; Wiitala, W.L.; Bahn, G.D.; Reda, D.J.; Ge, L.; McCarren, M.; Duckworth, W.C.; Emanuele, N.V.; VADT Investigators. Follow-up of glycemic control and cardiovascular outcomes in type 2 diabetes. *N. Engl. J. Med.* **2015**, *372*, 2197–2206. [CrossRef] [PubMed]
6. Reaven, G.M.; Lithell, H.; Landsberg, L. Hypertension and associated metabolic abnormalities-the role of insulin resistance and the sympathoadrenale. *N. Engl. J. Med.* **1996**, *334*, 374–381. [CrossRef]
7. Sun, D.; Zhou, T.; Heianza, Y.; Li, X.; Fan, M.; Fonseca, V.A.; Qi, L. Type 2 Diabetes and Hypertension: A Study on Bidirectional Causality. *Circ. Res.* **2019**, *124*, 930–937. [CrossRef]
8. He, J.; Whelton, P.K. Epidemiology and prevention of hypertension. *Med. Clin. N. Am.* **1997**, *81*, 1077–1097. [CrossRef]
9. Sharma, S.K.; Ruggeneti, P.; Remuzzi, G. Managing hypertension in diabetic patients-focus on trandolapril/verapamil combination. *Vasc. Health Risk Manag.* **2007**, *3*, 453–465.
10. Dunn, D.J.; Peters, D.H. Metformin. A review of is pharmacological properties and therapeutic use in non-insulin-dependent diabetes mellitus. *Drugs* **1995**, *49*, 721–749. [CrossRef]
11. Gong, L.; Goswami, S.; Giacomini, K.M.; Altman, R.B.; Klein, T.E. Metformin pathway: Pharmacokinetics and pharmacodynamics. *Pharm. Genom.* **2012**, *22*, 820–827. [CrossRef]
12. Scheen, A.J. Clinical pharmacokinetics of metformin. *Clin. Pharmacokinet.* **1996**, *30*, 359–371. [CrossRef] [PubMed]
13. Hermann, L.S. Clinical Pharmacology of Biguanides (*Oral antidiabetes*). In *Handbook of Experimental Pharmacology*; Kuhlmann, J., Puls, W., Eds.; Springer: New York, NY, USA, 1996; pp. 373–407.
14. Snorgaard, O.; Kober, L.; Carlsen, J. The effect of metformin on blood pressure and metabolism in nondiabetic hypertensive patients. *J. Intern. Med.* **1997**, *242*, 407–412. [CrossRef] [PubMed]
15. Nies, A.T.; Koepsell, H.; Winter, S.; Burk, O.; Klein, K.; Kerb, R.; Zanger, U.M.; Keppler, D.; Schwab, M.; Schaeffeler, E. Expression of organic cation transporters OCT1 (SLC22A1) and OCT3 (SLC22A3) is affected by genetic factors and cholestasis in human liver. *Hepatology* **2009**, *50*, 1227–1240. [CrossRef]

16. Nies, A.T.; Hofmann, U.; Resch, C.; Schaeffeler, E.; Ruis, M.; Schwab, M. Proton pump inhibitors inhibit metformin uptake by organic cation transporters (OCTs). *PLoS ONE* **2011**, *6*, e22163. [CrossRef] [PubMed]
17. Choi, Y.H.; Kim, S.G.; Lee, M.G. Dose-independent pharmacokinetics of metformin in rats: Hepatic and gastrointestinal first-pass effects. *J. Pharm. Sci.* **2006**, *95*, 2543–2552. [CrossRef] [PubMed]
18. Kimura, N.; Masuda, S.; Tanihara, Y.; Ueo, H.; Okuda, M.; Katsura, T.; Inui, K.I. Metformin is a superior substrate for renal organic cation transporter OCT2 rather than hepatic OCT1. *Drug Metab. Pharmacokinet.* **2005**, *20*, 379–386. [CrossRef]
19. Yang, S.; Dai, Y.; Liu, Z.; Wang, C.; Meng, Q.; Huo, X.; Sun, H.; Ma, X.; Peng, J.; Liu, K. Involvement of organic cation transporter 2 in the metformin-associated increased lactate levels caused by contrast-induced nephropathy. *Biomed. Pharmacother.* **2018**, *106*, 1760–1766. [CrossRef]
20. Abbasi, M.M.; Valizadeh, H.; Hamishehkar, H.; Zakeri-Milani, P. Inhibition of P-glycoprotein expression and function by anti-diabetic drugs gliclazide, metformin, and pioglitazone in vitro and in situ. *Res. Pharm. Sci.* **2016**, *11*, 177–186.
21. Krausova, L.; Stejskalova, L.; Wang, H.; Vrzal, R.; Dvorak, Z.; Mani*f*, S.; Pavek, P. Metformin suppresses pregnane X receptor (PXR)-regulated transactivation of CYP3A4 gene. *Biochem. Pharmacol.* **2011**, *82*, 1771–1780. [CrossRef]
22. Khodneva, Y.; Shalev, A.; Frank, S.J.; Carson, A.P.; Safford, M.M. Calcium channel blocker use is associated with lower fasting serum glucose among adults with diabetes from the REGARDS study. *Diabetes Res. Clin. Pract.* **2016**, *115*, 115–121. [CrossRef] [PubMed]
23. Yin, T.; Kuo, S.C.; Chang, Y.Y.; Chen, T.T.; Wang, K.W.K. Verapamil use is associated with reduction of newly diagnosed diabetes mellitus. *J. Clin. Endocrinol. Metab.* **2017**, *102*, 2604–2610. [CrossRef] [PubMed]
24. Andersson, D.E.H.; Rojdmark, S. Improvement of glucose tolerance by verapamil in patients with non-insulin dependent diabetes mellitus. *Acta Med. Scandina.* **2009**, *210*, 27–33. [CrossRef]
25. Cooper-Dehoff, R.; Cohen, J.D.; Bakris, G.L.; Messerli, F.H.; Erdine, S.; Hewkin, A.C.; Kupfer, S.; Pepine, C.J. Predictors of development of diabetes mellitus in patients with coronary artery disease taking antihypertensive medications (findings from the International Verapamil SR-Trandolapril Study [INVEST]). *Am. J. Cardiol.* **2006**, *98*, 890–894. [CrossRef] [PubMed]
26. Cooper-DeHoff, R.M.; Aranda, J.M., Jr.; Gaxiola, E.; Cangiano, J.L.; Garcia-Barreto, D.; Conti, C.R.; Hewkin, A.; Pepine, C.J. Blood pressure control and cardiovascular outcomes in high-risk Hispanic patients–findings from the International Verapamil SR/Trandolapril Study (INVEST). *Am. Heart J.* **2006**, *151*, 1072–1079. [CrossRef]
27. Hamann, S.R.; Blouin, R.A.; McAllister, R.G. Clinical pharmacokinetics of verapamil. *Clin. Pharmacokinet.* **1984**, *9*, 26–41. [CrossRef]
28. Hanada, K.; Ikemi, Y.; Kkita, K.; Mihara, K.; Ogata, H. Stereoselective first-pass metabolism of verapamil in the small intestine and liver in rats. *Drug Metab. Dispos.* **2008**, *36*, 2037–2042. [CrossRef]
29. Hong, S.P.; Chang, K.S.; Koh, Y.Y.; Choi, D.H.; Choi, J.S. Effects of lovastatin on the pharmacokinetics of verapamil and its active metabolite, norverapamil in rats: Possible role of p-glycoprotein inhibition by lovastatin. *Arch. Pharm. Res.* **2009**, *32*, 1447–1452. [CrossRef]
30. Uchida, Y.; Ohtsuki, S.; Terasaki, T. Pharmacoproteomics-based reconstruction of in vivo P-glycoprotein function at blood-brain barrier and brain distribution of substrate verapamil in pentylenetetrazole-kindled epilepsy, spontaneous epilepsy, and phenytoin treatment models. *Drug Metab. Dispos.* **2014**, *42*, 1719–1726. [CrossRef]
31. Zolk, O.; Solbach, T.F.; Konig, J.; Fromm, M.F. Functional characterization of the human organic cation transporter 2 Variant p.270Ala>Ser. *Drug Metab. Dispos.* **2009**, *37*, 1312–1318. [CrossRef]
32. Cho, S.K.; Kim, C.O.; Park, E.S.; Chung, J.-Y. Verapamil decreases the glucose-lowering effect of metformin in healthy volunteers. *Br. J. Clin. Pharmacol.* **2014**, *78*, 1426–1432. [CrossRef] [PubMed]
33. Han, S.Y.; Chae, H.S.; You, B.H.; Chin, Y.W.; Kim, H.; Choi, H.S.; Choi, Y.H. Lonicera japonica extract increases metformin distribution in the liver without change of systemic exposed metformin in rats. *J. Ethnopharmacol.* **2019**, *238*, 111892. [CrossRef] [PubMed]
34. You, B.H.; Chin, Y.W.; Kim, H.; Choi, H.S.; Choi, Y.H. Houttuynia cordata extract increased exposure and liver concentrations of metformin through OCTs and MATEs in rats. *Phytother. Res.* **2018**, *32*, 1004–1013. [CrossRef]
35. Liang, X.; Giacomini, K.M. Transporters involved in metformin pharmacokinetics and treatment response. *J. Pharm. Sci.* **2017**, *106*, 2245–2250. [CrossRef]

36. Tornio, A.; Filppula, A.M.; Niemi, M.; Backman, J.T. Clinical studies on drug-drug interactions involving metabolism and transport: Methodology, pitfalls, and interpretation. *Clin. Pharmacol. Ther.* **2019**, *105*, 1345–1361. [CrossRef]
37. Iwersen, S.; Schmoldt, A. A specific hydroxysteroid UGT is responsible for the conjugation of aliphatic alcohols in rats: An estimation of the importance of glucuronidation versus oxidation. *Alcohol* **1998**, *15*, 185–192. [CrossRef]
38. Peng, J.Z.; Remmel, R.P.; Sawchuk, R.J. Inhibition of murine cytochrome P4501A by tacrine: In vitro studies. *Drug Metab. Dispos.* **2004**, *32*, 805–812. [CrossRef]
39. Bradford, M.M. A rapid and sensitive method for the quantitation of microgram quantities of protein utilizing the principle of protein–dye binding. *Anal. Biochem.* **1976**, *72*, 248–254. [CrossRef]
40. Duggleby, R.G. Analysis of enzyme progress curves by nonlinear regression. *Methods Enzymol.* **1995**, *249*, 61–90.
41. Gibaldi, M.; Perrier, D. *Pharmacokinetics*, 2nd ed.; Marcel Dekker: New York, NY, USA, 1982.
42. Manitpisitkul, P.; Chiou, W.L. Intravenous verapamil kinetics in rats: Marked arteriovenous concentration difference and comparison with humans. *Biopharm. Drug Dispos.* **1993**, *14*, 555–566. [CrossRef]
43. US Food and Drug Administration, Center for Drug Evaluation and Research. Clinical Drug Interaction Studies-Study Design, Data Analysis, and Clinical Implications Guideline for Industry. 2017. Available online: https://www.fda.gov/downloads/drugs/guidances/ucm292362.pdf (accessed on 31 October 2017).
44. Davies, B.; Morris, T. Physiological parameters in laboratory animals and humans. *Pharm. Res.* **1993**, *10*, 1093–1095. [CrossRef] [PubMed]
45. Burt, H.J.; Neuhoff, S.; Almond, L.; Gaohua, L.; Harwood, M.D.; Jamei, M.; Rostami-Hodjegan, A.; Tucker, G.T.; Rowland-Yeo, K. Metformin and cimetidine: Physiologically based pharmacokinetic modelling to investigate transporter mediated drug-drug interactions. *Eur. J. Pharm. Sci.* **2016**, *88*, 70–82. [CrossRef] [PubMed]
46. Higgins, J.W.; Bedwell, D.W.; Zamek-Gliszczynski, M.J. Ablation of both organic cation transporter (Oct)1 and Oct2 alters metformin pharmacokinetics but has no effect on tissue drug exposure and pharmacodynamics. *Drug Metab. Dispos.* **2012**, *40*, 1170–1177. [CrossRef]
47. Zamek-Gliszczynski, M.J.; Bao, J.Q.; Day, J.S.; Higgins, J.W. Metformin sinusoidal efflux from the liver is consistent with negligible biliary excretion and absence of enterohepatic cycling. *Drug Metab. Dispos.* **2013**, *41*, 1967–1971. [CrossRef] [PubMed]
48. Lee, M.G.; Chiou, W.L. Evaluation of potential causes for the incomplete bioavailability of furosemide: Gastric first-pass metabolism. *J. Pharmacokinet. Biopharm.* **1983**, *11*, 623–640. [CrossRef] [PubMed]
49. Eichelbaum, M.; Mikus, G.; Vog Dunn, D.J.; Peters Elgesang, B. Pharmacokinetics of (+)-, (–)- and (+/–)-verapamil after intravenous administration. *Br. J. Clin. Pharmacol.* **1984**, *17*, 453–458. [CrossRef]
50. Wilkinson, G.R.; Shand, D.G. A physiological approach to hepatic drug clearance. *Clin. Pharmacol. Ther.* **1975**, *18*, 377–390. [CrossRef]
51. Scarpello, J.H.; Howlett, H.C. Metformin therapy and clinical uses. *Diabetes Vasc. Dis. Res.* **2008**, *5*, 157–167. [CrossRef]
52. US Food and Drug Administration, Center for Drug Evaluation and Reserach. Guidance for Industry: Estimating the Maximum Safe Starting Dose in Initial Clinical Trials for Therapeutics in Adult Healthy Volunteers. *Center Drug Eval. Res.* **2005**, *7*, 42346.

Permissions

All chapters in this book were first published by MDPI; hereby published with permission under the Creative Commons Attribution License or equivalent. Every chapter published in this book has been scrutinized by our experts. Their significance has been extensively debated. The topics covered herein carry significant findings which will fuel the growth of the discipline. They may even be implemented as practical applications or may be referred to as a beginning point for another development.

The contributors of this book come from diverse backgrounds, making this book a truly international effort. This book will bring forth new frontiers with its revolutionizing research information and detailed analysis of the nascent developments around the world.

We would like to thank all the contributing authors for lending their expertise to make the book truly unique. They have played a crucial role in the development of this book. Without their invaluable contributions this book wouldn't have been possible. They have made vital efforts to compile up to date information on the varied aspects of this subject to make this book a valuable addition to the collection of many professionals and students.

This book was conceptualized with the vision of imparting up-to-date information and advanced data in this field. To ensure the same, a matchless editorial board was set up. Every individual on the board went through rigorous rounds of assessment to prove their worth. After which they invested a large part of their time researching and compiling the most relevant data for our readers.

The editorial board has been involved in producing this book since its inception. They have spent rigorous hours researching and exploring the diverse topics which have resulted in the successful publishing of this book. They have passed on their knowledge of decades through this book. To expedite this challenging task, the publisher supported the team at every step. A small team of assistant editors was also appointed to further simplify the editing procedure and attain best results for the readers.

Apart from the editorial board, the designing team has also invested a significant amount of their time in understanding the subject and creating the most relevant covers. They scrutinized every image to scout for the most suitable representation of the subject and create an appropriate cover for the book.

The publishing team has been an ardent support to the editorial, designing and production team. Their endless efforts to recruit the best for this project, has resulted in the accomplishment of this book. They are a veteran in the field of academics and their pool of knowledge is as vast as their experience in printing. Their expertise and guidance has proved useful at every step. Their uncompromising quality standards have made this book an exceptional effort. Their encouragement from time to time has been an inspiration for everyone.

The publisher and the editorial board hope that this book will prove to be a valuable piece of knowledge for researchers, students, practitioners and scholars across the globe.

List of Contributors

Seung-Hyun Jeong, Ji-Hun Jang and Yong-Bok Lee
College of Pharmacy, Chonnam National University, 77 Yongbong-ro, Buk-Gu, Gwangju 61186, Korea

Hea-Young Cho
College of Pharmacy, CHA University, 335 Pangyo-ro, Bundang-gu, Seongnam-si, Gyeonggi-Do 13488, Korea

Won-Gu Choi, Dong Kyun Kim and Hye Suk Lee
BK21 PLUS Team for Creative Leader Program for Pharmacomics-based Future Pharmacy and Drug Metabolism and Bioanalysis Laboratory, College of Pharmacy, The Catholic University of Korea, Bucheon 420-743, Korea

Ju-Hyun Kim
BK21 PLUS Team for Creative Leader Program for Pharmacomics-based Future Pharmacy and Drug Metabolism and Bioanalysis Laboratory, College of Pharmacy, The Catholic University of Korea, Bucheon 420-743, Korea
College of Pharmacy, Yeungnam University, Gyeongsan 38541, Korea

Yongnam Lee, Ji Seok Yoo and Dae Hee Shin
Central R&D Institute, YUNGJIN PHARM. CO., LTD., Suwon 16229, Korea

Fakhrossadat Emami and Alireza Vatanara
College of Pharmacy, Tehran University of Medical Sciences, Tehran 1417614411, Iran

Eun Ji Park and Dong Hee Na
College of Pharmacy, Chung-Ang University, Seoul 06974, Korea

In Yong Bae, Min Sun Choi, Young Seok Ji and Hye Hyun Yoo
Institute of Pharmaceutical Science and Technology and College of Pharmacy, Hanyang University, Ansan, Gyeonggi-do 15588, Korea

Sang-Ku Yoo and Kyungil Kim
Glaceum Inc., Yeongtong-gu, Suwon, Gyeonggi-do 16675, Korea

Benoit Drolet, Jessica Virgili and Chantale Simard
Faculté de Pharmacie, Université Laval, 1050 Avenue de la Médecine, Québec, QC G1V 0A6, Canada
Centre de Recherche, Institut Universitaire de Cardiologie et de Pneumologie de Québec, 2725 Chemin Sainte-Foy, Québec, QC G1V 4G5, Canada

Carolanne Gélinas, Alida-Douce Kamaliza and Audrey Blais-Boilard
Faculté de Pharmacie, Université Laval, 1050 Avenue de la Médecine, Québec, QC G1V 0A6, Canada

Sylvie Pilote and Dany Patoine
Centre de Recherche, Institut Universitaire de Cardiologie et de Pneumologie de Québec, 2725 Chemin Sainte-Foy, Québec, QC G1V 4G5, Canada

Yiting Yang and Xiaodong Liu
Center of Drug Metabolism and Pharmacokinetics, China Pharmaceutical University, Nanjing 210009, China

Sherif Hanafy Mahmoud and Chen Shen
Faculty of Pharmacy and Pharmaceutical Sciences, University of Alberta, Edmonton, AB T6G 1C9, Canada

Ji-Hyeon Jeon, Sowon Lee and Im-Sook Song
College of Pharmacy and Research Institute of Pharmaceutical Sciences, Kyungpook National University, Daegu 41566, Korea

Bitna Kang, Sojeong Jin and Min-Koo Choi
College of Pharmacy, Dankook University, Cheon-an 31116, Korea

Jinfeng Chen, Xiaoyu Guo, Yingyuan Lu, Mengling Shi, Haidong Mu, Yi Qian, Jinlong Wang, Mengqiu Lu, Mingbo Zhao and Yong Jiang
State Key Laboratory of Natural and Biomimetic Drugs, School of Pharmaceutical Sciences, Peking University, Beijing 100191, China

Pengfei Tu
State Key Laboratory of Natural and Biomimetic Drugs, School of Pharmaceutical Sciences, Peking University, Beijing 100191, China
Modern Research Center for Traditional Chinese Medicine, Beijing University of Chinese Medicine, Beijing 100029, China

Yuelin Song
Modern Research Center for Traditional Chinese Medicine, Beijing University of Chinese Medicine, Beijing 100029, China

Steffen G. Oeser and Jon-Paul Bingham
Molecular Biosciences and Bioengineering, University of Hawaii, Manoa, 1955 East-West Rd. #218, Honolulu, HI 96822, USA

Abby C. Collier
Faculty of Pharmaceutical Sciences, 2405 Wesbrook Mall, University of British Columbia, Vancouver, BC V6T1Z3, Canada

Júlia T. Novaes, Ryan Lillico, Yufei Chen, Ana Luísa de P. Oliveira, Samaa Alrushaid and Ted M. Lakowski
The Rady Faculty of Health Sciences, College of Pharmacy, Pharmaceutical Analysis Laboratory, University of Manitoba, Winnipeg, MB R3E 0T5, Canada

Casey L. Sayre
College of Pharmacy, Roseman University of Health Sciences, South Jordan, UT 84096, USA

Kalyanam Nagabhushanam and Muhammed Majeed
Sabinsa Corporation, 20 Lake Drive, East Windsor, NJ 08520, USA

Emmanuel A. Ho
Faculty of Science, School of Pharmacy, University of Waterloo, Kitchener, ON N2G 1C5, Canada

Stephanie E. Martinez
Department of Veterinary Clinical Sciences, College of Veterinary Medicine, Washington State University, Pullman, WA 99164-6610, USA

Neal M. Davies
Faculty of Pharmacy and Pharmaceutical Sciences, University of Alberta, Edmonton, AB T6G 2R3, Canada

Hossain Mohammad Arif Ullah, Junhyeong Kim, Naveed Ur Rehman, Hye-Jin Kim, Mi-Jeong Ahn and Hye Jin Chung
College of Pharmacy and Research Institute of Pharmaceutical Sciences, Gyeongsang National University, Jinju 52828, Korea

Hamdah M. Al Nebaihi and Dion R. Brocks
Faculty of Pharmacy and Pharmaceutical Sciences, University of Alberta, Edmonton, AB T6G 2E1, Canada

Matthew Primrose and James S. Green
Department of Anesthesiology and Pain Medicine, Faculty of Medicine and Dentistry, University of Alberta, Edmonton, AB T6G 2B7, Canada

Seung Yon Han and Young Hee Choi
College of Pharmacy and Integrated Research Institute for Drug Development, Dongguk University_Seoul, 32 Dongguk-lo, Ilsandong-gu, Goyang-si 10326, Korea

Index

A
Albumin, 3, 7-8, 39, 42, 46, 101
Alkaline Phosphatase, 3, 40, 42
Amino Acids, 40, 45-46, 51, 53-54
Arachidonic Acid, 71, 79, 81-82, 94, 194
Atorvastatin, 84-86, 89, 91, 95, 101, 105, 107-108
Augmented Renal Clearance, 110-111, 125, 127, 131-136
Azosemide, 91, 106

B
Biliary Excretion, 84-85, 88, 100, 102, 107, 137, 146-147, 149-151, 194, 227, 231
Body Mass Index, 3, 8, 20, 166

C
Caffeic Acid, 21-22, 26, 33-34
Calcitonin, 41-42, 48, 54-55
Cardiovascular Disease, 71-72, 79-82, 102, 181, 216
Cardiovascular Tissue, 72
Carthamus Tinctorius Extract, 153-155, 158, 164
Cell Migration, 72
Chlorogenic Acid, 21-22, 26, 33-34
Compound K, 137-138, 140-152
Concentration Ratio, 67-68
Creatinine, 3, 7-8, 17-18, 20, 95, 110-111, 125-129, 131-136, 227

D
Diabetic Status, 83-86, 91, 95, 98, 100
Dog Plasma, 57, 59, 61, 67-69
Drug Disposition, 83-84, 100, 107, 109, 166
Drug Toxicity, 83-84

E
Endogenous Pathway, 71
Epoxyeicosatrienoic Acids, 71-72, 80-82
Ethidium Bromide, 4-5

F
Ferulic Acid, 21-23, 26, 32-33
Formic Acid, 21, 23-25, 31, 58, 60, 140-141, 181-182
Furosemide, 91, 93, 96, 98-99, 106-109, 231

G
Genetic Factors, 1-2, 13, 166, 229
Glabridin, 57-58, 68-69
Glucuronidases, 64, 68

H
Hepatitis B, 37
Hepatocytes, 84-86, 88, 96, 103, 106, 216, 227
Herbal Drugs, 22-23
Histone Deacetylase, 90, 179
Hydroxyl Group, 68
Hyperinsulinemia, 74, 216-217

I
Influx Transporters, 83-84, 89
Isoflurane, 25, 140

L
Lyophilization, 36-37, 43

M
Mean Residence Time, 25, 60, 141-142, 204, 221, 225
Metabolic Profile, 68
Metabolic Stability, 57-59, 62-64, 68
Metabolism Clearance, 88
Monocarboxylate Transporters, 83, 89, 100
Multidrug Resistance-associated Proteins, 83-84, 89, 92, 100
Multiple Reaction Monitoring, 59, 145, 148, 156, 158, 163, 182, 198-199, 206

N
Nifedipine, 87, 104
Notoginseng Total Saponins, 153-155, 158, 163-164

O
Oxidative Stress, 86, 92, 195

P
P-glycoprotein, 2, 83-84, 89, 92, 101-102, 105-106, 108, 137, 151, 181, 194, 217, 230
Parathyroid Hormone, 41, 47-48, 53
Peptide Transporters, 83, 89, 92, 101
Pharmacokinetic Model, 10, 13, 83-84, 96, 101, 109
Plasma Concentrations, 5-6, 8-10, 18-19, 29, 32, 57, 85, 87, 93, 97, 99, 101, 137-138, 141, 147, 149, 158, 199, 206, 212, 214
Polymerase Chain Reaction, 4, 165, 167-168, 176-177
Pregnane X Receptor, 91, 101, 106, 217, 230
Protein Degradation, 35, 40, 45
Protein Expression, 71, 73, 75-80, 82, 85-86, 93, 100, 102, 104-105, 166, 176
Protein Precipitation, 23, 26, 31, 196, 205
Protein Stability, 35-37, 39, 44-45, 48, 54-55

Protopanaxadiol, 137-138, 144, 151-152
Pulmonary Drug Delivery, 39, 41, 43-44, 53, 55

R
Rat Plasma, 21, 23-29, 31-32, 34, 57, 60, 65-69, 145-146, 148, 158, 163, 196-197, 199-201, 203-207, 220, 226
Renal Impairment, 108, 110
Rifampicin, 85, 101

S
Short Chain Fatty Acids, 90, 101
Simvastatin, 85-86, 89, 101
Single Nucleotide Polymorphism, 2, 19
Smooth Muscle Cell, 72, 80-81
Spray Freeze Drying, 35-36, 39-40, 52-54
Stauntonia Hexaphylla, 21-23, 32-33
Stereoselective Metabolism, 57, 68
Stereoselectivity, 57, 67-69
Streptozocin, 82, 85, 101-103
Systemic Exposure, 67-68, 152, 164, 216-217, 227, 229

T
Therapeutic Effect, 2
Therapeutic Proteins, 35-36, 49-53, 55
Tiropramide, 1-3, 5-20
Torasemide, 91, 93, 103

V
Vascular Endothelia, 72
Vascular Tone, 72, 80
Vasoconstriction, 72-73, 80

W
Western Blot, 73, 175

www.ingramcontent.com/pod-product-compliance
Lightning Source LLC
LaVergne TN
LVHW082154200926
848484LV00008B/2158